First Edition

Appleton & Lange's Review of

INTERNAL MEDICINE

First Edition

Appleton & Lange's Review of
INTERNAL MEDICINE

Barry J. Goldlist, MD, FRCPC, FACP
Associate Professor of Medicine
University of Toronto

Chief of Geriatric Medicine
Queen Elizabeth Hospital
Toronto, Ontario
Canada

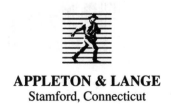

APPLETON & LANGE
Stamford, Connecticut

Copyright © 1996 by Appleton & Lange
A Simon & Schuster Company

96 97 98 99 00 / 10 9 8 7 6 5 4 3 2 1

Prentice Hall International (UK) Limited, *London*
Prentice Hall of Australia Pty. Limited, *Sydney*
Prentice Hall Canada, Inc., *Toronto*
Prentice Hall Hispanoamericana, S.A., *Mexico*
Prentice Hall of India Private Limited, *New Delhi*
Prentice Hall of Japan, Inc., *Tokyo*
Simon & Schuster Asia Pte. Ltd., *Singapore*
Editora Prentice Hall do Brasil Ltda., *Rio de Janeiro*
Prentice Hall, *Englewood Cliffs, New Jersey*

Library of Congress Cataloging-in-Publication Data

Goldlist, Barry J.
    Appleton & Lange's review of internal medicine / Barry J.
Goldlist. — 1st ed.
        p.   cm.
    ISBN 0-8385-0251-2 (pbk. : alk. paper)
    1. Internal medicine—Examinations, questions, etc.   I. Title.
    [DNLM: 1. Internal Medicine—examination questions.   WB 18.2
    G619a 1995]
    RC58.G59   1995
    616'.0076—dc20
DNLM/DLC
for Library of Congress   95-33372
                                                               CIP

ISBN 0-8385-0251-2

90000

9 780838 502464

Acquisitions Editor: Marinita Timban
Production Service: Rainbow Graphics, Inc.

PRINTED IN THE UNITED STATES OF AMERICA

Contents

PREFACE

The practice of internal medicine requires both breadth and depth of knowledge. To acquire mastery of the subject requires extensive reading and clinical experience. The knowledge base is also constantly expanding and changing as medicine enters the era of molecular biology and large randomized clinical trials. This textbook provides a review of the major issues in internal medicine by presenting a wide variety of typical examination questions and referenced answers.

The text is organized by topic to facilitate in-depth review, but contains a large comprehensive section that mimics the typical examination format. The content has been organized to reflect the areas tested on Step 2 of the USMLE. The questions are in the identical format as those used on the USMLE, making it an ideal study guide for individuals preparing for their licensing exams.

The questions and answers reflect the increasing growth of knowledge in the field of internal medicine. As a result, reviewing the answers gives the reader a "mini review" of basic concepts and pathophysiology in internal medicine, allowing the reader to approach clinical problems in an appropriate manner.

Barry J. Goldlist MD, FRCPC, FACP
January 1996

Acknowledgments

I would like to thank my family, particularly my wife Helen, for their support and understanding during those long hours I was absent in the library. Thanks also go to my secretary, Pamela Ayearst, for her patience during seemingly endless revisions and deadlines. I particularly owe a great debt to Professor Michael Baker, the original author of this text, whose encouragement and support made the entire task possible.

CHAPTER 1

Cardiology
Questions

DISEASES OF THE CARDIOVASCULAR SYSTEM

DIRECTIONS (Questions 1 through 32): Each of the questions or incomplete statements below is followed by five suggested answers or completions. Select the ONE that is best in each case.

1. Wenckebach's type AV block is recognized by

   (A) progressive P-R shortening
   (B) progressive lengthening of the P-R interval
   (C) tachycardia
   (D) dropped beat after P-R lengthening
   (E) fixed 2:1 block

2. An electrocardiographic sign of hypercalcemia is

   (A) shortened P-R interval
   (B) lengthened P-R interval
   (C) lengthened Q-U interval
   (D) shortening of the Q-T interval
   (E) shortening of the Q-U interval

3. A pacemaker that functions when the ventricular rate falls below a preset interval is called

   (A) asynchronous
   (B) atrial synchronous
   (C) ventricular synchronous
   (D) ventricular inhibited
   (E) atrial sequential

4. The electrocardiographic signs of pulmonary embolism include all of the following EXCEPT

   (A) a deep S_1
   (B) depressed ST in leads I and II
   (C) prominent Q_1, and inversion of T_3
   (D) left-axis deviation
   (E) clockwise rotation in the precordial leads

5. Angina pectoris and syncope are most likely to be associated with

   (A) mitral stenosis
   (B) mitral insufficiency
   (C) aortic stenosis
   (D) aortic insufficiency
   (E) tricuspid stenosis

6. Bacterial endocarditis may include all of the following complications EXCEPT

   (A) normocytic anemia
   (B) sudden peripheral gangrene
   (C) symmetrical peripheral neuropathy
   (D) hematuria
   (E) aortic insufficiency

7. Which of the following antiarrhythmic drugs mediates its effect by interfering with movement of calcium through the "slow channel"?

   (A) phenytoin
   (B) verapamil
   (C) lidocaine
   (D) amiodarone
   (E) bretylium

8. Chest pain and friction rub three days after admission to a coronary care unit probably indicate

   (A) misdiagnosis of infarction
   (B) chest trauma
   (C) viral infection
   (D) transmural infarction
   (E) dissecting aneurysm

9. The effect of calcium ions on the myocardium can best be described as

  (A) positively inotropic
  (B) negatively inotropic
  (C) positively chronotropic
  (D) negatively chronotropic
  (E) excitation–contraction uncoupling

10. Arterial hypertension in pregnancy

  (A) improves in the third trimester
  (B) leads to large birth-weight babies
  (C) should be rigorously controlled with drugs
  (D) spares the placenta
  (E) spares maternal kidney function

11. The temporary or standby pacemaker may be indicated in acute myocardial infarction (MI) with all of the following EXCEPT

  (A) persistent bradycardia
  (B) inferior infarction and block
  (C) first degree AV block
  (D) alternating right and left bundle branch block
  (E) Mobitz type 2 block

12. Which of the following is associated with an increased intensity of the pulmonic second heart sound?

  (A) pulmonary stenosis
  (B) aortic stenosis
  (C) myocardial infarction
  (D) pulmonary hypertension
  (E) systemic hypertension

13. A patient with a regular heart beat at a rate of 170/minute that abruptly changes to 75/minute after applying carotid sinus pressure most likely has

  (A) sinus tachycardia
  (B) paroxysmal atrial fibrillation
  (C) paroxysmal atrial flutter
  (D) paroxysmal atrial tachycardia
  (E) paroxysmal ventricular tachycardia

14. The Swan–Ganz catheter can be characterized by all of the following EXCEPT

  (A) measures pulmonary capillary wedge pressure
  (B) allows serial assessment of cardiac output
  (C) may induce arrhythmias

  (D) should be avoided in the presence of pulmonary embolism
  (E) may introduce sepsis

15. Angina pectoris, in the absence of coronary artery disease, occurs most frequently with

  (A) mitral stenosis
  (B) mitral insufficiency
  (C) pulmonary stenosis
  (D) aortic stenosis
  (E) aortic insufficiency

16. In aortic stenosis the second aortic sound at the base is characteristically

  (A) accentuated
  (B) diminished
  (C) normal in character
  (D) widely split due to delayed ventricular ejection
  (E) shows fixed splitting

17. Atrioventricular dissociation is defined as

  (A) surgical removal of an atrium
  (B) independent beating of atria and ventricles
  (C) congenital absence of atrial and ventricular septa
  (D) oxygen differential between chambers
  (E) heart rate under 60 beats/minute

18. Nitroprusside may be characterized as

  (A) primarily a vasoconstrictor
  (B) increases ventricular afterload
  (C) most effective with high cardiac output syndromes
  (D) causes change in heart rate and contractility
  (E) decreases afterload in heart failure

19. Of the following congenital lesions, which is the most frequently complicated by subacute bacterial endocarditis (SBE)?

  (A) ventricular septal defects
  (B) atrial septal defects
  (C) transposition of the great vessels
  (D) aortic stenosis
  (E) congenital mitral insufficiency

20. The most common primary cardiac tumor is a

  (A) myxoma
  (B) sarcoma
  (C) rhabdomyoma
  (D) fibroma
  (E) lipoma

21. Exercise electrocardiography

    (A) is an invasive procedure
    (B) is contraindicated in patients over 65 years of age
    (C) detects latent disease
    (D) has a morbidity of approximately 5%
    (E) is used in pulmonary embolism

22. Cardiac catheterization

    (A) is contraindicated in the presence of cyanosis
    (B) is considered noninvasive
    (C) is generally performed with cardiopulmonary bypass
    (D) may cause renal failure
    (E) requires carotid artery puncture

23. Pericarditis is known to occur with each of the following diseases EXCEPT

    (A) rheumatic fever
    (B) tuberculosis
    (C) pneumonia
    (D) myocardial infarction
    (E) scarlet fever

24. During cardiac catheterization, the pulmonary capillary "wedge" pressure is an approximation of pressure in the

    (A) pulmonary artery
    (B) pulmonary vein
    (C) left atrium
    (D) right atrium
    (E) vena cava

25. In atrial septal defects

    (A) pulmonary blood flow is greater than systemic blood flow
    (B) pulmonary blood flow is less than systemic blood flow
    (C) pulmonary blood flow is equal to systemic blood flow
    (D) the left ventricle is enlarged
    (E) the systemic blood pressure is elevated

26. Echocardiography is useful in the diagnosis of all of the following EXCEPT

    (A) mitral stenosis
    (B) coronary artery aneurysm
    (C) muscular subaortic stenosis
    (D) atrial septal defect
    (E) prosthetic valve dysfunction

27. A rapidly rising forceful pulse that collapses quickly is seen in which of the following lesions?

    (A) mitral stenosis
    (B) mitral regurgitation
    (C) aortic stenosis
    (D) aortic regurgitation
    (E) coarctation of the aorta

28. Mitral stenosis may be associated with all of the following clinical symptoms EXCEPT

    (A) angina pectoris
    (B) hoarseness
    (C) cough
    (D) hemoptysis
    (E) nausea and vomiting

29. The development of paroxysmal atrial tachycardia in a patient on digitalis indicates

    (A) an increase in digitalis dose
    (B) complete cessation of digitalis
    (C) withdrawal of digitalis for one dose
    (D) no change in digitalis, but other medication should be given
    (E) none of the above

30. Chronic constrictive pericarditis is found in association with all of the following EXCEPT

    (A) rheumatic fever
    (B) tuberculosis
    (C) unknown cause
    (D) previous acute pericarditis
    (E) neoplastic involvement of the pericardium

31. Digitalis given in atrial flutter frequently causes

    (A) atrial asystole
    (B) atrial bigeminy
    (C) atrial tachycardia
    (D) paroxysmal atrial tachycardia with block
    (E) atrial fibrillation

32. All of the following may lead to some fluid retention in heart failure EXCEPT

    (A) increased renin
    (B) increased aldosterone
    (C) increased estrogen
    (D) increased growth hormone
    (E) increased vasopressin

DIRECTIONS (Questions 33 through 37): The group of questions below consists of a list of lettered headings followed by a list of numbered words, phrases, or statements. For each numbered word, phrase, or statement, select the ONE lettered heading that is most closely associated with it. Each lettered heading may be selected once, more than once, or not at all.

(A) mitral stenosis
(B) acute rheumatic fever
(C) hypothyroidism
(D) hyperparathyroidism
(E) Wolff–Parkinson–White syndrome
(F) hypokalemia
(G) hyperkalemia
(H) aortic stenosis

33. Broad-notched P wave

34. Prolonged P-R interval

35. Short P-R interval

36. Short Q-T interval

37. Low-voltage QRS complexes

DIRECTIONS (Questions 38 through 46): For each numbered phrase select the ONE lettered heading that is most closely associated with it. Each lettered heading may be selected once, more than once, or not at all.

Questions 38 through 41

(A) true of propranolol but not verapamil
(B) true of verapamil but not propranolol
(C) true of *both* verapamil and propranolol
(D) true of *neither* verapamil nor propranolol

38. Well absorbed from the gastrointestinal (GI) tract with useful bioavailability

39. The effects on the heart result in a prominent negative inotropic effect

40. A treatment of choice in paroxysmal AV junctional tachycardias

41. Mechanism of action is calcium blockade

Questions 42 through 46

(A) true of hydralazine but not captopril
(B) true of captopril but not hydralazine
(C) true of *both* captopril and hydralazine
(D) true of *neither* captopril nor hydralazine

42. Direct action on vascular smooth muscle

43. Inhibition of angiotensin I converting enzyme

44. Myocardial stimulant

45. Used for pulmonary hypertension

46. Very few side effects

DIRECTIONS (Questions 47 through 58): Each of the questions or incomplete statements below is followed by five suggested answers or completions. Select the ONE that is best in each case.

47. The electrocardiographic sign most characteristic of a ventricular aneurysm is

   (A) ST elevation
   (B) RS-T depression in V_5 and V_6
   (C) inversion of T waves in one precordial lead
   (D) presence of an RS in a VL
   (E) tall, peaked T waves

48. X-ray examination of the heart in aortic stenosis is most likely to reveal

   (A) right ventricular dilatation
   (B) stenosis of the proximal ascending aorta
   (C) left atrial hypertrophy
   (D) normal overall cardiac size
   (E) displaced apex

49. All of the following are major risk factors for the development of cardiovascular disease EXCEPT

   (A) exercise over the age of 50
   (B) male sex
   (C) diabetes
   (D) cigarette smoking
   (E) high plasma LDL and low plasma HDL cholesterol

50. Blood pressure (BP) in the arms may differ significantly from pressure in the legs in the presence of

   (A) aortic insufficiency
   (B) coarctation of the aorta
   (C) normal children over the age of two years

(D) ventricular aneurysm

(E) severe juvenile diabetes

51. The electrocardiographic signs of left ventricular hypertrophy are most likely to include

(A) counterclockwise rotation of the electrical axis

(B) rSR pattern in V_1

(C) right axis deviation

(D) high voltage QRS complexes in V_5 and V_6

(E) prolonged P-R interval in the limb leads

52. Which of the following is most likely to occur in the presence of untreated, uncomplicated, congestive heart failure?

(A) increased urinary sodium content

(B) low urine specific gravity

(C) increased urinary chloride content

(D) anemia of chronic disease

(E) albuminuria

53. Cardiac findings secondary to hyperthyroid heart disease are most likely to include

(A) prolonged circulation time

(B) decreased cardiac output

(C) paroxysmal atrial fibrillation

(D) pericardial effusion

(E) aortic insufficiency

54. The retinopathy of accelerated hypertension is most likely to include

(A) retinitis obliterans

(B) cotton wool spots

(C) retinal detachment

(D) optic atrophy

(E) foveal blindness

55. Type II hyperlipoproteinemia may be associated with any of the following EXCEPT

(A) hyperthyroidism

(B) high risk of atherosclerosis

(C) myxedema

(D) nephrosis

(E) obstructive liver disease

56. The development of clinical symptomatology from a pericardial effusion depends most on the

(A) specific gravity of the fluid

(B) presence or absence of blood in the fluid

(C) rate of development of the effusion

(D) cellular count of the fluid

(E) viscosity of the fluid

57. Which of the following is LEAST likely to be informative in a diagnostic evaluation of patients with diastolic hypertension?

(A) renal ultrasound

(B) chest x-ray

(C) serum potassium

(D) magnetic resonance image of the brain

(E) family history

58. Mitral valve prolapse is most commonly associated with

(A) mitral stenosis

(B) absent first heart sound

(C) diastolic click

(D) aortic regurgitation

(E) late systolic murmur

DIRECTIONS (Questions 59 through 76): This section consists of clinical situations, each followed by a question or a series of questions. Study each situation, and select the ONE best answer to each question following it.

Questions 59 through 63: A 36-year-old man is seen because of palpitations. He admits to precordial discomfort, weakness, and anxiety. The pulse is 160. The blood pressure is 100/70. The heart sounds are normal. Carotid sinus pressure changes the rate to 80, but when released the pulse rate returns to 160.

59. The most likely diagnosis is

(A) atrial flutter with 2:1 block

(B) paroxysmal atrial tachycardia with 2:1 block

(C) sinus arrhythmia

(D) atrial fibrillation

(E) nodal tachycardia

60. Prior to the use of drugs, which of the following procedures were helpful in converting the above to a sinus rhythm?

(A) carotid sinus pressure

(B) gagging procedures

(C) Valsalva maneuver

(D) eyeball compression

(E) none of the above

61. Which of the following drugs is the best choice for treatment?

(A) digitalis

(B) mecholyl

(C) aminophylline

(D) ephedrine

(E) atropine

62. The tachycardia is commonly associated with all of the following EXCEPT

(A) hypertensive disease
(B) rheumatic heart disease
(C) syphilitic heart disease
(D) coronary disease
(E) hyperthyroidism

63. The common complications of the arrhythmia include all of the following EXCEPT

(A) right heart failure
(B) peripheral arterial embolization
(C) syncope
(D) left heart failure
(E) pericarditis

Questions 64 through 68: A 25-year-old man complains of left precordial chest pain that radiates to the left shoulder but not down the left arm. The pain is accentuated by inspiration and relieved by sitting up. The pain is accompanied by fever and chills. His blood pressure is 105/75, pulse 110/min and regular, and temperature 102°F. Aside from the tachycardia, there are no abnormal physical findings in the heart or lungs. The electrocardiogram shows ST segment elevation in all leads except aVR and VI. On the third hospital day, the blood pressure falls, the venous pressure rises, and the patient goes into congestive heart failure and shock.

64. The most likely diagnosis is

(A) pulmonary infarction
(B) myocardial infarction
(C) pericarditis
(D) myocardial infarction with secondary pericarditis
(E) viral pneumonitis

65. The underlying etiologic factor is

(A) coronary atherosclerosis
(B) thrombophlebitis
(C) neoplasm
(D) unknown but probably viral
(E) an arteritis

66. The events of the third hospital day were probably caused by

(A) a second pulmonary embolus
(B) extension of a myocardial infarct
(C) cardiac tamponade
(D) secondary bacterial infection
(E) rupture of a chorda tendineae

67. The correct treatment on the third hospital day would be

(A) ligation of the inferior vena cava
(B) pericardiocentesis
(C) anticoagulation and pressor amines
(D) penicillin and oxygen
(E) coronary endarterectomy

68. The chest roentgenogram on the third hospital day would probably reveal

(A) a wedge-shaped area of consolidation in the left lung field and a left pleural effusion
(B) no abnormal findings
(C) a "water-bottle" heart
(D) patchy areas of consolidation in the left lung field
(E) hypervascular lung fields

Question 69: The laboratory results shown in Table 1.1 are obtained from the investigation of a 37-year-old black woman who has a blood pressure at rest of 140/100 mm Hg. The most likely diagnosis is

(A) Cushing syndrome
(B) primary aldosteronism
(C) essential hypertension
(D) pyelonephritis
(E) bilateral renal artery stenosis

TABLE 1.1 LABORATORY INVESTIGATIONS

Urinalysis	
pH	5.2
Albumin	Negative to trace
Serum Na	140 mEq/L
K	3.5 mEq/L
Cl	100 mEq/L
CO_2	25 mEq/L
Creatinine	1.0 mg/100 mL
Fasting sugar	90 mg/100 mL
Calcium	9.0 mg/100 mL
Uric acid	5.0 mg/100 mL

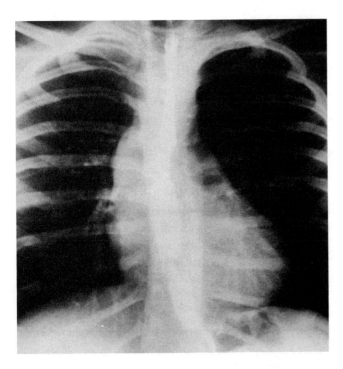

Figure 1.1

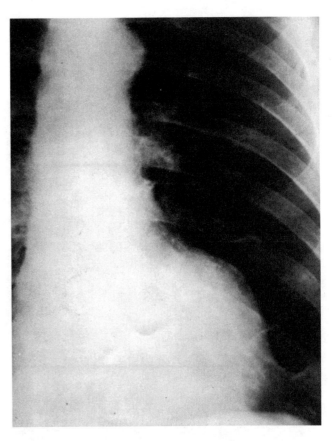

Figure 1.2

Question 70: Figure 1.1 is the x-ray of an 8-year-old boy who had easy fatigability and a soft, continuous murmur in the upper back. Electrocardiogram revealed minimal left ventricular hypertrophy. What is your diagnosis?

   (A) aortic stenosis

   (B) persistent ductus arteriosus

   (C) coarctation of the aorta

   (D) pulmonary valvular stenosis

   (E) peripheral pulmonary stenosis

Question 71: Figure 1.2 is an x-ray of an asymptomatic 48-year-old male executive coming in for his regular annual medical checkup. What is your diagnosis?

   (A) calcific pericarditis

   (B) left ventricular aneurysm

   (C) hydatid cyst

   (D) pleuropericarditis

   (E) normal

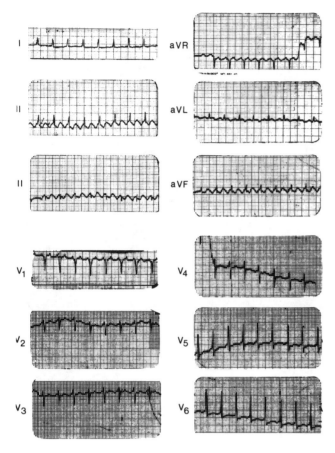

Figure 1.3

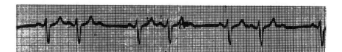

Figure 1.4

Question 73: What is the rhythm in the lead tracing shown in Figure 1.4?

    (A) first-degree heart block

    (B) second-degree heart block

    (C) third-degree heart block

    (D) ventricular premature beats

    (E) atrial premature beats

Question 74: The patient is a 42-year-old woman with a history of many years of anterior chest pain of a somewhat atypical nature. The patient's pain has been present and relatively stable for a number of years, and the electrocardiographic picture shown in Figure 1.5 is a stable one. What is the diagnosis?

    (A) inferior wall infarction

    (B) anterior wall infarction

    (C) ventricular aneurysm

    (D) nonspecific changes

    (E) pericarditis

Question 72: A 70-year-old man has dyspnea, orthopnea, and paroxysmal nocturnal dyspnea. He has generalized cardiomegaly and pulmonary and systemic venous hypertension. The ECG is shown in Figure 1.3 What is the cardiac rhythm?

    (A) ectopic atrial tachycardia

    (B) atrial flutter with 2:1 AV conduction

    (C) sinus tachycardia

    (D) supraventricular tachycardia

    (E) atrial fibrillation with rapid ventricular response

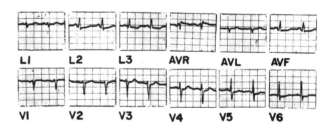

Figure 1.5

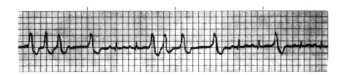

Figure 1.6

Question 75: This electrocardiogram shown in Figure 1.6 was obtained during the initial stages of an acute myocardial infarction. What is the rhythm?

   (A) atrial fibrillation
   (B) atrial flutter
   (C) second-degree heart block
   (D) Wenckebach phenomenon
   (E) ventricular tachycardia

Question 76: A 78-year-old man with advanced renal disease has the electrocardiogram shown in Figure 1.7 (lead II). What is the diagnosis?

   (A) hyperkalemia
   (B) hypercalcemia
   (C) hypernatremia
   (D) pericarditis
   (E) ventricular aneurysm

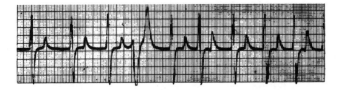

Figure 1.7

DIRECTIONS (Questions 77 through 113): For each numbered phrase select the ONE lettered heading that is most closely associated with it. Each lettered heading may be selected once, more than once, or not at all.

Questions 77 through 81

   (A) pulsus tardus
   (B) pulsus paradoxus
   (C) hyperkinetic pulse
   (D) bisferiens pulse
   (E) dicrotic pulse
   (F) pulsus alternans
   (G) delayed femoral pulse
   (H) pulsus bigeminus

   77. Patent ductus arteriosus

   78. Dilated cardiomyopathy

   79. Hypertrophic cardiomyopathy

   80. Aortic stenosis

   81. Superior vena cava obstruction

Questions 82 through 86

   (A) large "a" wave
   (B) prominent "x" descent
   (C) Kussmaul's sign
   (D) slow "y" descent
   (E) prominent "v" waves
   (F) positive abdominojugular reflux

   82. Tricuspid regurgitation

   83. Right atrial myxoma

   84. Right ventricular infarction

   85. Right-sided heart failure

   86. Complete heart block

Questions 87 through 91

    (A) true of aortic stenosis (AS) but not hypertrophic cardiomyopathy (HCM) with obstruction

    (B) true of HCM with obstruction but *not* AS

    (C) true of *both* HCM with obstruction and AS

    (D) true of *neither* HCM with obstruction nor AS

87. Exertional dyspnea, syncope, and angina pectoris are classical symptoms

88. Murmur increases with standing

89. Murmur decreases in intensity and length with Valsalva maneuver

90. Murmur increases with exercise

91. Double apical impulse often present

Questions 92 through 97

    (A) cardiac tamponade

    (B) constrictive pericarditis

    (C) restrictive cardiomyopathy

    (D) right ventricle myocardial infarction (RVMI)

92. Prominent "y" descent of neck veins, Kussmaul's sign, low voltage on ECG

93. Pulsus paradoxus, low ECG voltage, negative Kussmaul's sign

94. Elevated neck veins, abnormal ECG, third heart sound (S_3) present

95. Electrical alternans on ECG

96. Pericardial knock

97. No pulsus paradoxus, prominent "x" descent of neck veins, no Kussmaul's sign

Questions 98 through 102

    (A) diabetes mellitus (DM)

    (B) thiamine deficiency

    (C) hyperthyroidism

    (D) hypothyroidism

    (E) malignant carcinoid

    (F) pheochromocytoma

    (G) rheumatoid arthritis (RA)

    (H) seronegative arthropathies

    (I) systemic lupus erythematosus (SLE)

98. Endothelial plaques

99. Proximal aortitis

100. Focal myocardial necrosis

101. Systolic scratchy sound

102. Restrictive cardiomyopathy

Questions 103 through 107

    (A) fibric acid derivatives (clofibrate, gemfibrozil)

    (B) nicotinic acid

    (C) bile acid-binding resins (cholestyramine, colestipol)

    (D) HMG-CoA reductase inhibitors (lovastatin, simvastatin, pravastatin)

    (E) probucol

    (F) estrogens (premarin, estradiol)

103. Associated with malignancy

104. Can cause gallstones and myopathy

105. Minimal absorption and no systemic toxicity

106. Block the rate-limiting step in cholesterol synthesis

107. Can lower high-density lipoprotein (HDL) levels

Questions 108 through 112

    (A) thiazides

    (B) spironolactone

    (C) clonidine

    (D) prazosin

    (E) beta blockers

    (F) hydralazine

    (G) angiotensin-converting enzyme inhibitors (ACE inhibitors)

    (H) calcium channel blockers

108. Particularly useful in diabetes mellitus

109. Most extensively studied, with proven effect in morbidity and mortality

110. Drug of choice in unilateral renal artery stenosis

111. Older people and blacks respond particularly well

112. Edema without congestive heart failure

DIRECTIONS (Questions 113 and 114): Each of the questions or incomplete statements below is followed by five suggested answers or completions. Select the ONE that is best in each case.

113. Sudden death

    (A) is invariably due to cardiac cause

    (B) is rare in infants and children

    (C) has a bimodal distribution in the population

    (D) is defined as death within 24 hours of onset of symptoms

    (E) when caused by cardiac disease is most commonly characterized by coronary thrombi

114. Which of the following statements concerning essential hypertension is CORRECT?

    (A) over 95% of patients are salt sensitive

    (B) it comprises about 75% of hypertensives seen in a specialty clinic

    (C) renin levels are invariably high

    (D) women have a poorer prognosis

    (E) alcohol reduces risk

Cardiology

Answers and Explanations

1. **(D)** Wenckebach, or type I second-degree AV block, is characterized on ECG by progressive lengthening of the P-R interval until there is a nonconducted P wave. The magnitude of P-R lengthening declines with each beat, so the R-R intervals characteristically shorten prior to the dropped beat. It is almost always caused by abnormal conduction across the AV node, and the QRS complex is usually of normal duration. *(Ref. 9, p. 748)*

2. **(D)** The QRS complex may be insignificantly prolonged and the ST segment and QT intervals shortened in hypercalcemia. The T wave may actually start at the end of the QRS and there may be essentially no ST segment. The corrected QT interval (QT_c) although short, does not correlate with the level of hypercalcemia. Hypercalcemia rarely causes arrhythmias. *(Ref. 9, p. 768)*

3. **(D)** The ventricular inhibited (VVI) pacemaker functions when the heart rate falls below a present interval. If a QRS is detected, the pacemaker is inhibited. If a QRS is not sensed, the pacing stimulus is not inhibited and the ventricle is stimulated. *(Ref. 9, p. 826)*

4. **(D)** Occasionally there is right deviation of the electrical axis, but never left deviation during an acute episode. One of the most useful roles of the ECG is to rule out myocardial infarction when a massive embolism is present. The specific ECG signs of pulmonary embolism are rarely seen except in such cases of massive pulmonary embolism. In submassive pulmonary emboli, the ECG may show nonspecific ST changes and sinus tachycardia. On occasion, pulmonary embolism can precipitate atrial flutter or fibrillation. *(Ref. 9, p. 1881)*

5. **(C)** Aortic stenosis is most likely to be associated with angina pectoris and syncope. Increased oxygen requirement, myocardial hypertrophy, low diastolic aortic pressure, and shortening of diastole are contributory factors to the syncope. *(Ref. 9, p. 1459)*

6. **(C)** Peripheral neuropathy is not a complication of bacterial endocarditis. Many of the complications are thought to be embolic, but may include vasculitis. Autopsy studies reveal that many systemic emboli go unrecognized. Brain, lung, coronary arteries, spleen, extremities, gut, and eyes are common locations for emboli. *(Ref. 9, p. 1694)*

7. **(B)** The slow channel for calcium assumes considerable importance in the region of the sinus node and AV node. For verapamil, this results in both antiarrhythmic and negative inotropic effects. Different classes of calcium channel blockers have differential effects on these slow channels, explaining the different clinical properties of the various calcium channel-blocking drugs. *(Ref. 9, p. 1291)*

8. **(D)** Pericarditis secondary to transmural infarction is very common and most cases appear within four days. The most common manifestation of pericarditis is a friction rub along the left sternal border. It is evanescent, lasting only a few days. The pain is usually perceived by the patient to be different than that of the infarct. It is worsened by inspiration, swallowing, coughing, or lying down. It frequently is associated with a low-grade murmur. *(Ref. 9, p. 1151)*

9. **(A)** Positively inotropic is the best description of the effect of calcium ions on the myocardium. Calcium plays a role in excitation–contraction coupling and in possible drug effects and heart failure. *(Ref. 9, p. 769)*

10. **(C)** In the past, there was concern that rigorous drug treatment would harm the fetus. Studies now show benefit in controlling pressure with drugs, but ACE inhibitors are contraindicated. *(Ref. 9, p. 1440)*

11. **(C)** The temporary pacemaker is not required for first-degree block. For second-degree block of the Wenckebach type (usually with an inferior infarction), pacing is only required if symptoms of bradycardia and hypotension cannot be controlled medically. The necessity for temporary pacing during an acute MI does not necessarily indicate that permanent pacing will be required. *(Ref. 9, p. 1143)*

12. **(D)** Pulmonary hypertension is associated with an increased intensity of the second heart sound, which coincides with the end of the T wave on ECG. It is the pulmonic component of the second heart sound that is increased. As well, there may be prominent "a" waves in the jugular venous pulse, a right ventricular heave, an ejection click, and a right ventricular fourth heart sound. When signs and symptoms are apparent, the pulmonary hypertension is usually moderate to severe. *(Ref. 9, p. 1868)*

13. **(D)** The patient most likely has paroxysmal atrial tachycardia. Sinus tachycardia differs from atrial tachycardia in that it does not start or stop abruptly. In paroxysmal atrial tachycardia, the QRS is usually narrow without clearly discernible P waves. A wide QRS in paroxysmal supraventricular tachycardia can result from a pre-existing bundle branch block, or a functional bundle branch block secondary to the tachycardia. This can make the distinction from a ventricular arrhythmia quite difficult. *(Ref. 9, pp. 711, 715)*

14. **(D)** The Swan–Ganz catheter is valuable in monitoring fluid balance in patients with pulmonary embolism who have high levels of right atrial pressure and may require more fluids than apparent clinically. Although valuable for monitoring patients, Swan–Ganz catheters commonly precipitate nonsustained arrhythmias and local inflammations or infections. More serious complications such as sustained arrhythmias, pneumothorax, and major lung complications occur in 3 to 5 percent of patients, usually those who are already critically ill. *(Ref. 9, pp. 447–455)*

15. **(D)** In the absence of coronary artery disease, angina pectoris occurs most frequently with aortic stenosis. Acute myocardial infarction is usually due to associated atherosclerotic coronary occlusion. *(Ref. 9, pp. 460, 1459)*

16. **(B)** In aortic stenosis, the first sound is usually normal but may be faint and of low pitch; the second sound is characteristically diminished. *(Ref. 9, p. 1460)*

17. **(B)** Atrioventricular dissociation is the independent beating of atria and ventricles and is recognized on the electrocardiogram by fixed P-P and R-R intervals but variable P-R intervals. *(Ref. 9, p. 749)*

18. **(E)** With impaired myocardial function, stroke output is increased by nitroprusside as left ventricular end-diastolic pressure falls. *(Ref. 9, p. 613)*

19. **(A)** Of those listed, ventricular septal defect is most commonly involved with SBE, but patent ductus arteriosus may be more frequently involved. Less than 10% of cases of SBE occur in the setting of congenital cardiac disease. *(Ref. 9, p. 1683)*

20. **(A)** The myxoma is a solitary globular or polypoid tumor varying in size from that of a cherry to a peach. About 75% are found in the left atrium, and most of the remainder in the right atrium. The clinical presentation is with one or more of the classical triad of constitution symptoms (fatigue, fever, anemia), embolic events, or obstruction of the valve orifice. *(Ref. 9, p. 2008)*

21. **(C)** Exercise electrocardiography represents an increasingly popular noninvasive method for early detection of latent ischemic heart disease. As with other diagnostic tests, the exercise ECG is of most clinical value when the pretest probability of disease is moderate (i.e., 30 to 70%). *(Ref. 9, p. 1060)*

22. **(D)** Contrast media used in cardiac catheterization may result in renal impairment. The group at highest risk includes diabetics with renal disease and those with pre-existing renal failure. Good hydration is essential. Other manifestations of contrast media include nausea and vomiting (common), and anaphylactoid reactions characterized by low-grade fever, hives, itching, angioedema, bronchospasm, and even shock. *(Ref. 9, p. 2401)*

23. **(E)** Scarlet fever does not generally cause pericarditis. Pericarditis in clinical practice is commonly idiopathic and frequently assumed to be of possible viral origin. *(Ref. 9, p. 1650)*

24. **(C)** Left-heart catheterization is a more accurate measurement, but involves a slightly increased risk. End-expiratory pulmonary artery diastolic pressure is very close (2 to 4 mm) to wedge pressure as well. A discordance between wedge pressure and pulmonary artery diastolic pressure suggests the presence of pulmonary hypertension. *(Ref. 9, p. 2388)*

25. **(A)** Pulmonary blood flow is greater because of increased blood flow from the right atrium, which receives blood from the vena cava and left atrium. *(Ref. 9, pp. 1773–1774)*

26. **(B)** Echocardiography is not useful in the diagnosis of coronary artery aneurysm. These may be congenital or acquired. In addition to the conditions listed, this technique also detects ventricular hypertrophy, pericardial effusion, and atrial myxomas. *(Ref. 9, p. 1247)*

27. **(D)** This pulse is seen in aortic regurgitation. The pressure in diastole is usually 50 mm Hg or lower. This is known as a water-hammer or Corrigan's pulse. As well, a bisferiens pulse may be present. Systolic blood pressure is elevated. *(Ref. 9, p. 1471)*

28. **(E)** Nausea and vomiting are not associated with mitral stenosis. The positive symptoms are associated with isolated left atrial and pulmonary venocapillary hypertension. *(Ref. 9, p. 1485)*

29. **(B)** Atrioventricular dissociation and paroxysmal atrial tachycardia with block are distinctive manifestations of digitalis toxicity. Symptoms of digitalis toxicity include anorexia, nausea, fatigue, dizziness, and visual disturbances. The presence of hypokalemia increases the likelihood of digitalis toxicity. *(Ref. 9, p. 582)*

30. **(A)** Chronic constrictive pericarditis is not found in association with rheumatic fever, although isolated cases have been reported with rheumatoid arthritis. Acute rheumatic fever can produce a pancarditis which may involve the pericardium and produce a pericardial friction rub. However, it does not proceed to chronic pericardial disease. *(Ref. 9, pp. 1453, 1663–1665)*

31. **(E)** Digitalis given in atrial flutter frequently causes atrial fibrillation, and quinidine given in atrial fibrillation may induce atrial flutter. For acute management of atrial flutter, digoxin should be administered before other antiarrhythmias to prevent very rapid rates that might result if 1:1 AV conduction occurs. If hemodynamic instability is present, electrical cardioversion is the treatment of choice. *(Ref. 9, p. 724)*

32. **(D)** Retention of fluid is complex and not due to any one factor; however, hormones may contribute. Growth hormone does not have fluid-retaining properties. The exact mechanisms which initiate renal conservation of salt and water are not precisely understood, but may include arterial volume receptors sensing a decrease in the "effective" arterial blood volume. *(Ref. 9, p. 524)*

33. **(A)** ECG changes in mitral stenosis are due to enlargement and hypertrophy of the left atrium and asynchronous atrial activation. The notched P wave is most prominent in lead II. In lead V_1, the P wave has a negative terminal deflection. *(Ref. 9, p. 1486)*

34. **(B)** A prolonged P-R interval is the most frequent significant electrocardiographic abnormality in rheumatic fever. However, it is very nonspecific and seen in numerous other conditions. It is only a minor criterion for the diagnosis of acute rheumatic fever. *(Ref. 9, p. 1453)*

35. **(E)** In Wolff–Parkinson–White syndrome, the P-R interval is short, the QRS is widened, and there is slurring of the upstroke of the R wave. The shortened P-R interval reflects faster than normal conduction through an accessory pathway. The ventricular complex represents a fusion beat. The blurred upstroke of the QRS (delta wave) represents ventricular activation via the accessory pathway. The normal end portion of the QRS represents activation via the normal route through the AV node. *(Ref. 9, p. 337)*

36. **(D)** In hyperparathyroidism, hypercalcemia may prolong the QRS and shorten the ST and QT intervals. Serious arrhythmias rarely occur with hypercalcemia. Patients with hyperparathyroidism might also have a higher prevalence of hypertension. *(Ref. 9, pp. 768, 1913)*

37. **(C)** The ECG in hypothyroidism may exhibit sinus bradycardia, low amplitude P and QRS waves, conduction disturbances, nonspecific ST and T-wave changes, and QT prolongation. The reduced cardiac output and enlarged cardiac silhouette on chest x-ray often lead to confusion between hypothyroidism and heart failure. *(Ref. 9, p. 1911)*

38. **(C)** Propranolol is well absorbed in the GI tract, but undergoes extensive metabolism on its first pass through the liver, so that only 20 to 50% of the dose is bioavailable. Despite only 10 to 20% bioavailability, verapamil is still a useful drug taken orally. *(Ref. 9, p. 1295)*

39. **(C)** Both can result in severe hypotension, left ventricular failure, and cardiogenic shock in patients with left ventricular dysfunction. Unlike beta blockers, the various calcium channel blockers have varying effects on cardiac function. Some, such as amlodipine, rarely cause congestive heart failure. *(Ref. 9, pp. 1289, 1303)*

40. **(B)** Verapamil exerts a potent effect on the region of the sinus node and AV node, so that intravenous verapamil is highly effective in junc-

tional tachycardias. Verapamil can be used acutely, as well as chronically, for prophylaxis against paroxysmal supraventricular tachycardia. *(Ref. 9, p. 1299)*

41. **(B)** Verapamil appears to mediate its effect by interfering with movement of calcium through the so-called slow channel. These slow channels predominantly allow calcium to enter, in contrast to the fast channels where sodium enters. Various classes of calcium channel blockers have differential effects on these slow channels, explaining their differential clinical effects. *(Ref. 9, p. 1291)*

42. **(A)** Hydralazine has a greater dilator effect on arterioles than veins. Reflex tachycardia is common in patients with hypertension, but less so in heart failure. Tachycardia may precipitate angina. *(Ref. 9, p. 614)*

43. **(B)** Captopril may exert its effect by inhibiting formation of angiotensin II. This lowers systemic vascular resistance. In addition, ACE inhibitors have a natriuretic effect by inhibition of aldosterone secretion. *(Ref. 9, p. 618)*

44. **(D)** Hydralazine and captopril increase cardiac output by decreasing impedance to left ventricular ejection. The combination of hydralazine and isosorbide dinitrate prolongs life in patients with heart failure. However the ACE inhibitor enalapril provides even greater survival benefit. *(Ref. 9, pp. 615, 618)*

45. **(D)** Although they have been used, neither drug is very useful in pulmonary hypertension. Even low doses of vasodilators can cause untoward reactions in patients with pulmonary hypertension. Lung transplants have provided a major therapeutic modality for managing severe pulmonary hypertension. *(Ref. 9, p. 1870)*

46. **(D)** Hydralazine causes flushing, nasal congestion, conjunctivitis, and a lupus-like syndrome. Captopril causes hypotension, proteinuria, neutropenia, and urticaria. *(Ref. 9, pp. 614, 618)*

47. **(A)** ST elevation persisting two weeks after an infarct, an abnormal pericardial impulse, and a bulge on the left ventricular border on x-ray are characteristic of an aneurysm. Ventricular aneurysms are most often a result of a large anterior infarct. The poor prognosis associated with these aneurysms is due to the associated left ventricular dysfunction, rather than to the aneurysm itself. *(Ref. 9, p. 1153)*

48. **(D)** There is normal overall cardiac size, but dilatation of the proximal ascending aorta and blunt rounding of the lower left cardiac contour. Calcification of the valve is often difficult to determine on plain films. Although left atrial enlargement can occur, its presence on the chest x-ray should raise other diagnostic possibilities, such as mitral valve disease. *(Ref. 9, p. 1461)*

49. **(A)** Exercise is not a major risk factor in fit individuals and may be protective. Lesser risk factors also include overweight, sedentary way of life, and hardness of water. A family history of premature coronary artery disease is also important, suggesting genetic factors. *(Ref. 9, pp. 1206–1208)*

50. **(B)** Besides coarctation of the aorta, aortic occlusive disease, dissection of the aorta, and abdominal aneurysm may lead to differential BP in arms and legs. Coarctation is the third most common form of congenital cardiac disease. One-third of patients will be hypertensive. The femoral pulses are weak, delayed, and even absent. *(Ref. 9, p. 1786)*

51. **(D)** ECG signs include left-axis deviation, high-voltage QRS complexes in V_5 and V_6, deep S in V_1 and V_2, and prolonged QRS in the left precordial leads. Age, orientation of the heart in the chest, and noncardiac factors make the ECG an imperfect tool for diagnosing or excluding left ventricular hypertrophy. The echocardiogram is more accurate, and better for following progression or regression of LVH. *(Ref. 9, p. 342)*

52. **(E)** High urinary specific gravity, nocturia, and daytime oliguria occur in addition to albuminuria in uncomplicated, untreated, congestive heart failure. *(Ref. 9, p. 214)*

53. **(C)** Thyroid disease may affect the heart muscle directly or there may be excessive sympathetic stimulation. Common symptoms of thyrotoxic heart disease include palpitations, exertional dyspnea, and worsening angina. Atrial fibrillation is particularly common in older individuals. *(Ref. 9, p. 1909)*

54. **(B)** Cotton wool spots, hemorrhage, and papilledema are common. Fibrinoid necrosis occurs on the arterioles of many organs. Earlier manifestations of arteriosclerosis include thickening of the vessel wall. This is manifested by obscuration of the venous column at arterial crossings. *(Ref. 9, p. 316)*

55. **(A)** A high risk of atherosclerosis and coronary artery disease is associated with type II hyperlipoproteinemia regardless of associated cause. It is not as common as type IIB, but the manifestations are more severe. LDL levels are character-

istically elevated two- or three-fold. *(Ref. 9, p. 1747)*

56. **(C)** The diagnostic triad for pericardial tamponade is rising venous pressure, falling arterial pressure, and a small quiet heart. Unless hypotension is extreme, pulsus paradoxus is usually present. In severe cases consciousness may be impaired. *(Ref. 9, p. 1658)*

57. **(D)** Essential hypertension is commonly associated with a strong family history, but absence does not rule it out. Onset is usually in the fourth decade of life and blacks are more frequently affected. *(Ref. 9, p. 1413)*

58. **(E)** In mitral valve prolapse, the first heart sound is usually preserved followed by a systolic click and late systolic murmur. Regurgitation may occur. *(Ref. 9, p. 1505)*

59. **(A)** The symptoms and signs are like any sudden paroxysmal tachycardia, but the ventricular rate is the clue, after carotid pressure, to the diagnosis of atrial flutter with 2:1 block. *(Ref. 9, pp. 722–724)*

60. **(E)** The maneuvers listed increase the block and are useful for diagnosis, not for converting the atrial flutter to a sinus rhythm. *(Ref. 9, pp. 722–724)*

61. **(A)** Digitalis slows the ventricular rate and controls or prevents heart failure. Verapamil may be of help in both acute paroxysms of atrial flutter and chronic management. At times surgical or catheter ablation of the flutter pathway is required in chronic atrial flutter. *(Ref. 9, p. 724)*

62. **(C)** The tachycardia is not commonly associated with syphilitic heart disease. The sudden change to half rate on vagal stimulation is diagnostic of atrial flutter with 2:1 block. *(Ref. 9, pp. 722–724)*

63. **(E)** All of the first four complications are common in arrhythmia, but pericarditis is not seen. The attacks of flutter are often more complicated than atrial tachycardia because of their tendency to persist. *(Ref. 9, pp. 722–724)*

64. **(C)** Pericarditis is the most likely diagnosis. The pain may be sternal or parasternal, and radiate to posterior or anterior cervical areas, to either trapezius, or to either shoulder. *(Ref. 9, pp. 1649–1651)*

65. **(D)** Viruses include coxsackie B virus, ECHO, adenovirus, and infectious mononucleosis. The erythrocyte sedimentation rate is usually elevated, and an early leukocytosis is common. Cardiac enzymes are usually normal. Rising viral titers are required to confirm the exact causative virus. *(Ref. 9, p. 1650)*

66. **(C)** Management of acute viral or idiopathic pericarditis includes analgesia (usually aspirin every 3 to 4 hours initially) and rest if the pain is severe. Occasionally nonsteroidal anti-inflammatory drugs are required, e.g., ibuprofen or indomethacin. Careful observation for increasing effusion and tamponade are essential. *(Ref. 9, pp. 1651, 1658)*

67. **(B)** Pericardiocentesis would be the correct treatment. Open pericardial biopsy is performed if there is uncertainty as to diagnosis or there is no response to therapy. *(Ref. 9, p. 1661)*

68. **(C)** A water-bottle heart would probably be revealed. The association of clear lung fields with a large cardiac silhouette distinguishes pericardial effusion from heart failure. *(Ref. 9, p. 914)*

69. **(C)** Essential hypertension is the most likely diagnosis. A secondary cause for hypertension is found in only 10% of patients, with 90% labelled as "essential." *(Ref. 9, p. 1413)*

70. **(C)** Coarctation of the aorta is the diagnosis. There is a "reverse 3" deformity of the esophagus, the belly of which represents the dilated aorta after the coarctation. The border of the descending aorta shows a medial indentation called the "3" or "tuck" sign, the belly of the "3" representing the poststenotic dilation and the upper portion by the dilated subclavian artery and small transverse aortic arch. *(Ref. 9, p. 1786)*

71. **(B)** Note the abnormal humped contour of the left ventricular border, with a curvilinear calcification following the abnormal cardiac contour. The presence of calcification in the ventricular wall and the abnormal left ventricular contour alert one to the consideration of a ventricular aneurysm. *(Ref. 9, p. 1153)*

72. **(B)** The cardiac rhythm is atrial flutter with 2:1 AV conduction. QRS complexes occur with perfect regularity at a rate of about 150/minute. Their normal contour and duration indicate that ventricular activation occurs normally via the AV junction–His–Purkinje system. *(Ref. 9, p. 722)*

73. **(B)** The P-R interval of the first two complexes is normal at 0.20 seconds. The QRS duration is 0.16 seconds. The third P wave is nonconducted. This cycle recurs in the remainder of the strip. This is second-degree heart block of the Mobitz type II variety. Note the wide QRS. When this

type of heart block develops, either de novo or in the course of an acute myocardial infarction, a cardiac pacemaker is usually recommended, as the incidence of complete heart block is high in this situation. *(Ref. 9, p. 749)*

74. **(D)** The ST is depressed in leads II, III, aVF, and V$_{4-6}$. These nonspecific abnormalities do not indicate significant coronary heart disease, especially in an apprehensive young patient. *(Ref. 9, pp. 322–325)*

75. **(E)** The rhythm is regular sinus rhythm with a rate of 85 beats/minute. The sinus rhythm is interrupted frequently by bursts of irregular ventricular, premature beats. Sinus rhythm is uninterrupted as can be determined by plotting the P-P intervals, which are regular. The rhythm may be termed a chaotic ventricular arrhythmia or ventricular tachycardia. Its gross irregularity is unusual. Antiarrhythmic therapy is indicated. *(Ref. 9, p. 736)*

76. **(A)** No atrial activity is detected. The ventricular rate is slightly irregular. Beat no. 4 is a ventricular premature contraction. The T waves are tall and markedly peaked. This type of T wave is characteristic of hyperkalemia, as is absence of visible atrial activity. The potassium level was 8.2 mmol/L. *(Ref. 9, pp. 761–762)*

77. **(C)** A hyperkinetic pulse occurs in the setting of an elevated stroke volume (anemia, fever, anxiety, or an abnormally rapid run-off from the arterial system (patent ductus, arteriovenous fistula). *(Ref. 2, p. 948)*

78. **(E)** A dicrotic pulse has a peak in systole and another in diastole. It occurs in patients with very low stroke volume, especially dilated cardiomyopathy. *(Ref. 2, p. 948)*

79. **(D)** The bisferiens pulse, two systolic peaks, occurs in hypertrophic cardiomyopathy and aortic regurgitation. In aortic regurgitation, the bisferiens pulse can occur both in the presence or absence of aortic stenosis. *(Ref. 2, p. 948)*

80. **(A)** The pulsus tardus of aortic stenosis is the result of mechanical obstruction to left ventricular ejection and often has an accompanying thrill. The characteristic feel of the pulse is caused by a delayed systolic peak. *(Ref. 2, p. 948)*

81. **(B)** Pulsus paradoxus, a drop of greater than 10 mm Hg in systolic blood pressure during inspiration, is caused by pericardial tamponade, airways obstruction, or superior vena cava ob-

struction. At times, the peripheral pulse may disappear completely during inspiration. *(Ref. 2, p. 948)*

82. **(E)** Tricuspid regurgitation increases the size of the "v" wave. When tricuspid regurgitation becomes severe, the combination of a prominent "v" wave and obliteration of the "X" descent results in a single large positive systolic wave. *(Ref. 2, p. 949)*

83. **(D)** Right atrial myxoma, or tricuspid stenosis, will slow the "y" descent by obstructing right ventricular filling. The "y" descent of the JVP is produced mainly by the tricuspid valve opening and the subsequent rapid inflow of blood into the right ventricle. *(Ref. 2, p. 949)*

84. **(C)** Right ventricular infarction and constrictive pericarditis frequently result in an increase in jugular venous pressure during inspiration (Kussmaul's sign). Severe right-sided failure can also be a cause. *(Ref. 2, p. 949)*

85. **(F)** Right-sided heart failure is the most common cause of a positive abdominojugular reflux (normal JVP at rest, increases during 10 seconds of firm mid-abdominal compression, and rapidly drops when pressure is released). *(Ref. 2, p. 949)*

86. **(A)** Large "a" waves occur with increased resistance to filling (tricuspid stenosis, pulmonary hypertension) or when the right atrium contracts against a tricuspid valve closed by right ventricular systole ("cannon a" waves) in complete heart block or other arrhythmias. *(Ref. 2, p. 949)*

87. **(C)** Both HCM and valvular aortic stenosis can present with dyspnea, angina, or syncope. Other causes of obstruction to left ventricular outflow include discrete subvalvular aortic stenosis or supravalvular aortic stenosis. Both conditions are congenital anomalies and quite uncommon. *(Ref. 2, pp. 1059, 1092)*

88. **(B)** The murmur of HCM increases with standing while AS murmur decreases. With squatting, the murmur of HCM decreases, AS increases. During the initial relative hypotension following amyl nitrate administration, the murmur of AS will increase while that of HCM will decrease. *(Ref. 2, p. 950)*

89. **(A)** Like most murmurs, that of AS decreases in intensity and length with Valsalva. The murmur of HCM (and mitral valve prolapse) increases with Valsalva. *(Ref. 2, p. 950)*

90. **(A)** The murmur of AS increases with exercise, whereas that of HCM decreases. In particular, the murmur of HCM will often decrease with near-maximum handgrip exercise. *(Ref. 2, p. 950)*

91. **(C)** Both AS and HCM often have double apical impulses. In aortic stenosis the first impulse occurs during atrial contraction and reflects the important contribution of atrial contraction to ventricular filling. In HCM there can even be a triple apical impulse. *(Ref. 2, pp. 1060, 1092)*

92. **(B)** Constrictive pericarditis is characterized by a prominent "y" descent of the neck veins, and low voltage on ECG. The presence of a positive Kussmaul's sign helps differentiate the syndrome from cor pulmonale and restrictive cardiomyopathies. *(Ref. 2, pp. 1097–1101)*

93. **(A)** Cardiac tamponade can occur with as little as 200 mL of fluid if the accumulation is rapid. Physical exam reveals a pulsus paradoxus (a greater than 10 mm Hg inspiratory decline in systolic arterial pressure), a prominent "x" descent of the jugular veins, but no Kussmaul's sign. The ECG may show low voltage. *(Ref. 2, pp. 1096–1097)*

94. **(D)** RVMI is characterized by high neck veins, ECG abnormalities, and often a right-sided S_3. The low cardiac output associated with right ventricular myocardial infarction can often be treated by volume expansion. Although a third of patients with inferoposterior infarctions have some degree of right ventricular necrosis, extensive RVMI is uncommon. *(Ref. 2, pp. 1076, 1097)*

95. **(A)** Electrical alternans (a beat-to-beat alternation in one or more components of the ECG signal) can occur in pericardial effusion and numerous other conditions. Total electrical alternans (P-QRS-T) and sinus tachycardia is relatively specific for pericardial effusion (often with tamponade). *(Ref. 2, pp. 965, 1097)*

96. **(B)** A pericardial knock is characteristic of constrictive pericarditis. It is in fact an early S_3, occurring 0.06 to 0.12 seconds after aortic closure. S_1 and S_2 are frequently distant. *(Ref. 2, p. 1100)*

97. **(C)** The combination of absent pulsus and absent Kussmaul's sign with prominent "x" descent favors a restrictive cardiomyopathy. Unlike constrictive pericarditis, restrictive cardiomyopathies frequently present with an enlarged heart, orthopnea, left ventricular hypertrophy, and bundle branch blocks. *(Ref. 2, pp. 1097, 1100)*

98. **(E)** The cardiac lesions of gastrointestinal carcinoids are almost exclusively in the right side of the heart and occur only when there are hepatic metastases. Fibrous plaques are found on the endothelium of the cardiac chambers, valves, and great vessels. These plaques can distort cardiac valves; tricuspid regurgitation and pulmonic stenosis are the most common valvular problems. *(Ref. 2, p. 1104)*

99. **(H)** The proximal aortitis of seronegative arthritis (ankylosing spondylitis, Reiter syndrome, psoriatic arthritis, or associated with inflammatory bowel disease) can result in aortic regurgitation and AV block. *(Ref. 2, p. 1105)*

100. **(F)** Focal myocardial necrosis and inflammatory cell infiltration caused by high circulating levels of catecholamines are seen in about 50% of patients who die with pheochromocytoma. As well, hypertension can further impair left ventricular function. *(Ref. 2, p. 1105)*

101. **(C)** The Means–Lerman scratch, a systolic scratchy sound, heard at the left second intercostal space during expiration, is thought to result from the rubbing of the hyperdynamic pericardium against the pleura. Palpitations, atrial fibrillation, hypertension, angina, and heart failure are more common cardiac manifestations of hyperthyroidism. *(Ref. 2, p. 1104)*

102. **(A)** Diabetes mellitus can result in a restrictive cardiomyopathy in the absence of large vessel coronary artery disease. Histology reveals increased collagen, glycoprotein, triglycerides, and cholesterol in the myocardial interstitium. Abnormalities may be present in small intramural arteries. *(Ref. 2, p. 1103)*

103. **(F)** Estrogens are effective in decreasing low-density lipoprotein (LDL) levels in postmenopausal women. They have been associated with endometrial cancer, and can also raise VLDL levels. *(Ref. 2, pp. 1112–1113)*

104. **(A)** Fibric acid derivatives decrease VLDL, but have been associated with gallstones and myopathy. They act by decreasing VLDL synthesis and enhancing lipoprotein lipase action. They have been shown to decrease risk from ischemic heart disease. *(Ref. 2, p. 1113)*

105. **(C)** The minimal absorption and lack of systemic toxicity of the resins make them good choices for use in children with familial hypercholesterolemia and for primary prevention in young adults. They act by promoting sterol excretion and increasing LDL receptor-mediated removal. *(Ref. 2, pp. 1112–1113)*

106. **(D)** The HMG-CoA reductase inhibitors block cholesterol synthesis and increase LDL receptor-

mediated catabolism of LDL. They are very effective in lowering LDL with minimal side effects. Gastrointestinal symptoms and myopathy have been reported, however. *(Ref. 2, pp. 1112–1113)*

107. **(E)** Probucol lowers levels of high-density lipoproteins (HDL), an important "antirisk factor" for atherosclerosis. Its mechanism of action is unknown, and it has not yet been definitely shown to decrease the risk from ischemic heart disease. It can also cause diarrhea. *(Ref. 2, p. 1113)*

108. **(G)** ACE inhibitors have no adverse effects on glucose or lipid metabolism and may actually minimize the development of diabetic nephropathy by reducing renal vascular resistance and renal perfusion pressure. *(Ref. 2, p. 1130)*

109. **(A)** Thiazides have been a cornerstone in most trials of antihypertensive therapy. Their adverse metabolic consequences include renal potassium loss leading to hypokalemia, hyperuricemia from uric acid retention, carbohydrate intolerance, and hyperlipidemia. *(Ref. 2, p. 1125)*

110. **(G)** Although contraindicated in bilateral stenosis, ACE inhibitors are the drug of choice in unilateral renal artery stenosis. When ACE inhibitors are used in patients with impaired renal function, renal function should be monitored twice a week for the first three weeks. *(Ref. 2, p. 1130)*

111. **(A)** Thiazides seem to work particularly well in blacks and the elderly. Younger individuals and whites respond well to beta blockers, ACE inhibitors, and calcium channel antagonists. *(Ref. 2, p. 1129)*

112. **(H)** Calcium channel blockers, particularly nifedipine, can cause edema. Nifedipine can also cause tachycardia, flushing, gastrointestinal disturbances, hyperkalemia, and headache. Constipation can be a troublesome side effect. Some calcium channel blockers have a negative inotropic effect, and should be used with caution in patients with left ventricular dysfunction. *(Ref. 2, p. 1127)*

113. **(C)** Sudden death, defined as death within one hour of onset of symptoms, is usually caused by cardiac disease in middle age and elderly patients, but in younger age groups noncardiac causes predominate. There is a bimodal distribution in the population, with the first peak before six months of age (sudden infant death syndrome). The most common coronary artery finding is extensive chronic coronary atherosclerosis, although acute syndromes do occur. *(Ref. 2, pp. 193–194)*

114. **(B)** Although over 90% of hypertensives in the general population have essential hypertension, the referral bias of a hypertension clinic results in only 65% to 85% prevalence of essential hypertension. Only about 60% of hypertensives are very sensitive to salt. About 20% of hypertensives have low-renin essential hypertension. This is more common in blacks. Male sex, black race, youth, smoking, diabetes mellitus, excess alcohol ingestion, hypercholesterolemia, more severe hypertension, and evidence of end-organ damage are among the factors that suggest a poor prognosis. *(Ref. 2, pp. 1117–1119)*

CHAPTER 2

Skin

Questions

DIRECTIONS (Questions 115 through 132): Each of the questions or incomplete statements below is followed by five suggested answers or completions. Select the ONE that is best in each case.

115. Koebner's phenomenon (lesions at the site of trauma) is typically seen in

    (A) psoriasis
    (B) eczema
    (C) hypersensitivity reactions
    (D) hyperkeratosis
    (E) toxic erythemas

116. Kaposi's sarcoma often manifests as

    (A) multiple blue dermal plaques
    (B) melanotic nodules
    (C) eczema
    (D) maculopapular rash
    (E) serum-filled bullae

117. Psoriasis may present all of the following clinical manifestations EXCEPT

    (A) sharp demarcation of lesions at the hairline
    (B) progression of lesions unless therapy is applied
    (C) drop-shaped lesions
    (D) extensive large plaques
    (E) pitting of the nails

118. Which of the following does NOT occur in dermatomyositis?

    (A) discoloration of the upper eyelids
    (B) loss of pigmentation
    (C) sensitivity to light
    (D) calcification of subcutaneous tissue
    (E) dermatitis herpetiformis

119. The best treatment of atopic dermatitis includes

    (A) psychoanalysis
    (B) warm clothing
    (C) dry environment
    (D) a change of environment
    (E) vigorous exercise

120. Keratoacanthoma is best characterized by

    (A) slow growth
    (B) slow involution
    (C) usual occurrence on the trunk
    (D) a malignant potential
    (E) a dark brown color

121. An 85-year-old woman has large blistering lesions on the abdomen and thighs that come and go without therapy. The Nikolsky sign is negative. She most likely has

    (A) pemphigus vulgaris
    (B) dermatitis herpetiformis
    (C) pemphigoid
    (D) herpes gestationis
    (E) erythema multiforme

122. Patients with acanthosis nigricans should be studied for

    (A) a visceral carcinoma
    (B) lymphoma
    (C) diabetes mellitus
    (D) sarcoidosis
    (E) an allergy

123. Treatment of acute contact dermatitis during the bullous, oozing stage should include

    (A) bland compresses and baths
    (B) corticosteroid ointments
    (C) topical anesthetics
    (D) systemic antibiotics
    (E) antihistamines

124. Characteristic of ringworm fungi as compared with other fungi is their

    (A) ability to digest and hydrolyze keratin
    (B) high degree of contagiousness
    (C) ability to invade the dermis
    (D) sensitivity to penicillin
    (E) ability to spread to other organs

125. Verrucae (warts)

    (A) are viral in etiology
    (B) may be premalignant lesions
    (C) are found mainly in patients with a lymphoma
    (D) are contagious in children only
    (E) may be treated with griseofulvin

126. For skin disease to be considered occupational, the history should reveal all of the following EXCEPT

    (A) other workmen affected
    (B) no dermatitis preceding occupation
    (C) worsening eruption during weekend
    (D) list of chemicals contacted
    (E) reappearance on return to work

127. Following the appearance of the primary chancre, the serologic test for syphilis (STS) may remain negative for a period not longer than

    (A) one week
    (B) two weeks
    (C) one month
    (D) three months
    (E) six months

128. Skin manifestations associated with chronic ulcerative colitis include all of the following EXCEPT

    (A) maculopapular eruptions
    (B) erythema nodosum
    (C) pyoderma gangrenosum
    (D) erythema multiforme
    (E) necrobiosis lipoidica

129. Mycosis fungoides is best described as a

    (A) fungal infection of the epidermis
    (B) benign skin lesion
    (C) cutaneous lymphoma
    (D) dermatitis
    (E) form of eczema

130. Rhinophyma is a complication of

    (A) acne vulgaris
    (B) pemphigus
    (C) acne rosacea
    (D) psoriasis
    (E) seborrheic dermatitis

131. The cutaneous complex of signs that includes pallor, jaundice, glossitis, cheilitis, and vitiligo is most likely to indicate a diagnosis of

    (A) sickle cell anemia
    (B) cold agglutinin syndrome
    (D) methemoglobinemia
    (D) pernicious anemia
    (E) polycythemia

132. von Recklinghausen's disease is characterized by all of the following EXCEPT

    (A) areas of skin pigmentation
    (B) pedunculated skin tumors
    (C) multiple neural tumors
    (D) tumors most frequently appearing during puberty
    (E) viral etiology

DIRECTIONS (Questions 133 through 142): For each numbered phrase select the ONE lettered heading that is most closely associated with it. Each lettered heading may be selected once, more than once, or not at all.

Questions 133 through 137

    (A) true of erythema multiforme but *not* pemphigus
    (B) true of pemphigus but *not* erythema multiforme
    (C) true of *both* pemphigus and erythema multiforme
    (D) true of *neither* pemphigus nor erythema multiforme

133. Fatal in many instances, especially if untreated

134. Sharply demarcated macular lesion with a tendency to develop "target" lesions

135. Involvement of mucous membranes

136. Responds very well to sulfadiazine

137. Corticosteroids are the treatment of choice

Questions 138 through 142

    (A) true of squamous cell carcinoma of the skin but not basal cell carcinoma of the skin

    (B) true of basal cell carcinoma of the skin but not squamous cell carcinoma of the skin

    (C) true of *both* basal cell and squamous cell carcinomas of the skin

    (D) true of *neither* basal cell nor squamous cell carcinomas of the skin

138. Does not metastasize beyond the skin

139. May be caused by excessive exposure to sunlight

140. May be treated with x-ray therapy

141. Keratin pearls are seen pathologically

142. May develop in long-standing scars

DIRECTIONS (Questions 143 through 153): Each of the following questions or incomplete statements below is followed by five suggested answers or completions. Select the ONE that is best in each case.

143. The skin lesion pictured in Figure 2.1 suggests a diagnosis of

    (A) erythema nodosum

    (B) acanthosis nigricans

    (C) herpes zoster

    (D) alopecia variegata

    (E) pemphigoid

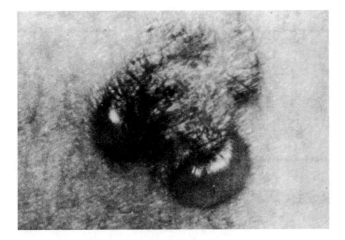

Figure 2.1

144. All of the following are characteristic of neurofibromatosis EXCEPT

    (A) dominant inheritance

    (B) viral etiology

    (C) subcutaneous nodules along nerve sheaths

    (D) association with pheochromocytoma

    (E) pigmentary abnormalities

145. Benefit to patients with severe acne is usually obtained with

    (A) dietary controls

    (B) radiotherapy

    (C) ultraviolet light

    (D) psychotherapy

    (E) low-dose antimicrobials

146. All of the following are characteristic of Sezary syndrome EXCEPT

    (A) response to electron beam therapy

    (B) exfoliative erythroderma

    (C) folded cerebriform nuclei

    (D) T cell markers

    (E) resistance to cyclophosphamide

147. Which of the following features indicate a more negative prognosis for patients with malignant melanoma?

    (A) female sex

    (B) location on the leg

    (C) dark pigmentation of the lesion

    (D) nodularity of the lesion

    (E) level A invasion

148. Zinc deficiency associated with inadequate nutrition in malabsorption syndromes may lead to

    (A) ichthyosis

    (B) acrodermatitis enteropathica

    (C) Paget's disease

    (D) candidiasis

    (E) herpes simplex

149. Acanthosis nigricans may be associated with all of the following EXCEPT

    (A) adenocarcinoma

    (B) adrenal insufficiency

    (C) porphyria cutanea tarda

    (D) Cushing syndrome

    (E) response to local therapy

150. Erythema nodosum is associated with

(A) aspergillosis

(B) children younger than five years

(C) males more than females

(D) malignant disease only

(E) chronic ulcerative colitis

151. A patch differs from a macule because

(A) it is more easily palpable

(B) a patch is erythematous

(C) a patch can contain fluid

(D) the etiology is very different

(E) it is larger

152. A potassium hydroxide (KOH) preparation

(A) is done on skin obtained via a punch biopsy

(B) is useful in diagnosing herpes virus infections

(C) is used in skin testing for allergies

(D) is prepared from skin scrapings

(E) will turn color in the presence of fungal elements

153. Impetigo is a skin disorder that is

(A) caused by fungi of the *Microsporum* species

(B) caused exclusively by staphylococcal infections

(C) characterized by premalignant changes

(D) treated by improved hygiene

(E) characterized by papulosquamous lesions

DIRECTIONS (Questions 154 through 164): The group of questions below consists of lettered headings followed by a list of numbered phrases. For each numbered phrase, select the ONE lettered heading that is most closely associated with it. Each lettered heading may be selected once, more than once, or not at all.

Questions 154 through 159

(A) generalized vitiligo

(B) localized vitiligo

(C) telangiectasia

(D) erythroderma

(E) papulosquamous lesions of palms and soles

(F) scarring alopecia

(G) yellow-colored papules

(H) acanthosis nigricans

154. Tuberculoid leprosy

155. Scleroderma

156. Sulfa drugs

157. Hyperlipoproteinemia

158. Secondary syphilis

159. Obesity

Questions 160 through 164

(A) dystrophic nail changes

(B) gram-negative folliculitis

(C) black pigmentation of face

(D) erythema nodosum

(E) morbilliform eruption in patients with AIDS

(F) gingival hyperplasia

(G) reactions in patients with nasal polyps

160. Bleomycin

161. Chloroquine

162. Birth control pills

163. Tetracycline

164. Sulfamethoxazole and trimethoprim

Skin

Answers and Explanations

115. (A) Koebner's phenomenon is typically seen in psoriasis. The kind of injury eliciting the phenomenon is usually mechanical, but ultraviolet light or allergic damage to the skin may be provocative. Koebner's phenomenon can also occur in lichen planus, lichen nitidus, keratosis follicularis, and pemphigoid. The Koebner phenomenon has been used to study early skin changes in these diseases. *(Ref. 5, p. 587)*

116. (A) Kaposi's sarcoma often manifests as multiple blue dermal plaques. Lesions have two prominent features: accumulation of spindle cells and presence of vascular elements. Classical Kaposi's sarcoma is an indolent disease of later life, and is much more common in men than women. Kaposi's sarcoma in association with HIV infection is a much more aggressive disorder. *(Ref. 5, p. 2468)*

117. (B) Psoriasis does not present a progression of lesions unless therapy is applied. Lesions vary in size and configuration from patient to patient and in the same patient from time to time. *(Ref. 5, p. 1469)*

118. (E) In dermatomyositis, the dermatitis may be the most striking feature of the illness or so minor as to be easily overlooked. The classic manifestation is a purplish-red heliotrope erythema of the eyelids, upper cheeks, forehead, and temples, often with edema of eyelids and periorbital tissue. The typical hand changes involve scaly, bluish-red plaques around the base of the nails and backs of the joints of the fingers. There is an association with visceral malignancy. *(Ref. 5, p. 1376)*

119. (D) A change of environment is among the best treatments for atopic dermatitis. The patient should be kept in as dust-free an environment as possible and should not wear rough garments. *(Ref. 5, p. 419)*

120. (B) This tumor as a rule occurs on exposed, hairy skin. It grows rapidly but involutes slowly, occasionally up to one year. It is more common in white-skinned males. The lesion starts as a small, rounded, flesh-colored or reddish papule. It grows rapidly and may reach 10 to 20 mm in a few weeks. There are telangiectasias just below the surface and the center contains a horny plug or is covered by a crust concealing a keratin-filled crater. *(Ref. 5, p. 2395)*

121. (C) There are antibodies to skin basement membrane, but unlike pemphigus, antibody levels do not correlate with disease activity. Bullous pemphigoid is most common in the elderly, and the disease often starts with urticaria-like and pruritic erythematous lesions before classic blisters occur. Unlike pemphigus, mucosal lesions are minimal or absent. *(Ref. 5, p. 1639)*

122. (A) Patients with acanthosis nigricans should be studied for a visceral carcinoma. Other dermatoses associated with malignancy include dermatomyositis, flushing, acquired ichthyosis, and thrombophlebitis migrans. *(Ref. 5, p. 1461)*

123. (A) Ointments are not used, but wet dressings are applied several times a day, using Burow's solution or boric acid, and baths are also included in the treatment. The key aspect of care is prevention. When contamination does occur, washing the affected area is the first mode of treatment. *(Ref. 5, p. 435)*

124. (A) The ability to digest and hydrolyze keratin is characteristic of ringworm fungi. As dermatophytes fluoresce, an ultraviolet light with a Wood's filter may be used to identify infected hair. The spectrum of infection depends on the exact species, and can range from a few dull gray, broken-off hairs to a severely painful inflammatory mass. Host response is also an important factor. *(Ref. 5, p. 911)*

125. **(A)** Verrucae are viral in etiology. The human papillomavirus is a DNA-containing virus of the papovavirus group that includes animal tumor viruses. Although most warts are not felt to be premalignant, there is evidence to show that genital warts are correlated with malignancy. *(Ref. 5, p. 668)*

126. **(C)** The history should not reveal worsening eruption during the weekend. Allergy, acne, diabetes, psoriasis, xeroderma, or seborrheic dermatitis may all be mistaken for occupational disorders. The list of possible occupational skin hazards is long. At times, a site visit to the workplace is required to confirm the diagnosis. *(Ref. 5, p. 569)*

127. **(C)** The STS may remain negative for a period not longer than one month after the appearance of the primary chancre. The STS usually becomes positive about one week after the chancre appears. With therapy the chancre heals in a week. *(Ref. 5, p. 839)*

128. **(E)** Skin manifestations do not include necrobiosis lipoidica. Unlike the arthritis of ulcerative colitis, the dermatologic lesions respond to therapy to control the bowel disease. Necrobiosis lipoidica is associated with diabetes and the lesion is found on the anterior aspect of the leg. *(Ref. 5, p. 2354)*

129. **(C)** Mycosis fungoides is best described as a cutaneous lymphoma. Lesions may remain confined to the skin for years, and internal organ involvement occurs when the disease advances into late stages. It is a disorder involving T lymphocytes. Treatment is usually palliative rather than curative. *(Ref. 5, p. 1736)*

130. **(C)** Rhinophyma is a complication of acne rosacea. It can be treated surgically by shaving off the excessive tissue with a scalpel, but regrowth occurs in time. There is very little evidence to support the association between alcoholism and rhinophyma. *(Ref. 5, p. 1609)*

131. **(D)** Jaundice results from hemolysis, and glossitis and cheilitis from the vitamin deficiency affecting rapidly turning over tissues. Patients may complain of a burning tongue, and examination reveals atrophy of papillae, a deep red mucosa, and a "cobblestone" appearance. B_{12} administration rapidly relieves these symptoms. The vitiligo is caused by an associated autoimmune disorder. *(Ref. 5, p. 2093)*

132. **(E)** The disorder is inherited in an autosomal manner. Incomplete forms are frequent. The skin manifestations include café au lait spots (more

than 6 required for diagnosis), axillary freckles, cutaneous neurofibromas, and pigmented iris hamartomas (Liech nodules). There are numerous other manifestations as well. *(Ref. 5, p. 119)*

133. **(B)** Pemphigus is fatal in many instances, especially if untreated. Glucocorticoid administration is the mainstay of treatment; antibiotics may be required for secondary infection. *(Ref. 5, pp. 1085, 1631)*

134. **(A)** In erythema multiforme, vivid red blots appear suddenly in symmetrical distribution, favoring the extensor surfaces and distal limbs. *(Ref. 5, pp. 1085, 1631)*

135. **(C)** The mucous membranes are involved in both conditions. Oral lesions often occur in erythema multiforme, leading first to blisters, and then to erosions of the cheeks, gums, and tongue. *(Ref. 5, pp. 1085, 1631)*

136. **(D)** Neither condition responds to sulfadiazine. Oral antihistamines may hasten recovery in erythema multiforme. *(Ref. 5, pp. 1085, 1631)*

137. **(B)** Corticosteroids are the treatment of choice for pemphigus. Methotrexate may be used in patients with pemphigus in the early, localized stage of the disease. *(Ref. 5, pp. 1085, 1631)*

138. **(B)** Basal cell tumors have a substantial capacity for local destruction but metastasize very rarely. *(Ref. 5, pp. 2414, 2431)*

139. **(C)** Sunlight is only one of many factors causing both, as carcinomas frequently appear in areas not maximally irradiated. *(Ref. 5, pp. 2414, 2431)*

140. **(C)** In both carcinomas, early detection may lead to cure by surgical removal, but radiotherapy may be curative if used in high dosage. *(Ref. 5, pp. 2414, 2431)*

141. **(A)** Invasive squamous cell carcinoma consists of malignant epidermal cells extending beyond the dermoepidermal junction. *(Ref. 5, pp. 2414, 2431)*

142. **(A)** In squamous cell carcinoma of the skin, other early lesions include solar keratoses, cutaneous horns, arsenical keratoses, and Bowen's disease. *(Ref. 5, pp. 2414, 2431)*

143. **(E)** Pemphigus is characterized histologically by acantholysis, whereas pemphigoid causes bullae without acantholysis. The initial presentation may be with oral lesions which can precede cutaneous lesions by several months. Diagnosis may

be difficult in these cases because intact bullae are rarely seen in the mouth. *(Ref. 5, p. 1631)*

144. **(B)** Neurofibromatosis is associated with systemic manifestations in the nervous system, bone, soft tissues, and skin. About 90% of patients have pigmentary abnormalities. *(Ref. 5, p. 119)*

145. **(E)** Tetracyclines are commonly used in the treatment of acne, but may be associated with risk of dental discoloration or photosensitivity. Clindamycin is equally effective. Topical benzoyl peroxide, retinoic acid, and topical antibiotics are also frequently used. *(Ref. 5, p. 1920)*

146. **(A)** Sezary syndrome resembles mycosis fungoides in many respects, but does not respond well to chemotherapy with alkylating agents or to electron beam therapy. The diagnosis requires the presence of the classic triad: erythroderma, lymphadenopathy, and 10% or more of mononuclear cells in the peripheral blood being abnormal. The majority of patients are elderly males, and the prognosis is poor. *(Ref. 5, p. 1748)*

147. **(D)** Nodular melanoma is invasive from the start. Women do better than men; trunk lesions and depigmented lesions carry a worse prognosis. Prognosis is directly related to depth of the lesion. *(Ref. 5, p. 2445)*

148. **(B)** It is a persistent dermatitis around the mouth, with acral involvement that begins as vesicles but is soon crusted. The syndrome can rarely be inherited as an autosomal recessive. It has been described after prolonged parenteral alimentation as well. *(Ref. 5, p. 2336)*

149. **(C)** There is no local therapy, but the early recognition of this cutaneous sign warrants a thorough search for underlying pathology. The earliest changes are usually pigmentation, dryness, and roughness of the skin. The skin is gray-brown or black, palpably thickened, and covered by small papillomatous elevations which give it a velvety texture. The most common sites are axillae, back, neck, anogenital region, and the groins. *(Ref. 5, p. 1461)*

150. **(E)** It is a hypersensitivity vasculitis associated with many infections, and is more common in females. The lesions are rare in children. It is a nodular erythematous eruption, usually on the extensor aspects of the legs, less commonly on thighs and forearms. It regresses by bruise-like color changes in 3 to 6 weeks without scarring. *(Ref. 5, p. 1156)*

151. **(E)** A macule is a flat, colored lesion not raised above the surface of the surrounding skin. It is less than 2 cm in diameter. A patch differs from a macule only in size, being greater than 2 cm in diameter. *(Ref. 2, p. 271)*

152. **(D)** A potassium hydroxide preparation is useful when performed on scaling skin lesions when a fungal etiology is suspected. The scraped scales are placed on a microscope slide, treated with 1 or 2 drops of KOH solution and examined for hyphae, pseudohypha, or budding yeast. *(Ref. 2, p. 272)*

153. **(D)** Impetigo is a superficial bacterial infection of skin caused by group A beta-hemolytic streptococci or *S. aureus*. It is characterized by superficial pustules that rupture resulting in a honey-colored crust. The bullous variant is more likely staphylococcal in origin. Treatment requires improving hygiene and soaking the crust as well as oral antibiotics. *(Ref. 2, p. 277)*

154. **(B)** Localized areas of vitiligo can be seen in numerous primary skin disorders. As well, it can be caused by systemic disorders such as sarcoidosis and tuberculoid leprosy. In the latter disorder there is associated anesthesia, anhidrosis, and alopecia of the lesions. Biopsy of the palpable border will reveal granulomas. *(Ref. 2, p. 297)*

155. **(C)** Scleroderma is characterized by typical fibrotic and vascular lesions. These lesions may be periungual telangiectasia that are found in lupus erythematosus and dermatomyositis. Another form of telangiectasia, mat telangiectasia, is seen only in scleroderma. These lesions are broad macules 2 to 7 mm in diameter. They are found on the face, oral mucosa, and hands. The nail beds of scleroderma patients often reveal loss of capillary loops with dilatation of the remaining loops when examined under magnification. *(Ref. 2, p. 295)*

156. **(D)** Drug reactions most frequently result in papulosquamous reactions or diffuse erythroderma. Sulfa drugs frequently cause erythroderma. *(Ref. 2, pp. 290–291)*

157. **(G)** Hyperlipoproteinemia is frequently associated with xanthomas, yellow-colored cutaneous papules or plaques. Xanthomas associated with hypertriglyceridemia are frequently eruptive; these yellow papules have an erythematous halo and are most frequently found on exterior surfaces of the extremities and buttocks. *(Ref. 2, p. 302)*

158. **(E)** Secondary syphilis often involves the palms and soles. Associated findings that help make the diagnosis include annular plaques on the face, nonscarring alopecia, condylomalata, mucous patches, lymphadenopathy, malaise, fever, headache, and myalgia. *(Ref. 2, p. 291)*

159. **(H)** Obesity is the most common cause of acanthosis nigricans, a velvety, localized hyperpigmentation. Other causes include gastrointestinal malignancy and endocrinopathy such as acromegaly, Cushing syndrome, Stein–Leventhal syndrome, or insulin-resistant diabetes. *(Ref. 2, p. 297)*

160. **(A)** Cancer chemotherapy most frequently involves rapidly proliferating elements of the skin resulting in stomatitis and alopecia. Bleomycin, hydroxyurea, and 5-Fluorouracil can cause dystrophic nail changes. Other skin manifestations of cancer drugs include sterile cellulitis, phlebitis, ulceration of pressure areas, urticaria, angioedema, and exfoliative dermatitis. The underlying malignancy often makes diagnoses of skin disease more difficult. *(Ref. 2, p. 284)*

161. **(C)** Chloroquine is used for certain skin diseases such as lupus and polymorphous light eruption, but can also cause skin reactions and exacerbate porphyria cutanea tarda. Black pigmentation can involve the face, mucous membrane, and pretibial and subungual areas. *(Ref. 2, p. 284)*

162. **(D)** Birth control pills and gold are two of the drugs that can cause erythema nodosum. This is a panniculitis characterized by tender, subcutaneous, erythematous nodules characteristically found on the anterior portion of the legs. *(Ref. 2, pp. 283, 284)*

163. **(B)** Tetracycline can cause a gram-negative folliculitis with long-term use. It looks like acne. Other common skin reactions with tetracyclines include photosensitivity, onycholysis, fixed drug reactions, and lichenoid eruptions. If used during pregnancy or early childhood, tetracyclines can stain teeth. *(Ref. 2, p. 284)*

164. **(E)** The combination of sulfamethoxazole and trimethoprim causes two distinct cutaneous reactions; a urticarial eruption in the first few days of therapy and a morbilliform eruption occurring a week or more after therapy has begun. This latter reaction is particularly common in patients with AIDS. *(Ref. 2, p. 284)*

CHAPTER 3

Endocrine
Questions

DISEASES OF NUTRITION, METABOLISM, AND ENDOCRINES

DIRECTIONS (Questions 165 through 194): Each of the questions or incomplete statements below is followed by five suggested answers or completions. Select the ONE that is best in each case.

165. The most common cause of hypothyroidism in the adult is

    (A) trauma
    (B) radioactive iodine ingestion
    (C) pimary hypothyroidism
    (D) parathyroid surgery
    (E) antithyroid chemicals

166. Nephropathy secondary to gout is most likely to manifest as

    (A) nephrotic syndrome
    (B) isosthenuria and moderate albuminuria
    (C) acute renal failure
    (D) acute tubular necrosis
    (E) malignant hypertension

167. All of the following are characteristics of panhypopituitarism EXCEPT

    (A) occurrence of myxedema
    (B) decreased melanin pigmentation
    (C) emaciation and cachexia
    (D) loss of axillary and pubic hairs
    (E) moderate normocytic and normochromic anemia

168. The receptors for these hormones are intracellular

    (A) protein kinases
    (B) growth hormone/prolactin
    (C) steroid hormones
    (D) acetylcholine/GABA
    (E) LH/TSH/parathyroid

169. The cutaneous manifestations of protoporphyria are best treated with

    (A) phenobarbital
    (B) corticosteroids
    (C) high carbohydrate diet
    (D) beta-carotene
    (E) chlorpromazine

170. In the human menstrual cycle, follicle-stimulating hormone (FSH) can be said to

    (A) cause ovulation
    (B) encourage progesterone secretion
    (C) cause the secretory phase of the uterine mucosa
    (D) inhibit estrogen secretion
    (E) encourage maturation of the follicle

171. Findings in hyperparathyroidism include all of the following EXCEPT

    (A) renal colic
    (B) bone pain
    (C) gastrointestinal symptoms
    (D) mental confusion
    (E) dyspnea

172. The most common cause of hypoparathyroidism is

    (A) idiopathic
    (B) familial
    (C) postradiation
    (D) end-organ resistance
    (E) surgical removal

173. In adrenocortical insufficiency

    (A) the skin is shiny and pale
    (B) a diabetic glucose tolerance is characteristic
    (C) water diuresis is impaired
    (D) the urinary steroids are high
    (E) none of the above

174. Grossly overweight patients with "essential obesity" can be expected to have

(A) normal mortality risk
(B) hypothyroidism
(C) low P_{CO_2} values
(D) hypertriglyceridemia
(E) hyperadrenocorticism

175. Hemachromatosis is characterized by

(A) diabetes mellitus as the most frequent presentation
(B) arrhythmias as the most common cardiac manifestation
(C) phlebotomy improving the arthropathy
(D) arthritis involving the hands
(E) pigmentation of skin by iron

176. Patients with hepatic porphyria should avoid

(A) chlorpromazine
(B) barbiturates
(C) a high calcium diet
(D) narcotics
(E) steroids

177. Obesity is associated with all of the following EXCEPT

(A) diabetes mellitus
(B) hyperlipoproteinemia
(C) abnormal growth hormone response
(D) atherosclerosis
(E) increased peripheral vascular resistance causing hypertension

178. Tay–Sachs disease is characterized by all of the following EXCEPT

(A) glycogen storage
(B) ganglioside accumulation
(C) spasticity
(D) macular degeneration
(E) ballooning of cerebral ganglion cells

179. The characteristic neurologic findings in amyloidosis include

(A) peripheral motor and sensory neuropathy
(B) spinal cord compression in the lumbar region
(C) spinal cord compression in the thoracic region
(D) a peripheral neuropathy associated with cerebral manifestations
(E) a Guillain–Barré-type syndrome

180. One finds increased levels of 5-hydroxyindoleacetic acid in the urine in

(A) phenylketonuria
(B) alkaptonuria
(C) malignant melanoma
(D) carcinoid syndrome
(E) disseminated carcinomatosis

181. Familial hyperbetalipoproteinemia (type II hyperlipoproteinemia) is characterized by

(A) milky serum
(B) severe diabetes
(C) aggravation with ingestion of polyunsaturated fats
(D) an increased incidence of coronary artery disease
(E) high serum triglycerides

182. The syndrome of congenital absence of beta-lipoproteins includes all of the following EXCEPT

(A) ataxic neuropathy
(B) crenated red blood cells (acanthocytosis)
(C) renal disease
(D) hypocholesterolemia
(E) retinopathy

183. An adult patient with hepatosplenomegaly and large reticulated cells in the bone marrow containing glucocerebrosides can be diagnosed as having

(A) metachromatic leukodystrophy
(B) Gaucher's disease
(C) reticulum cell sarcoma associated with diabetes
(D) glycogen storage disease
(E) familial hyperchylomicronemia

184. Glycogen storage diseases

(A) do not affect the liver
(B) may cause xanthomas
(C) are always autosomal dominant
(D) are due to a single enzyme defect
(E) are corrected by surgery

185. Cystinuria is commonly associated with

(A) severe mental retardation
(B) homocystinuria
(C) hexagonal crystals in the urine
(D) malnutrition due to urine loss of cystine
(E) hydrocephalus

186. Magnesium deficiency may be seen in all of the following EXCEPT

(A) alcoholism
(B) chronic malabsorption
(C) diabetes mellitus
(D) kwashiorkor
(E) hypervitaminosis E

187. The syndrome of hepatomegaly, splenomegaly, leukopenia, anemia, periosteal changes, sparse and coarse hair, and increased serum lipids occurs in chronic

(A) vitamin D intoxication
(B) vitamin D deficiency
(C) vitamin A deficiency
(D) vitamin A intoxication
(E) acarotenemia

188. The patient whose hands are shown in Figure 3.1 is mentally retarded with a short stocky build. What is the most likely diagnosis?

(A) achondroplastic dwarf
(B) Down syndrome
(C) Klinefelter syndrome
(D) pseudohypoparathyroidism
(E) Turner syndrome

189. Which of the following laboratory values is the patient in Figure 3.1 likely to show?

(A) hypercalcemia, hypophosphatemia
(B) hypocalcemia, low parathormone
(C) hypocalcemia, high parathormone
(D) hypocalcemia, hypophosphatemia
(E) hyperphosphatemia, low parathormone

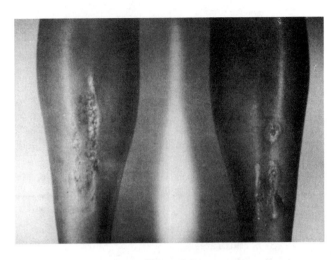

Figure 3.2

190. A 28-year-old woman with diabetes has leg lesions shown in Figure 3.2. What is the most likely diagnosis?

(A) eruptive xanthomas
(B) necrobiosis lipoidica diabeticorum
(C) gangrene
(D) staphylococcal infection
(E) erythema nodosum

191. Allopurinol is useful in the prevention of gout because of which of the following mechanisms of action?

(A) inhibition of xanthine oxidase
(B) solubilization of uric acid
(C) reactivity with hypoxanthine
(D) anti-inflammatory effect on joint tissue
(E) increased renal tubular secretion of uric acid

192. Hypomagnesemia may result in all of the following EXCEPT

(A) lethargy
(B) neuromuscular irritability
(C) anorexia
(D) tachyarrhythmias
(E) hyperkalemia

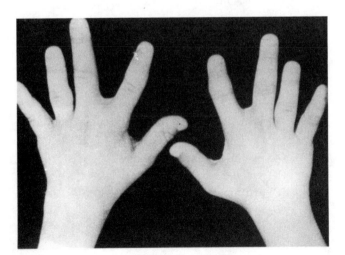

Figure 3.1

193. A 22-year-old man with arm span greater than height, subluxed lenses, flattened corneas, and dilation of the aortic ring is most likely to have

(A) Ehlers–Danlos syndrome
(B) Marfan syndrome
(C) Werner syndrome
(D) Laurence–Moon–Biedl syndrome
(E) Hunter syndrome

194. Which of the following drugs suppresses the release of antidiuretic hormone (ADH)?

(A) phenytoin
(B) cyclophosphamide
(C) barbiturates
(D) nicotine
(E) morphine

DIRECTIONS (Questions 195 through 207): The group of questions below consists of five lettered headings followed by a list of numbered words, phrases, or statements. For each numbered word, phrase, or statement, select the ONE lettered heading that is most closely associated with it. Each lettered heading may be selected once, more than once, or not at all.

(A) palmar plane xanthomas
(B) triglycerides greater than 1000
(C) subcutaneous extensor tendon xanthomas
(D) low serum cholesterol
(E) cholesterol normal

195. Hyperchylomicronemia

196. Hyperbetalipoproteinemia

197. Type III hyperlipoproteinemia

198. Hyperprebetalipoproteinemia

199. Hypertriglyceridemia

Questions 200 through 203

(A) true of diabetes mellitus (DM) but *not* diabetes insipidus (DI)
(B) true of DI but *not* DM
(C) true of *both* DM and DI
(D) true of *neither* DM nor DI

200. Polyuria and polydipsia

201. Does not cause renal disease in adults

202. Does not occur as a result of tumors

203. Related in some manner to obesity

Questions 204 through 207

(A) associated with increased LDL (type IIA hyperlipoproteinemia) but *not* increased VLDL (type IV hyperlipproteinemia)
(B) associated with increased VLDL but *not* increased LDL
(C) associated with *both* increased LDL and increased VLDL
(D) associated with *neither* increased LDL nor increased VLDL

204. Increased risk of heart disease

205. Tendon xanthomas

206. Pattern seen in diabetes mellitus

207. Hyperchylomicronemia

DIRECTIONS (Questions 208 through 234): Each of the questions or incomplete statements below is followed by five suggested answers or completions. Select the ONE that is best in each case.

208. Which of the following cardiac changes is most characteristic of thyrotoxicosis?

(A) atrial fibrillation
(B) systolic murmurs
(C) bradycardia
(D) decrease in heart size
(E) pericardial effusion

209. Needle biopsy of the thyroid is commonly used in diagnosis in

(A) chronic thyroiditis
(B) thyroid storm
(C) nontoxic multinodular goiter
(D) subacute thyroiditis
(E) malignant neoplasms

210. All of the following may result from primary idiopathic hemochromatosis EXCEPT

(A) insulin-dependent diabetes
(B) iron deposits in renal glomeruli
(C) arthropathy
(D) hypogonadism
(E) skin pigmentation

211. The release of vasopressin is controlled by

(A) toxicity of the blood perfusing the liver
(B) phosphate levels in the renal plasma
(C) cerebrospinal fluid pressure
(D) calcium levels in the cerebral inflow
(E) volume receptors in the left atrium

212. The differential diagnosis of hypoglycemia includes

(A) excess growth hormone
(B) Cushing's disease
(C) thyrotoxicosis
(D) tumor of the pancreatic beta cells
(E) gastrin deficiency

213. Amyloid resulting from light chain-related deposition is likely to be deposited in all of the following EXCEPT

(A) tongue
(B) red cells
(C) heart
(D) lymph nodes
(E) spleen

214. Glucagon can be best described as a hormone that is

(A) secreted by the alpha cells of the pancreas
(B) a carbohydrate in structure
(C) effective in lowering blood sugar levels
(D) antigenically similar to insulin
(E) effective in decreasing cyclic AMP in target cells

215. Hyperparathyroidism may be associated with all of the following EXCEPT

(A) the Zollinger–Ellison syndrome
(B) an adrenal adenoma
(C) a testicular carcinoma
(D) acromegaly
(E) hypercalcemia

216. Administration of estrogen most likely results in

(A) development of the secretory phase of the endometrium
(B) a decrease of sebaceous gland activity
(C) thinning of the vaginal mucosa
(D) development of secondary sexual characteristics
(E) hirsutism

217. Feminizing adrenocortical tumors

(A) can be benign or malignant
(B) are associated with hypertension
(C) are common in girls with early breast development
(D) are associated with an increase in the size of the phallus
(E) are associated with hypothyroidism

218. Excessive growth hormone affects the muscles by causing

(A) enlargement
(B) spasm
(C) increased strength
(D) myositis
(E) rhythmic contraction

219. Which of the following is LEAST likely to be associated with vitamin D-resistant rickets?

(A) hypophosphatemia
(B) decreased calcium absorption
(C) osteomalacia
(D) osteoporosis
(E) bony deformities

220. Risk of death in anorexia nervosa is most often associated with

(A) renal failure
(B) ventricular tachyarrhythmias
(C) diabetes mellitus
(D) hyperthermia
(E) pernicious anemia

221. Gouty patients are most likely to have associated

(A) pernicious anemia
(B) diabetes insipidus
(C) Alzheimer's disease
(D) anorexia
(E) renal disease

222. All of the following are likely to occur in osteomalacia EXCEPT

(A) bending of long bones
(B) Milkman syndrome (pseudofractures)
(C) absence of lamina dura
(D) hypercalcemia
(E) nephrocalcinosis

223. Which of the following is NOT likely to be a complication of Paget's disease of bone?

(A) renal calculi
(B) osteogenic sarcoma
(C) primary hyperparathyroidism
(D) hypercalcemia
(E) radiologic abnormalities

224. A deficiency of vitamin D can lead to all of the following EXCEPT

(A) decreased renal excretion of phosphorus
(B) decreased gastrointestinal absorption of calcium
(C) hypocalcemia
(D) decreased renal excretion of calcium
(E) hypophosphatemia

225. Ammonia levels in the blood are determined by all of the following EXCEPT

(A) glomerular function
(B) protein catabolism
(C) amino acid catabolism
(D) absorption from the gut
(E) hepatocellular function

226. In phenylketonuria, the best management includes all of the following EXCEPT

(A) a gluten-free diet to age 12 years
(B) a total elimination of phenylalanine from the diet
(C) early detection by mass screening
(D) long-term dietary control
(E) a low carbohydrate diet

227. Which of the following is most likely to be a feature of Wilson's disease

(A) renal failure
(B) cirrhosis of the liver
(C) elevated ceruloplasmin
(D) neurological long tract signs
(E) increased plasma copper

228. Insulin acts at the cellular receptor level by

(A) stimulating tyrosine kinase
(B) binding to ion channels
(C) binding to intracellular erb A receptors
(D) stimulating guanylate cyclase
(E) activating G-proteins

229. The metabolic effects of insulin on adipose tissue are most likely to include

(A) decrease of glucose transport
(B) decrease in glucose phosphorylation
(C) decrease in cyclic AMP
(D) decrease in lipoprotein lipase
(E) enhancement of glucagon effect

230. The management of patients with thyroid storm should NOT include

(A) propylthiouracil
(B) hydrocortisone
(C) beta-adrenergic blockade
(D) parenteral fluids
(E) salicylates

231. All of the following features are characteristic of noninsulin-dependent diabetes EXCEPT

(A) onset usually over age 40 years
(B) most patients are obese
(C) no circulating islet cell antibodies
(D) no associated autoimmune phenomena
(E) insulin resistance does not develop

232. Delayed adolescence in the male is most commonly due to

(A) inadequate diet
(B) normal variation
(C) pituitary tumor
(D) Leydig cell dysfunction
(E) drug side effects

233. Response to hormone treatment of carcinoma of the breast is most improved in

(A) metastases confined to liver
(B) patient more than five years premenopausal
(C) androgen receptors on the tumor cell membrane
(D) disease-free interval in excess of two years
(E) metastases confined to brain

234. Which of the following represents an increased risk factor for carcinoma of the breast?

(A) castration before age 40 years
(B) late first pregnancy
(C) long-term nursing
(D) history of breast cancer in an aunt
(E) multiparity

235. Which of the following statements is correct?

(A) resting metabolic rate (RMR) is identical in men and women when corrected for weight and height

(B) virtually all nitrogen loss is through the urine in the form of urea

(C) increasing the proportion of protein in the diet increases the efficiency of protein production in the body

(D) generally physical activity accounts for only one-third of total energy expenditure over most conditions

(E) recommended levels of adult protein ingestion should be decreased by 30% for the very elderly

DIRECTIONS (Questions 236 through 242): This section consists of clinical situations, each followed by a series of questions. Study each situation and select the ONE best answer to each question following it.

Questions 236 through 240: A 35-year-old obese woman complains of recent weight loss in spite of a large appetite, vulvar pruritus, and waking up frequently at night to urinate.

236. The most likely diagnosis is

(A) diabetes mellitus

(B) diabetes insipidus

(C) vaginitis and cystitis

(D) myxedema

(E) pheochromocytoma

237. The diagnosis may be established by any of the following EXCEPT

(A) a urine glucose and acetone

(B) an insulin tolerance test

(C) a fasting blood sugar

(D) a glucose tolerance test

(E) a two-hour postprandial blood glucose

238. The disease process might cause the eye examination to reveal any of the following EXCEPT

(A) central microaneurysm

(B) retinal exudates

(C) retinal hemorrhages

(D) retinitis proliferans

(E) open-angle glaucoma

239. Which of the following renal diseases is this patient most likely to develop?

(A) acute glomerulonephritis

(B) obstructive uropathy

(C) glomerulosclerosis with mesangial thickening

(D) renal infarction

(E) polycystic kidneys

240. All of the following cutaneous manifestations may be found EXCEPT

(A) necrobiosis lipoidica

(B) xanthomas

(C) pyoderma gangrenosum

(D) candidiasis

(E) dermatophytosis

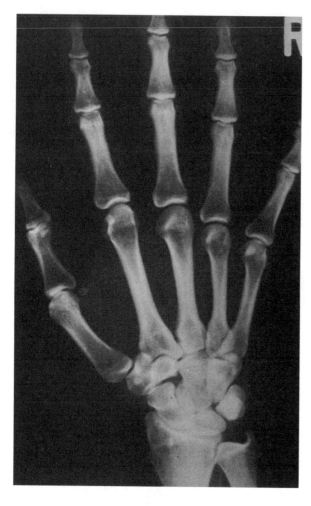

Figure 3.3

TABLE 3.1 CASE WORK-UP

	Normal	Patient
Plasma ACTH pg/mL	< 150	< 50
Plasma cortisol Eg/mL	17	35
Urine 17-OH mg/24 hr	2 to 10	25
Urine 17-Ks mg/24 hr	5 to 15	10
Urine 17-OH response to:		
ACTH IV	Increase X 5	No response
Dexamethasone 0.5 mg	< 3.0	No response
2.0 mg	< 95 3.0	No response
Metyrapone 750 mg	Increase X 2	No response

Question 242:   The case work-up shown in Table 3.1 is of a 35-year-old woman presenting with hypertension, central obesity, and skin striae. The most likely diagnosis is

(A) adrenal hyperplasia secondary to hypothalamic dysfunction

(B) adrenal adenoma with complete autonomy

(C) exogenous steroids, iatrogenic

(D) pituitary tumor

(E) carcinoma of the adrenal

DIRECTIONS (Questions 243 through 246): Each lettered heading below describes an alteration in male sexual function. Each numbered phrase gives a possible cause for an alteration of male sexual function. For each numbered phrase select the ONE lettered heading that is most closely associated with it. Each lettered heading may be selected once, more than once, or not at all.

(A) loss of desire

(B) failure of erection with absent nocturnal penile tumescence (NPT)

(C) absence of emission

(D) absence of orgasm with normal libido and erectile function

(E) failure of detumescence

243.   Can be caused by high prolactin level

244.   Rarely indicates organic disease

245.   Can be caused by hematological disease

246.   Can be caused by vascular disease

Question 241:   Figure 3.3 is the x-ray of a 35-year-old woman with chronic renal disease complaining of pain in the hand after dialysis. What is your diagnosis?

(A) scleroderma

(B) gout

(C) hyperparathyroidism

(D) pseudogout

(E) Paget's disease

DIRECTIONS (Questions 247 through 250). Each lettered heading below describes a condition associated with hirsutism in women. Each numbered phrase contains clinical information related to hirsutism. For each numbered phrase select the ONE lettered heading that is most closely associated with it. Each lettered heading may be selected once, more than once, or not at all.

(A) drugs

(B) adrenal tumor

(C) polycystic ovarian disease

(D) adrenal hyperplasia

(E) idiopathic hirsutism

(F) ovarian tumor

247. Slight elevation of plasma testosterone and androstenedione

248. Can be associated with anovulation, obesity, amenorrhea

249. May stimulate surrounding tissue to secrete androgens

250. Often associated with elevated 17-hydroxyprogesterone levels

DIRECTIONS (Questions 251 through 256): For each numbered phrase select the ONE lettered heading that is most closely associated with it. Each lettered heading may be selected once, more than once, or not at all.

(A) true of anorexia nervosa but *not* bulimia

(B) true of bulimia but *not* anorexia nervosa

(C) true of *both* anorexia nervosa and bulimia

(D) true of *neither* anorexia nervosa nor bulimia

251. Markedly decreased weight at diagnosis

252. Vomiting present

253. Antisocial behavior common

254. Skin changes usually occur

255. Exercise very common

256. May evolve into the other eating disorder

DIRECTIONS (Questions 257 through 262) Each lettered heading below describes a condition for which dietary modification is frequently prescribed. Each numbered phrase describes a dietary modification. For each numbered phrase select the ONE lettered heading that is most closely associated with it. Each lettered heading may be selected once, more than once, or not at all.

(A) diabetes mellitus

(B) obesity

(C) hypertension

(D) anorexia nervosa

(E) gastroesophageal reflux

(F) postgastrectomy

(G) marathon running

(H) hepatic encephalopathy

(I) Crohn's disease

(J) osteoporosis

(K) celiac disease

(L) monoamine oxidase (MAO) inhibitor therapy

(M) hyperlipidemia

257. Low fiber

258. Tyramine controlled

259. Low sodium

260. Low simple sugar

261. Low protein

262. High carbohydrate (65% to 70% of energy intake)

DIRECTIONS (Questions 263 through 267): Each lettered heading below describes an essential vitamin. Each numbered phrase describes a syndrome of vitamin deficiency or excess. For each numbered phrase select the ONE lettered heading that is most closely associated with it. Each lettered heading may be selected once, more than once, or not at all.

(A) niacin
(B) thiamine
(C) pyridoxine
(D) vitamin C
(E) vitamin A
(F) vitamin E
(G) vitamin K

263. Perifollicular hemorrhage, splinter hemorrhages

264. Papilledema

265. Flushing and pruritus secondary to histamine release

266. High output cardiac failure

267. Dermatitis, dementia, diarrhea

Endocrine

Answers and Explanations

165. (C) Primary hypothyroidism is the most common cause of hypothyroidism in adults. Primary hypothyroidism is several times more common in women than in men and occurs most often between the ages of 40 and 60. Postablative hypothyroidism (radiation or surgery induced) is also very common. *(Ref. 7, p. 453)*

166. (B) Diminished concentrating ability and proteinuria occur even when GFR is near normal. The severity of renal involvement correlates with the duration and magnitude of serum uric acid elevation. Uric acid and monosodium urate deposit in the renal parenchyma. These deposits can cause intrarenal obstruction and elicit an inflammatory response as well. Hypertension, nephrolithiasis, and pyelonephritis can also contribute to the nephropathy of gout. *(Ref. 2, p. 1316)*

167. (C) Patients with panhypopituitarism are found to have a normal distribution of body weight and are rarely cachectic or even undernourished. Patients with pituitary tumors present with symptoms of a mass, or either hyperfunction or hypofunction or both. *(Ref. 7, pp. 248–249)*

168. (C) Receptors for steroid hormones, thyroid hormones, and vitamin A are intracellular. Disease states due to abnormal intracellular receptors include testicular feminization, cortisol resistance, vitamin D-dependent rickets, type II, thyroid hormone resistance, and pseudohypoaldosteronism. There are several different types of cell membrane receptors. *(Ref. 2, p. 1886)*

169. (D) Beta-carotene increases the patient's tolerance for sunlight, apparently by quenching active intermediates. Beta-carotene is an effective scavenger of free radicals. While many affected individuals can tolerate sun exposure while taking beta-carotene, it has no effect on the basic metabolic defect in porphyrin-heme synthesis. *(Ref. 2, p. 311)*

170. (E) FSH is said to encourage maturation of the follicle in the human menstrual cycle. The cardinal hormonal change in phase one is a rise in FSH caused by a decrease in the level of estrogens and a waning activity of the corpus luteum. In men, FSH stimulated Sertoli cells, which have an important role in spermatogenesis. *(Ref. 7, p. 244)*

171. (E) The first four signs listed are findings in hyperparathyroidism. Dyspnea is not usually seen. Most patients with hyperparathyroidism have a simple adenoma that functions autonomously, so that hormone is secreted with high calcium. In about 20% of cases, hyperplasia of all the parathyroid glands (chief cell hyperplasia) is the cause. Differentiation from adenoma is important to determine the correct surgical approach, but is unfortunately very difficult. *(Ref. 7, pp. 1430–1431)*

172. (E) Surgical removal is the most common cause of hypoparathyroidism. When the glands or their blood vessels have merely been damaged and not removed, tissue often regenerates. Hypoparathyroidism can frequently follow thyroid surgery. The incidence varies, and depends on the extent of resection, the skill of the surgeon, and the degree of diligence in diagnosing hypocalcemia. *(Ref. 7, p. 1457)*

173. (C) Water diuresis is impaired in adrenocortical insufficiency. Lack of aldosterone also favors the development of hyperkalemia and mild acidosis. The decreased circulating volume secondary to aldosterone deficiency is one of the factors resulting in elevated basal antidiuretic hormone (ADH) levels and thus hyponatremia. *(Ref. 7, p. 524)*

174. (D) Hypertriglyceridemia may result in part from hyperinsulinism because insulin is one of the factors involved in lipoprotein secretion by the liver. With massive obesity there is an increased prevalence of cardiovascular disease, hypertension, diabetes, pulmonary disorders, and gallstones. Young men with morbid obesity have a 12-fold higher mortality risk than the general population. Even in old age (65 to 74 years) the mortality is doubled in obese men. Cardiovascular disease is the most important factor. *(Ref. 7, p. 1347)*

175. **(D)** The arthritis is characterized by chondrocalcinosis, but unlike idiopathy chondrocalcinosis the hands are usually involved first. The arthropathy often progresses despite phlebotomy. Liver disease is usually the presenting feature. Skin pigmentation is predominantly by melanin. Heart failure is the most common cardiac problem. *(Ref. 2, p. 2071)*

176. **(B)** In patients with hepatic porphyria, oral phenothiazines may be used for abdominal or muscle pains, and Demerol may also be used, but barbiturates should be avoided. Other unsafe medications include alcohol, sulfonamide, carbamazepine, valproic acid, and synthetic estrogens and progestogens. Most heterozygotes remain asymptomatic unless a precipitating factor such as a drug or weight loss is present. Poorly localized abdominal pain is the most common symptom. *(Ref. 2, p. 2076)*

177. **(E)** Obesity causes hypertension by unknown mechanisms, but peripheral vascular resistance is usually normal. Growth hormone response to numerous stimuli is reduced. Insulin resistance and consequent hyperinsulinism is common in obese individuals. Both receptor and postreceptor defects have been identified. *(Ref. 2, p. 449)*

178. **(A)** Glycogen storage is not characteristic of Tay–Sachs disease. Ganglioside accumulation can now be diagnosed by decreased hexosaminidase in peripheral leukocytes. Tay–Sachs is characterized as a lysosomal storage disease. Mental retardation, seizures, blindness, and a retinal cherry red spot are characteristic. It is most common in Ashkenazi Jews. *(Ref. 2, p. 2092)*

179. **(A)** In addition to peripheral motor and sensory neuropathy, cardiac involvement, tongue enlargement, gastrointestinal manifestations, and carpal tunnel syndrome are also seen in amyloidosis. The specific diagnosis requires tissue biopsy with presence of amyloid with specific stains. In primary amyloidosis and myeloma, the amyloid protein is of the AL type. In reactive amyloidosis the protein is of the AA type. *(Ref. 2, p. 1629)*

180. **(D)** Carcinoid syndrome is characterized by increased levels of 5-hydroxyindoleacetic acid. The syndrome occurs in relation to malignant tumors that have metastasized, usually with hepatic implants. Gastrointestinal carcinoids are most commonly found in the appendix. They are very slow growing, thus the 5-year survival rate is 99%. Many carcinoids are discovered as incidental findings on autopsy. *(Ref. 7, p. 1619)*

181. **(D)** In type II hyperlipoproteinemia there is an increased incidence of coronary artery disease, and hypercholesterolemia occurs along with tuberous xanthomas, arcus senilis, and atheromas. Most affected individuals are heterozygotes for the mutant gene. The beta-lipoproteins accumulate because of impaired catabolism. It is expressed early in life, and has been found in cord blood samples. *(Ref. 7, p. 1382)*

182. **(C)** In congenital absence of beta-lipoproteins, there is an inability to manufacture the beta-globulin required for beta-lipoprotein formation. Renal disease is not associated with this syndrome. The disease is caused by a rare autosomal recessive syndrome. Malnutrition, steatorrhea, and pigmentary retinal degeneration are other manifestations. Vitamin E has been used successfully for symptomatic therapy. *(Ref. 7, p. 1386)*

183. **(B)** The diagnosis is Gaucher's disease. The glucocerebrosides are derived from lipid catabolites from the membranes of senescent leukocytes and erythrocytes. While the juvenile form may have severe neurological symptoms (mental retardation, spasticity, ataxia), the adult form usually has no neurologic symptoms. Like Tay–Sachs, it is a lysosomal storage disease with a predilection for Ashkenazi Jews. *(Ref. 2, p. 2092)*

184. **(B)** Xanthomas may be caused by glycogen storage diseases. There are many types of glycogen storage diseases, each caused by a different enzymatic abnormality. The best known types of glycogen storage disease are those that have hepatic–hypoglycemic pathophysiology (e.g., von Gierke disease) or those that have muscle–energy pathophysiology (McArdle's disease). *(Ref. 2, p. 2102)*

185. **(C)** Cystinuria is commonly associated with hexagonal crystals in the urine. Cystine, lysine, arginine, and ornithine are excreted in great excess by patients homozygous for the disease. The tissues manifesting the transport defect of cystinuria are the proximal renal tubule and the jejunal mucosa. It is inherited as an autosomal recessive. Cystine kidney stones are the major clinical manifestation. *(Ref. 2, p. 2128)*

186. (E) Magnesium deficiency is not seen in hypervitaminosis E. Causes of magnesium deficiency also include milk diets in infants, the diuretic phase of acute tubular necrosis, chronic diuretic therapy, acute pancreatitis, and inappropriate ADH. The symptoms of hypomagnesemia include anorexia, nausea, tremor, and mood alteration. As well, symptoms can be caused by the associated hypocalcemia or hypokalemia. *(Ref. 7, p. 1466)*

187. (D) Symptoms of vitamin A intoxication occur in infants or adults ingesting from 75,000 to 500,000 international units of vitamin A. The prognosis is good when vitamin A intake ceases. Rare occurrence of hypercalcemia with vitamin A intoxication have been reported. *(Ref. 7, p. 1453)*

188. (D) The deformity of the hands is due to short metacarpals. Other deformities include short metatarsals, round facies, and thickening of the calvarium. The syndrome is caused by target organ unresponsiveness to PTH, and was the first hormone-resistance syndrome described. *(Ref. 7, pp. 1459–1460)*

189. (C) The findings of hypocalcemia and hyperphosphatemia are the same as in hypoparathyroidism, but the serum parathyroid hormone levels are appropriately increased. As well, the normal urinary rise in cyclic AMP does not occur when these patients are injected with exogenous (normal) PTH. *(Ref. 7, p. 1459)*

190. (B) This lesion is more frequent in females and may antedate other clinical signs and symptoms of diabetes. The plaques are round, firm, and reddish brown to yellow in color. They most commonly involve the legs but can also involve hands, arms, abdomen, and head. *(Ref. 7, p. 1294)*

191. (A) Allopurinol inhibits the enzyme xanthine oxidase, resulting in decreased uric acid production. Allopurinol is particularly useful in the treatment of uric acid nephrolithiasis in gouty individuals. Even if the gouty individual has calcium oxalate stones, allopurinol may be helpful. *(Ref. 2, p. 2086)*

192. (E) Magnesium deficiency results in hypokalemia because of a tendency toward renal potassium wasting. As well, intracellular potassium is depleted, and ventricular irritability is increased (particularly when digoxin is administered). These effects may be caused by dysfunction of Na^+, K^+–ATPase, which is a magnesium-dependent enzyme. *(Ref. 7, p. 1466)*

193. (B) The severe form is caused by a mutation in a single allele of the fibrillin gene (FBN1). The gene product is a major component of elastin-associated microfibrils. Long, thin extremities, ectopia lentis, and aortic aneurysms are the classical triad. Milder forms of the disease probably also occur, but are hard to classify. *(Ref. 2, pp. 2115–2116)*

194. (A) Other drugs that suppress ADH release are alcohol and alpha-adrenergic agents. ADH secretion is also influenced by osmotic and nonosmotic (pressure and volume) factors. Numerous chemical mediators are known to increase ADH secretion. *(Ref. 7, p. 319)*

195. (B) In the familial form, the defect is believed to be a deficiency of lipoprotein lipase, with low release of this enzyme with heparin. It is a rare autosomal recessive syndrome, and usually presents in childhood with typical eruptive xanthoma and abdominal pain secondary to acute pancreatitis. Secondary hyperchylomicronemia (diabetes, hypothyroidism, uremia) is a much more common syndrome. *(Ref. 7, p. 1379)*

196. (C) Subcutaneous xanthomas begin to appear at about age 20 and may involve Achilles tendons, elbows, and tibial tuberosities. Familial hypercholesterolemia may be monogenic or polygenic in its inheritance. The disorder is common, and heterozygous familial hypercholesterolemia is felt to affect 1 in 500 individuals. It can be secondary to other diseases such as hypothyroidism, nephrotic syndrome, or even porphyria. *(Ref. 7, p. 1379)*

197. (A) In the rare familial form, raised, yellow plaques appear on palms and fingers, and reddish-yellow xanthomas occur on the elbows. This disorder is felt to be secondary to accumulation of remnants after lipoprotein lipase acts on triglyceride rich lipoproteins. It is probably due to inherited homozygous defects in apo E structure. *(Ref. 7, p. 1379)*

198. (E) Triglycerides are over 150 and are raised by alcohol intake, estrogens, stress, insulin, and physical activity. If more than one factor is apparent elevation in chylomicrons as well as pre-betalipoproteins (VLDL) may occur. *(Ref. 7, p. 1379)*

199. (B) Hypertriglyceridemia is usually secondary to diabetes mellitus or drugs, rather than a genetic disorder. It can be a normal response to caloric excess or alcohol ingestion, and is common in the third trimester of pregnancy. *(Ref. 7, pp. 1379–1380)*

200. (C) In DM, there is an obligatory osmotic diuresis, but in DI there is lack of water resorption in the tubules. Both result in polyuria, but in diabetes mellitus there will be substantial glucosuria as well. Central diabetes insipidus can be inherited as an autosomal dominant disorder or acquired later in life (idiopathic, postsurgical, post-traumatic, etc.). *(Ref. 7, pp. 334, 1286)*

201. (B) Renal involvement is a characteristic of diabetes mellitus. The characteristic course of the disease is that the kidneys are initially enlarged with supernormal function and microalbuminuria. After a few years, thickened glomerular basement membranes and an increase in mesangial matrix occur. By 10 to 20 years after onset, proteinuria and decline in renal function occur. Diabetes insipidus starting in early life can result in dilatation of the collecting system and permanent renal damage, but in most cases DI does not cause renal impairment. *(Ref. 7, pp. 335, 1295).*

202. (D) Diabetes mellitus can result from glucagon or somatostatin producing tumors of the pancreas as well as pancreatic carcinoma. DI may follow metastatic carcinoma, especially breast. Lymphomas, meningiomas, and craniopharyngiomas have also been associated with DI. *(Ref. 7, pp. 333, 1568)*

203. (A) Four-fifths of diabetes mellitus cases occur as maturity onset, and many patients are obese at diagnosis. Obesity and insulin resistance are positively correlated, and may play pathogenetic roles in noninsulin-dependent diabetes mellitus. *(Ref. 7, p. 1348)*

204. (C) An increased death rate at an early age is seen in both types, with incidence possibly improved on treatment. The patterns of hyperlipidemia are not specific, and the plasma lipoprotein pattern may change with time in any individual. *(Ref. 7, pp. 1272, 1379)*

205. (A) In type II, xanthomas are located on tendons. The xanthomas of type IV are eruptive. *(Ref. 7, p. 1379)*

206. (B) Glucose intolerance is seen in many patients with familial type IV, but hypertriglyceridemia of this pattern occurs in diabetes as well. *(Ref. 7, p. 1383)*

207. (D) Increased chylomicrons are seen in type I and type V and have a high triglyceride content. *(Ref. 7, p. 1379)*

208. (A) Atrial fibrillation and cardiomegaly are characteristic. Other symptoms include palpitation, tachycardia, nervousness, sweating, and dyspnea. Sinus tachycardia is the most common cardiac manifestation. *(Ref. 7, p. 415)*

209. (E) Needle biopsy can be used in numerous diseases, but the main rationale is to differentiate benign from malignant nodules. The specimen must be read by an experienced cytologist. It is difficult to diagnose differentiated follicular carcinoma or to differentiate lymphoma from Hashimoto's thyroiditis. Papillary carcinoma is the easiest diagnosis to make by needle biopsy. *(Ref. 7, p. 408)*

210. (B) Arthropathy usually involves the second and third metacarpophalangeal joints, then knees, hips, and shoulders. It occurs in one-quarter to one-half of patients. Diabetes occurs in 65% of patients and is more common in those with a family history of diabetes. Cardiac disease is the presenting symptom in 15% of patients with heart failure being the usual manifestation. Hypogonadism may manifest as loss of libido, impotence, amenorrhea, testicular atrophy, and sparse body hair. Skin pigmentation is present in 90% of symptomatic patients at presentation, but renal involvement is not characteristic of the disease. *(Ref. 2, p. 2071)*

211. (E) Regulation of vasopressin is by osmotic stimuli and nonosmotic stimuli such as neural stimuli arising outside the hypothalamus. As little as 15% of cells remaining in the posterior hypothalamus are sufficient to prevent permanent diabetes insipidus. *(Ref. 7, p. 333)*

212. (D) Classification of hypoglycemia includes spontaneous causes such as reactive or fasting hypoglycemia and pharmacologic or toxic causes. The diagnosis of hypoglycemia is most certain when Whipple's triad is fulfilled; symptoms consistent with hypoglycemia, low plasma glucose, and relief of symptoms with elevation of plasma glucose to normal. *(Ref. 7, p. 1234)*

213. (B) Cardiac failure, arrhythmias, carpal tunnel syndrome, peripheral neuropathy, and ecchymoses are more frequent in the light chain type than in the secondary type of amyloid. The precursors of the AL amyloid protein found in primary amyloidosis and myeloma are kappa and lambda light chains. Serum amyloid A protein (SAA) is the precursor for the AA amyloid found in secondary amyloidosis. *(Ref. 2, p. 1628)*

214. (A) Glucagon exerts a marked effect on carbohydrate, fat, and lipid metabolism, and increases cyclic AMP in many tissues. Glucagonomas of the pancreas present with features such as mild diabetes mellitus, psychiatric disturbances, diarrhea, venous thromboses, and skin findings (necrolytic migratory erythema). *(Ref. 7, p. 1568)*

215. **(C)** Polyendocrine adenomatosis type I frequently includes islet cell tumors of the pancreas, leading to the Zollinger–Ellison syndrome, insulinomas, and glucagonomas. Inheritance is via an autosominal dominant pattern. Hypercalcemia does not usually occur until after the first decade. *(Ref. 7, p. 1443)*

216. **(D)** Estrogens cause thickening of vaginal mucosa with cornification. The age of onset of pubertal changes and their rates of progression are subject to a number of variables. *(Ref. 7, p. 1141)*

217. **(A)** Ultrasound can usually differentiate the two. Breast development alone is usually just premature thelarche and rarely needs investigation. Feminizing adrenocortical tumors can occur in boys, and cause gynecomastia. *(Ref. 7, p. 1206)*

218. **(A)** Growth hormone produces hypertrophy with functional impairment in many tissues and may cause high glycogen content in the muscle. Short-term administration of growth hormone results in increased nitrogen retention. This is not maintained with continued administration. *(Ref. 7, pp. 234–236)*

219. **(D)** This is a familial disorder with an X-linked recessive pattern treated with pharmacologic doses of vitamin D. Rickets and osteomalacia are characterized by impaired mineralization of bone. Osteoporosis is a disorder with a diminished amount of normally mineralized bone. *(Ref. 7, p. 1492)*

220. **(B)** Risk of death in anorexia nervosa is also associated with hypothermia, suicide, or pneumonia with emaciation. Because of the danger of ventricular tachyarrhythmias, patients should be followed with electrocardiograms. A prolonged Q-T interval is a sign of danger. In addition, severe weight loss can lead to both systolic and diastolic dysfunction of the ventricles. *(Ref. 7, p. 1355)*

221. **(E)** In gouty patients, nephrolithiasis and uric acid nephropathy may occur. The association of cardiovascular disease, hypertension, pyelonephritis, and hyperlipoproteinemia with gout contribute to the high prevalence of renal disease in these individuals. *(Ref. 2, p. 2086)*

222. **(D)** In severe cases, there is bowing of the long bones, inward deformity of the long bones, and wide osteoid borders on bone surfaces. Hypocalcemia is characteristic of osteomalacia, however secondary hyperparathyroidism often raises the serum calcium to low normal levels. The PTH

mediated increase in phosphate clearance often produces hypophosphatemia. *(Ref. 2, p. 2178)*

223. **(C)** The sacrum and pelvis are most frequently involved, followed closely by the tibia and femur. Hypercalcemia can complicate immobilization. The etiology is not known, but a viral agent has been postulated. Symptoms may be absent, or be severe (pain, deformity). *(Ref. 7, p. 1498)*

224. **(A)** Many affected persons with vitamin D deficiency have no demonstrable abnormality except for hypophosphatemia. There is a decreased renal threshold for phosphate excretion. This is mediated by secondary hyperparathyroidism. This is caused by decreased calcium absorption with subsequent mild hypocalcemia. The filtered load of calcium in the kidneys is low, so despite the hyperparathyroidism renal excretion of calcium is low. *(Ref. 7, p. 1490)*

225. **(A)** The normal blood ammonia is less than 150% μ but may rise as high as 500% μ in liver disease. Ammonia is freely diffusible across cell membranes and levels are not affected by glomerular filtration. Other substances possibly implicated in the pathogenesis of hepatic encephalopathy include mercaptans, short-chain fatty acids, and phenol. Excessive GABA (gamma aminobutyric acid), an inhibitory neurotransmitter, in the central nervous system may result in decreased level of consciousness. *(Ref. 2, pp. 1493–1494)*

226. **(E)** In phenylketonuria, a low-phenylalanine diet and a gluten-free diet to age 12 are required, with relentless attention to details of diet for a good outcome. The diet should be started by one month of age. Children of mothers with phenylketonuria can be affected if exposed to phenylalanine in utero. Therefore women with the disorder should stay on a restricted diet until they complete childbearing. *(Ref. 2, p. 2122)*

227. **(B)** Wilson's disease includes cirrhosis of the liver, signs of basal ganglia disease, and a brownish pigmented ring at the corneal margin. Cerulosplasm levels are low. The gene for Wilson's disease is located on the long arm of chromosome 13. In some cases it is possible to identify carrier states and make prenatal diagnoses. The relationship between the abnormal gene and the metabolic defect (inability to regulate copper balance) is unclear. *(Ref. 2, p. 2088)*

228. **(A)** Other stimulators of protein kinases include platelet-derived growth factor, and epidermal growth factor. Tyrosine phosphorylation results from this interaction. Insulin-resistant states can be caused by prereceptor resistance

(mutated insulin, anti-insulin antibodies) or receptor and postreceptor resistance. *(Ref. 2, p. 1998)*

229. **(C)** Insulin lowers cyclic AMP, probably via an increase in phosphodiesterase activity. This probably inactivates cyclic AMP-dependent protein kinase. This promotes glycogen formation, and stimulates glycolysis and inhibits gluconeogenesis. Pyruvate becomes available for lipogenesis, ketone formation slows, and fatty acid synthesis increases. As well, in the presence of glucose, insulin enhances the activity of lipoprotein lipase. *(Ref. 7, pp. 1283–1286)*

230. **(E)** Do not use salicylates in thyroid storm as they cause an increase in free thyroid hormones and oxygen consumption. Management usually includes propylthiouracil, iodide, and dexamethasone. In the absence of cardiac insufficiency, beta blockers may be used. *(Ref. 7, p. 445)*

231. **(E)** Patients ultimately develop insulin resistance due to receptor and postreceptor defects. It is not clear which is the initiating problem, insulin resistance or hyperinsulinemia. *(Ref. 7, p. 1282)*

232. **(B)** All the causes listed may delay puberty, but the most common cause by far is normal variation in growth pattern. There is often a family history of delayed puberty in parents or siblings. In these individuals, bone age often correlates better with the onset and progression of puberty than does chronological age. *(Ref. 7, p. 1170)*

233. **(D)** Response to hormone therapy can be predicted in patients with metastases confined to bone, skin, lung, and nodes, and in those at least five years postmenopausal. Presence of estrogen receptors indicates a better response. *(Ref. 7, p. 1582)*

234. **(B)** A generally increased risk of breast cancer is associated with nulliparity, late first pregnancy, and especially a history of maternal breast cancer. Prior history of breast cancer is of course a powerful risk factor. *(Ref. 7, p. 1578)*

235. **(D)** Although the variation is great depending on occupation, hobbies, etc, generally only one-third of energy is utilized for physical activity. Height is not used at all in calculating RMR, and RMR is higher in men than women of identical weight. Amino acids ingested without other energy sources are inefficiently incorporated into protein. Current recommendations are to encourage full adult levels of protein, vitamins, and minerals in the elderly. *(Ref. 2, pp. 437–439)*

236. **(A)** Diabetes mellitus is a syndrome consisting of hyperglycemia, large vessel disease, microvascular disease, and neuropathy. The classic presenting symptoms are increased thirst, polyuria, polyphagia, and weight loss. In noninsulin-dependent diabetes the presentation can be more subtle, and is often made when the patient is asymptomatic. *(Ref. 7, p. 1255)*

237. **(B)** An insulin tolerance test does not establish the diagnosis of diabetes mellitus. Blood analysis of glucose may rely on the glucose oxidase method, but the autoanalyzer uses the ferricyanide reagent. With typical symptoms even an elevated random sugar is diagnostic. The gold standard is still a fasting plasma glucose ≥ 7.8 mmol/L (140 mg/dL) on two separate occasions. *(Ref. 7, p. 1256)*

238. **(E)** Open-angle glaucoma is not revealed on eye examination. The earliest eye changes may be a functional disturbance of the blood vessels. Increased vascular permeability and ischemia are felt to be factors in the development of diabetic retinopathy. Laser therapy has proven to be an effective tool. Despite this, diabetes is a major cause of adult blindness in the United States. *(Ref. 7, p. 1299)*

239. **(C)** The patient is most likely to develop glomerulosclerosis. This can be diffuse or nodular (Kimmelstiel–Wilson nodules). Poor metabolic control is probably a major factor in the progression of diabetic nephropathy. *(Ref. 7, p. 1296)*

240. **(C)** Pyoderma gangrenosum is not a cutaneous manifestation. Perineal pruritus in a diabetic is almost always associated with *Candida* albicans. A severe external otitis can occur in older patients. It is caused by *Pseudomonas aeruginosa* and is characterized by ear pain, drainage, fever, and leukocytosis. Facial nerve paralysis can occur and is a poor prognostic sign. *(Ref. 2, pp. 562, 1997)*

241. **(C)** The diagnosis is hyperparathyroidism. Calcium deposits are seen in the periarticular areas of the fourth and fifth metacarpophalangeal, third proximal interphalangeal, and fourth distal interphalangeal joints. There is slight soft tissue swelling, especially of the fourth and fifth metacarpophalangeal joints. Calcification in scleroderma is subcutaneous in location. In gout, if monosodium urate is deposited it could appear as a soft tissue mass. *(Ref. 7, p. 1444)*

242. **(B)** Autonomous adrenal tumors are ACTH-insensitive and fail to demonstrate a brisk rise in urinary 17-hydroxycorticoids. In Cushing syndrome secondary to an autonomous renal tumor,

onset is usually gradual, and hirsutism, other androgenic effects, and hyperpigmentation are absent. *(Ref. 7, p. 558)*

243. (B) High prolactin level suppresses luteinizing hormone-releasing hormone (LHRH) and can result in low plasma gonadotropin and testosterone levels. It may not be obvious on physical examination. Therapy with a dopamine agonist, bromocriptine, may lower prolactin levels and reverse impotence. *(Ref. 2, p. 263)*

244. (D) An absent orgasm when libido and erectile function are normal invariably indicates that organic disease is absent. Loss of desire can also be caused by psychological disturbance, but may also indicate androgen deficiency or drug effect. *(Ref. 2, pp. 263–264)*

245. (E) Failure of detumescence, priapism, can be caused by sickle cell anemia or chronic granulocytic leukemia. Priapism must be treated promptly to preserve future erectile functioning. *(Ref. 2, p. 264)*

246. (B) Vascular disease, by itself or in conjunction with peripheral neuropathy in diabetes mellitus, is a common cause of erectile dysfunction. The lesions can be in large vessels (aortic occlusion, Leriche syndrome), small arteries, or even in the sinusoidal spaces. *(Ref. 2, pp. 263–264)*

247. (E) Idiopathic hirsutism may simply represent an extreme of normal androgen production. It is diagnosed by demonstrating minimal elevation of androgens and exclusion of other causes. Management is primarily by cosmetic therapy, although drugs to suppress androgen production and/or androgen effects on the hair follicle can be used. *(Ref. 2, pp. 268–270)*

248. (C) The most severe form of polycystic ovarian disease, Stein–Leventhal syndrome, is associated with chronic anovulation, hirsutism, enlarged cystic ovaries, obesity, and amenorrhea. The spectrum of disease, however, is quite wide and some patients have only mild hirsutism. *(Ref. 2, p. 269)*

249. (F) Krukenberg tumors of the ovary stimulate surrounding ovarian stromal tissue to produce excess androgen. When onset of hair growth (with or without frank virilization) is very rapid, a neoplastic source of androgen is suggested. As well as ovarian tumors, the potential neoplasms include adenomas and carcinomas of the adrenal gland. *(Ref. 2, p. 269)*

250. (D) Attenuated forms of adrenal hyperplasia can present with hirsutism at puberty or in adulthood. Elevated levels of a precursor of cortisol biosynthesis such as 17-hydroxyprogesterone, 17-hydroxypregnenolone, or 11 deoxycortisol. ACTH infusion will increase the precursor level, and dexamethasone will suppress it. *(Ref. 2, pp. 269, 1969)*

251. (A) Anorexia nervosa requires a weight loss of 25% of original body weight for diagnosis. Bulimics are usually within 15% of body weight, but fluctuations are common. *(Ref. 2, pp. 452–455)*

252. (B) Patients with anorexia nervosa control intake, whereas bulimics binge and vomit. Secrecy is common, and often family and friends are unaware of the syndrome. *(Ref. 2, pp. 452–455)*

253. (B) Anorectic patients are much less commonly involved in antisocial behavior. Stealing is common in bulimia and food is the item most often taken. There is a high rate of alcohol and drug abuse as well. *(Ref. 2, p. 454)*

254. (A) In anorexia, skin is often dry and scaly, and yellow due to carotenemia. Body hair can be increased. Bulimia is not characteristically associated with skin findings. *(Ref. 2, p. 454)*

255. (A) Ritualized exercise is characteristic, particularly following food intake. Frenzied calisthenics or running is common. Patients usually deny hunger, thinness, or fatigue. *(Ref. 2, p. 453)*

256. (A) Although overlap syndromes occur, pure bulimia rarely evolves into anorexia whereas the transformation of anorexia to bulimia is not uncommon. *(Ref. 2, p. 453)*

257. (I) Low fiber diets are frequently prescribed during flares of inflammatory bowel disease to reduce diarrhea and pain. Similar diets are often prescribed for diverticulitis or other conditions associated with narrowed or stenosed colon. It may be prescribed for patients with a new ostomy. *(Ref. 2, p. 458)*

258. (L) Limiting foods with high tyramine content for patients on MAO inhibitors might prevent elevations of blood pressure. Such foods include old cheeses and red wine. *(Ref. 2, p. 458)*

259. (C) Some patients with hypertension are salt-sensitive, and will lower their blood pressure with salt restriction. Low sodium diets are also recommended in patients with congestive heart failure, ascites, or chronic renal failure. *(Ref. 2, p. 458)*

260. (F) After gastrectomy, avoiding simple sugars, and limiting liquids can ameliorate symptoms of dumping. Early dumping occurs within 30 minutes of eating and is characterized by vasomotor symptoms such as palpitations, tachycardia, lightheadedness, and diaphoresis. Late dumping includes similar symptoms plus dizziness, confusion, and even syncope. It occurs 1 1/2 to 3 hours after eating. (Ref. 2, pp. 457, 1374)

261.   **(H)**   The symptoms of hepatic encephalopathy are improved with protein restriction. It is presumed that this results in lower levels of serum ammonia, but other substances in the serum may be implicated. These include mercaptans, short-chain, fatty acids and phenol. GABA levels in the brain are also increased. (Ref. 2, pp. 457, 1493–1494)

262.   **(G)**   Carbohydrate loading a week or more before an endurance event may improve performance by increasing muscle glycogen stores and energy reserves. This might be relevant in events that require long, sustained activity. (Ref. 2, p. 457)

263.   **(D)**   Scurvy is characterized by a tendency to hemorrhage and perifollicular hyperkeratotic papules in which hairs become fragmented and buried. Gums are involved only if teeth are present. The peak incidence is in infants of 6 to 12 months of age who are on processed milk formulas without citrus fruit or vegetable supplementation. Another peak occurs later in life, particularly in edentulous men who live alone and cook for themselves. It is frequently associated with other nutritional deficiencies (e.g., folic acid). (Ref. 2, p. 476)

264.   **(E)**   Excessive vitamin A ingestion can cause abdominal pain, nausea, vomiting, headache, dizziness, and papilledema. Deficiency of vitamin A can cause night blindness and progress to visual loss. It is common in children in developing countries and is a major cause of blindness. (Ref. 2, p. 478)

265.   **(A)**   Pharmacologic doses of niacin for hypercholesterolemia may cause histamine release which results in flushing, pruritus, and gastrointestinal disturbance. As well, asthma may be aggravated, acanthosis nigricans can occur, and in high doses elevation of uric acid and fasting blood sugar can occur. Hepatic toxicity, including cholestatic jaundice, has been described with large doses. (Ref. 2, p. 479)

266.   **(B)**   Thiamine deficiency can cause high output cardiac failure (wet beriberi) or neurologic symptoms (dry beriberi). In North America thiamine deficiency occurs in alcoholics or food faddists. In alcoholics deficiency is secondary to low intake, impaired absorption and storage, and accelerated destruction. Genetic factors are important as clinical manifestations occur only in a small proportion of chronically malnourished individuals. Beriberi heart disease is characterized by peripheral vasodilatation, sodium and water retention, and biventricular failure. (Ref. 2, pp. 474–475)

267.   **(A)**   Diarrhea, dementia and dermatitis are the classic triad for pellagra (niacin deficiency). There is no biochemical test to confirm the diagnosis, and diagnosis is based on clinical suspicion and response to therapy. Small doses of niacin (10 mg/day) with adequate dietary tryptophan will cure pellagra secondary to nutritional deficiency. (Ref. 2, p. 474)

Gastroenterology
Questions

DIRECTIONS (Questions 268 through 291): Each of the questions or incomplete statements below is followed by five suggested answers or completions. Select the ONE that is best in each case.

268. Diverticulosis coli is best treated with

    (A) stool softeners
    (B) prophylactic surgery
    (C) phenolphthalein laxatives
    (D) increasing stool bulk
    (E) psychotherapy

269. Characteristically, carcinoid tumors of the GI tract

    (A) are more common in women
    (B) produce hypertension
    (C) produce jaundice
    (D) produce steatorrhea
    (E) are multiple in up to 40% of cases

270. Extra-intestinal manifestations of inflammatory bowel disease include all of the following EXCEPT

    (A) fatty liver
    (B) pneumonitis
    (C) pyoderma gangrenosum
    (D) anemia
    (E) conjunctivitis

271. Characteristically, cancer of the esophagus

    (A) usually occurs in the upper third
    (B) is more common in females
    (C) has a five-year cure rate of 20%
    (D) may be either adenocarcinoma or squamous cell carcinoma
    (E) always presents with early dysphagia

272. The most reliable method of measuring steatorrhea is

    (A) xylose absorption
    (B) Schilling test
    (C) x-ray studies
    (D) stool fat quantitation
    (E) small intestinal biopsy

273. Acquired lactase deficiency is seen in association with all of the following EXCEPT

    (A) nontropical sprue
    (B) tropical sprue
    (C) regional enteritis
    (D) ulcerative colitis
    (E) hypersensitivity reactions

274. Clinical characteristics of Whipple's disease include all of the following EXCEPT

    (A) women are usually affected
    (B) arthritis
    (C) diarrhea
    (D) progressive wasting
    (E) skin pigmentation

275. Celiac sprue includes all of the following features EXCEPT

    (A) decrease in intestinal disaccharidases
    (B) weight loss
    (C) mononuclear infiltrate in mucosa
    (D) increase in pancreatic enzymes
    (E) response to gluten-free diet

276. The presence of antibody to hepatitis B surface antigen (anti-HBs) is indicative of

    (A) previous hepatitis B infection
    (B) chronic active hepatitis
    (C) acute hepatitis B infection
    (D) poor prognosis
    (E) need for vaccine to hepatitis B

277. Which of the following conditions may be associated with impaired hepatic uptake of bilirubin?

(A) Crigler–Najjar syndrome
(B) Dubin–Johnson syndrome
(C) Rotor syndrome
(D) Gilbert syndrome
(E) pregnanediol therapy

278. Dark brown spots in the lips and palate associated with Peutz–Jeghers syndrome may indicate

(A) intestinal polyposis
(B) Addison's disease
(C) lead poisoning
(D) malignant melanoma
(E) gastric ulcers

279. Carcinoma of the large bowel occurs most frequently in the

(A) cecum
(B) sigmoid
(C) transverse colon
(D) appendix
(E) ascending colon

280. Postprandial postgastrectomy syndromes may be associated with all of the following EXCEPT

(A) symptoms 20 minutes after eating
(B) palpitation and sweating
(C) functional hypoglycemia
(D) relief with frequent small meals
(E) prolonged vomiting

281. Characteristics of hepatoma include all of the following EXCEPT

(A) commonly metastasize
(B) poor prognosis
(C) predisposing cirrhosis
(D) markedly elevated alkaline phosphatase
(E) more common in males

282. Ascitic fluid in cirrhosis of the liver would be expected to show

(A) hemorrhage
(B) protein greater than 2.5 gm per 100 mL
(C) positive malignant cytology
(D) specific gravity less than 1.016
(E) more than 1000 white cells per cubic mm

283. Which of the following is true of common duct stones?

(A) all originate in the gallbladder
(B) they always produce jaundice

(C) jaundice is always constant
(D) jaundice can be painless
(E) none of the above

284. Patients with anorexia nervosa may manifest all of the following EXCEPT

(A) extreme emaciation
(B) loss of pubic/axillary hair
(C) decreased blood pressure
(D) signs of vitamin deficiency
(E) psychiatric disturbance

285. Diarrhea and cramping with postprandial vasomotor phenomena with concomitant cardiovascular findings should suggest

(A) abdominal angina
(B) pheochromocytoma
(C) carcinoid syndrome
(D) hyperlipemia
(E) congestive heart failure and small bowel ulceration

286. The diagnosis of achalasia (cardiospasm) includes all of the following EXCEPT

(A) symptoms of dysphagia
(B) symptoms of regurgitation
(C) hyposensitive Mecholyl test
(D) smooth narrowing of lower esophagus
(E) lack of resistance to passage of esophagoscope through the narrowed segment

287. Mechanical narrowing of the esophageal lumen causing dysphagia is commonly caused by any of the following EXCEPT

(A) squamous cell carcinoma of the esophagus
(B) adenocarcinoma of the cardia of the stomach
(C) reflux esophagitis
(D) lye ingestion
(E) motor system disease

288. Zollinger–Ellison syndrome is associated with all of the following EXCEPT

(A) 12-hour nocturnal secretion of gastric juice more than 2 liters
(B) diffusion of 50% of tumors throughout the pancreas
(C) malignancy of 50% of tumors
(D) recurrent peptic ulcerations
(E) small incidence of hypoglycemia

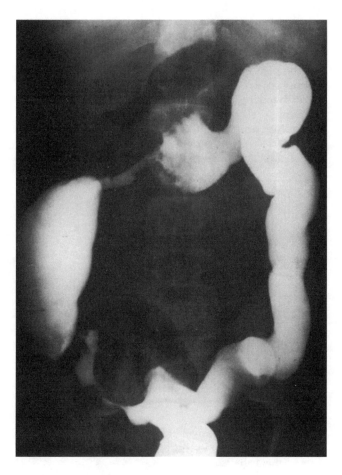

Figure 4.1

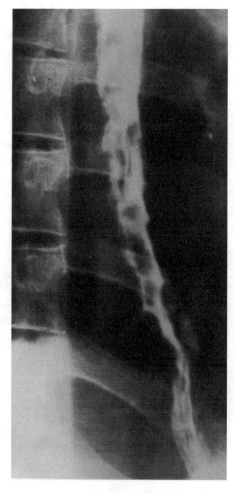

Figure 4.2

289. A 35-year-old white man presents with a long history of fulminant diarrhea and rectal bleeding (Figure 4.1). What is your diagnosis?

(A) toxic megacolon

(B) amoebic colitis

(C) appendicitis

(D) ischemic colitis

(E) annular carcinoma

290. A 45-year-old man with a long history of alcoholic intake comes into the emergency room with upper gastrointestinal bleeding (Figure 4.2). What is your diagnosis?

(A) esophageal varices

(B) esophageal carcinoma

(C) foreign body

(D) tertiary waves

(E) Barrett's esophagus

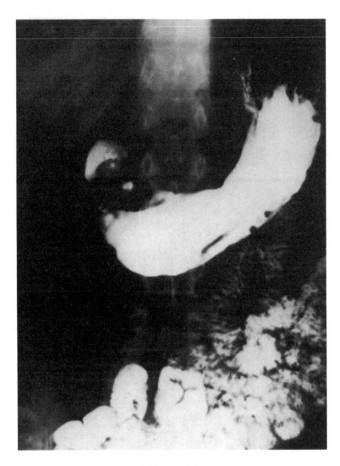

Figure 4.3

291. A 40-year-old taxicab driver presents with worsening epigastric pain (Figure 4.3). What is your diagnosis?

    (A) benign gastric ulcer
    (B) malignant gastric ulcer
    (C) duodenal ulcer
    (D) normal
    (E) hiatus hernia

DIRECTIONS (Questions 292 through 301): The group of questions below consists of a list of lettered headings followed by a list of numbered words, phrases, or statements. For each numbered word, phrase, or statement, select the ONE lettered heading that is most closely associated with it. Each lettered heading may be selected once, more than once, or not at all.

Questions 292 through 296

    (A) hepatitis A
    (B) hepatitis B
    (C) hepatitis C
    (D) chronic persistent hepatitis
    (E) chronic active hepatitis

292. Associated with α-$_1$-antitrypsin deficiency

293. Causative agent appears to be a 27 nm RNA particle

294. The major cause of post-transfusion hepatitis

295. Commonly transmitted among the sexually promiscuous, especially male homosexuals

296. A nonprogressive inflammatory process largely confined to portal areas with no significant stromal collapse

Questions 297 through 301

    (A) associated with benign gastric ulcer but not malignant gastric ulcer
    (B) associated with malignant gastric ulcer but not benign gastric ulcer
    (C) associated with both malignant and benign gastric ulcers
    (D) associated with neither malignant nor benign gastric ulcers

297. Associated with bezoars

298. Achlorhydria

299. Extension of the tumor beyond the contour of the curvature

300. Prepyloric ulcer

301. Frequently complete healing in four to six weeks

DIRECTIONS (Questions 302 through 315): Each of the questions or incomplete statements below is followed by five suggested answers or completions. Select the ONE that is best in each case.

302. Acute pancreatitis tends to occur in patients with any of the following EXCEPT

(A) alcoholism

(B) peptic ulcer

(C) mumps

(D) multiple endocrine neoplasia

(E) lysinuria

303. Any of the following would be suitable for initial therapy of duodenal ulcer EXCEPT

(A) cimetidine

(B) verapamil

(C) sucralfate

(D) ranitidine

(E) magnesium hydroxide

304. The actions of pure gastrin include all of the following EXCEPT

(A) stimulation of intrinsic factor

(B) stimulation of pepsin secretion

(C) stimulation of gastric motility

(D) increased volume of output by the pancreas

(E) increased flow of hepatic bile

305. Cholestatic jaundice is frequently associated with

(A) unconjugated hyperbilirubinemia

(B) a moderate to marked increase in alkaline phosphatase

(C) a marked increase in acid phosphatase

(D) a moderate increase in SGOT

(E) severe parenchymal liver damage

306. All of the following may be associated with protein-losing enteropathy EXCEPT

(A) gastric carcinoma

(B) nontropical sprue

(C) ulcerative colitis

(D) congestive heart failure

(E) ischemic infarction of the colon

307. The association of diarrhea and arthritis is most suggestive of

(A) lymphoma of the bowel

(B) amyloid infiltration

(C) chronic pancreatitis

(D) ulcerative colitis

(E) tropical sprue

308. Which of the following is most characteristic of hepatitis C?

(A) caused by RNA virus

(B) spread by oral–fecal route

(C) no carrier state occurs

(D) incubation 2 to 20 weeks

(E) not detectable in serum

309. Acute necrotizing (membranous) enterocolitis is most typically associated with

(A) spontaneous regression

(B) streptococcal invasion

(C) previous antibiotic therapy

(D) vesicular rash

(E) bowel infarction

310. Total parenteral nutrition for patients with malabsorption syndrome should include all of the following EXCEPT

(A) fat emulsion

(B) dextrose

(C) vitamin E

(D) amino acids

(E) trace minerals

311. Which of the following is most commonly associated with biliary cirrhosis?

(A) malignant clinical course

(B) nonobstructive-type jaundice

(C) decreased serum lipids

(D) hepatitis C infection

(E) marked hepatomegaly

312. The small bowel mucosal biopsy is mostly likely to be normal in

(A) tropical sprue

(B) postgastrectomy steatorrhea

(C) Whipple's disease

(D) nontropical sprue

(E) a betalipoproteinemia

313. The radiologic "string sign" in ileitis is most often seen

(A) in the stenotic or nonstenotic phase of the disease

(B) in the stenotic phase only

(C) as a rigid, nondistensible phenomenon

(D) with gastric involvement

(E) with rectal involvement

314. Volvulus of the intestines most frequently involves the

(A) cecum

(B) stomach

(C) rectum

(D) sigmoid flexure

(E) jejunum

315. The following statements concerning *Helicobacter pylori* gastric colonization are true EXCEPT

(A) the majority of persons with gastric ulcer are colonized

(B) the majority of persons with duodenal ulcer are colonized

(C) the majority of patients with colonization have peptic ulcer disease

(D) colonization rates increase with advancing age

(E) social circumstances influence colonization rates

DIRECTIONS (Questions 316 through 336): For each numbered phrase select the ONE lettered phrase that is most closely associated with it. Each lettered phrase may be selected once, more than once, or not at all.

Questions 316 through 320

(A) associated with dysphagia secondary to mechanical obstruction of the esophagus but *not* motor dysfunction

(B) associated with dysphagia secondary to motor dysfunction of the esophagus but *not* mechanical obstruction

(C) associated with *both* dysphagia secondary to motor dysfunction and mechanical obstruction of the esophagus

(D) associated with *neither* dysphagia secondary to mechanical obstruction nor motor dysfunction of the esophagus

316. Severe weight loss out of proportion to the degree of dysphagia

317. Hoarseness following the onset of dysphagia

318. Episodic dysphagia to solids of several years' duration

319. Dysphagia to solids and liquids

320. A prolonged history of heartburn and reflux preceding dysphagia

Questions 321 through 326

(A) associated with predominantly unconjugated hyperbilirubinemia *not* conjugated

(B) associated with predominantly conjugated hyperbilirubinemia *not* unconjugated

(C) associated with *both* conjugated and unconjugated hyperbilirubinemia

(D) associated with *neither* conjugated nor unconjugated hyperbilirubinemia

321. Biliary colic

322. Sepsis

323. Hereditary disorders

324. Breast milk jaundice

325. Prolonged fasting

326. Chlorpromazine

Questions 327 through 331

(A) chronic gastritis type A

(B) chronic gastritis type B

(C) Menetrier's disease

(D) eosinophilic gastritis

(E) granulomatous gastritis

(F) gastritis following gastric surgery

(G) acute erosive gastritis

327. Ischemia of the gastric mucosa implicated in the pathogenesis

328. Associated with *H. pylori* infection

329. Immune or autoimmune pathogenesis suspected

330. Commonly associated with protein-losing enteropathy

331. Bile reflux implicated in pathogenesis

Questions 332 through 336

    (A) associated with ulcerative colitis but *not* Crohn's disease

    (B) associated with Crohn's disease but *not* ulcerative colitis

    (C) associated with *both* Crohn's disease and ulcerative colitis

    (D) associated with *neither* Crohn's disease nor ulcerative colitis

332. Transmural involvement

333. Lymph node involvement

334. Frequent rectal involvement

335. Rarely associated with malignancy

336. The interphalangeal joints are a common site for involvement with associated arthritis

Gastroenterology
Answers and Explanations

268. **(D)** Diverticula are present in over 50% of octogenarians. Most patients remain asymptomatic. They are most common in the sigmoid colon and decrease in frequency in the proximal colon. The relative scarcity of diverticulae in underdeveloped nations has led to the hypothesis that low fiber diets result in decreased fecal bulk, narrowing of the colon, and an increased intraluminal pressure to move the small fecal mass. This results in thickening of the muscular coat and eventually herniations or diverticulae of the mucosa at the points where nutrient arteries penetrate the muscularis. *(Ref. 2, p. 1419)*

269. **(E)** Carcinoid tumors are multiple in up to 40% of cases. Primary carcinoid tumors of the appendix are common but rarely metastasize. Those in the large colon may metastasize but do not function. Carcinoids are the most common gastrointestinal endocrine tumors. They arise from neuroendocrine cells most commonly in the GI tract, pancreas, or bronchi. GI carcinoids cause abdominal pain, bleeding, or even obstruction (usually via intussusception). Carcinoid syndrome is characterized by flushing, diarrhea, and valvular heart disease. *(Ref. 2, p. 1537)*

270. **(B)** Other extra-intestinal manifestations include hypoalbuminemia, erythema nodosum, cirrhosis of the liver, and kidney stones. Joint manifestations occur in 25% of IBD patients. The peripheral, nondeforming arthritis involves knees, ankles, and wrists most commonly. Typically this arthritis correlates with activity of the underlying bowel disease. The ankylosing spondylitis associated with IBD in contrast, is unassociated with activity of the underlying bowel disease and is strongly associated with HLA-B27. *(Ref. 2, p. 1412)*

271. **(D)** Lesions in the upper two-thirds of the esophagus are squamous, but in the distal esophagus over half are adenocarcinomas. In total, over 85% are squamous cell carcinomas. The adenocarcinomas develop more commonly from columnar epithelium in the distal esophagus (Barrett's esophagus). Adenocarcinomas of the esophagus have the biologic behavior of gastric cancers. *(Ref. 2, pp. 1382–1383)*

272. **(D)** Greater than 6 gm of stool fat per 24 hours indicates malabsorption or maldigestion. The Schilling test is useful in testing for B_{12} absorption. X-rays can be helpful in diagnosing underlying disorders, but are nonspecific. Small intestinal biopsy is useful in determining the cause of malabsorption. *(Ref. 2, p. 1390)*

273. **(E)** Lactase intolerance is not a hypersensitivity reaction but rather a malabsorption syndrome caused by a disaccharidase (lactase) deficiency in the brush border of intestinal epithelial cells. Acquired lactase deficiency can be caused by numerous gastrointestinal diseases that affect the mucosa. *(Ref. 2, pp. 1400–1401)*

274. **(A)** Whipple's disease is unusual in women and occurs predominantly in men of middle age. The classical symptoms are arthritis (the most common), diarrhea, malabsorption, and weight loss. This disease is caused by a PAS-staining bacillus. The organism has been found in synovium, lymph nodes, pericardium, brain, and many other tissues. Prolonged antibiotic therapy is required. *(Ref. 2, p. 1703)*

275. **(D)** Severe mucosal damage leads to decrease in secretin and cholecystokinin and decreased pancreatic secretion. This results in decreased stimulation of the pancreas with lower than normal levels of pancreatic enzymes in response to a meal. The gallbladder becomes resistant to cholecystokinin, resulting in sequestration of bile salts in a noncontracting gallbladder. These defects in intraluminal fat digestion add to the mucosal defect. *(Ref. 2, p. 1399)*

276. **(A)** The antibody can be demonstrated in 80 to 90% of patients, usually late in convalescence, and indicates relative or absolute immunity. In

contrast, surface antigen (HB_sA_g) occurs very early and disappears in less than 6 months. Persistence of HB_sA_g indicates chronic infection. *(Ref. 2, p. 1461)*

277. **(D)** Gilbert syndrome may be associated with impaired hepatic uptake of bilirubin. Uptake of bilirubin by the liver cell involves dissociation of the pigment from albumin and binding to cytoplasmic proteins (Y and Z). Impairment of bilirubin conjugation is a more common cause. *(Ref. 2, p. 1454)*

278. **(A)** Intestinal polyposis is a possible indication of Peutz–Jeghers syndrome associated with dark brown spots on the lips and palate. There is characteristic distribution of pigment around lips, nose, eyes, and hands. *(Ref. 2, p. 1425)*

279. **(B)** Despite some decline, distal tumors are still the most common. The fact that up to 60% of tumors are located in the rectosigmoid is the rationale for screening via sigmoidoscopy. Flexible, fiberoptic sigmoidoscopes probably enhance cancer detection. *(Ref. 2, p. 1426)*

280. **(E)** Prolonged vomiting is not associated with postprandial postgastrectomy syndromes. The early syndrome may be due to fluid loss into the intestine, release of serotonin or kinins, or enteric glucagon release. *(Ref. 2, p. 1374)*

281. **(A)** Hepatomas usually do not metastasize. More common reasons for nonresectability include cirrhosis or involvement of both lobes. In contrast, many malignancies metastasize to the liver. At autopsy, hepatic metastases have been found in 30% to 50% of patients dying from malignant disease. Metastatic liver disease is second only to cirrhosis as a cause of fatal liver disease. *(Ref. 2, p. 1497)*

282. **(D)** Ascitic fluid in cirrhosis of the liver shows a specific gravity less than 1.016. Protein is less than 2.5%, and the gross appearance is straw colored. In spontaneous bacterial peritonitis the fluid may be cloudy and the number of white cells (neutrophils) increased. In uncomplicated ascites, the difference between plasma albumin and ascitic fluid albumin is greater than 1.1 g/dL. *(Ref. 2, p. 233)*

283. **(D)** Jaundice can be painless, or it may give rise to severe pain, chills, and fever. The jaundice is generally conjugated hyperbilirubinemia. Partial obstruction of the common duct produces variable amounts of jaundice and is influenced by the presence of concurrent hepatocellular disease or cholangitis. *(Ref. 2, pp. 230–231)*

284. **(B)** Anorexia nervosa occurs 20 times more often in females than males. It does not cause loss of pubic/axillary hair. *(Ref. 2, p. 454)*

285. **(C)** These signs suggest carcinoid syndrome. Flushing, lacrimation, tachycardia, and telangiectasia may also be associated. *(Ref. 2, p. 1538)*

286. **(C)** Severe achalasia may have minimal dysphagia, delayed regurgitation, persistent substernal pain, and cachexia. A hyposensitive Mecholyl test is not diagnostic of achalasia. The underlying problem in achalasia is a motor disorder of the esophageal smooth muscle in which the lower esophageal sphincter does not relax appropriately. Esophageal peristalsis is also impaired. *(Ref. 2, p. 1358)*

287. **(E)** Squamous cell carcinoma accounts for 95% of true esophageal tumors, but often adenocarcinoma of the stomach causes esophageal symptoms. Motor system disease is not a cause of mechanical narrowing of the esophageal lumen. *(Ref. 2, pp. 1358–1359)*

288. **(B)** Diffusion of 50% of tumors throughout the pancreas is not a feature of the Zollinger–Ellison syndrome. In 20% of cases, multiple endocrine adenomas are present in parathyroid, pituitary adrenal, or thyroid. *(Ref. 2, p. 1375)*

289. **(E)** The carcinoma has occurred in a patient with ulcerative colitis. The barium enema shows a long, constricting lesion in the transverse colon, with the whole colon devoid of haustral markings. Some pressure effects are seen in the ileum due to metastases. The diagnosis of ulcerative colitis is made from the clinical symptoms and proctosigmoidoscopic examination of an abnormally inflamed colonic mucosa. *(Ref. 2, p. 1412)*

290. **(A)** In esophageal varices, the esophageal folds are thick and tortuous, giving rise to a wormy or worm-eaten appearance. The radiographic picture would vary with the severity of the varices, as well as the distention of the esophagus. When varices are severe, they should be appreciated in any projection. The left anterior oblique projection is most ideal for its demonstration. *(Ref. 2, pp. 1489–1490)*

291. **(A)** In benign gastric ulcer, an ulcer niche is present in the prepyloric area, with folds radiating to and extending up to the margin of the niche with a halo around it. The differentiation between benignity and malignancy may be difficult at times, but proper use of radiographic criteria could boost the accuracy to 98%. In the presence of an ulcer niche, a Hampton line,

which is an ulcer collar, or a mound should be sought on a profile view. *(Ref. 2, pp. 1371–1372)*

292. **(E)** Chronic active hepatitis requires a biopsy for diagnosis as it is essential to establish a specific cause if possible, such as α-₁-antitrypsin deficiency, Wilson's disease, or ethanol. *(Ref. 2, pp. 1478, 1499)*

293. **(A)** The causative agent of hepatitis A virus is a 27-nm diameter RNA virus which, although similar to other picornaviruses, is not cytopathogenic in tissue culture. Hepatitis B is associated with the 42-nm DNA particle. *(Ref. 2, p. 1459)*

294. **(C)** Hepatitis C is the major cause of post-transfusion hepatitis. It occurs in approximately 5 to 10 cases per 1,000 transfusions and is especially transmitted in clotting factor concentrates. Testing of blood products is now available. *(Ref. 2, p. 1463)*

295. **(B)** The hepatitis B virus is present in virtually all body fluids and excreta and is, therefore, transmitted by sexual contact, as well as by transfusion or exposure of health care workers. *(Ref. 2, p. 1466)*

296. **(D)** There is little or no periportal or lobular hepatitis, and fibrosis and cirrhosis are absent. This condition may be entirely asymptomatic or associated with nonspecific symptoms. *(Ref. 2, p. 1478)*

297. **(D)** The vast majority of gastric ulcers are benign, about 7% with no clear diagnosis will prove malignant. Neither benign nor malignant gastric ulcers are associated with bezoars. *(Ref. 2, pp. 1371–1372)*

298. **(B)** True achlorhydria (with pentagastrin stimulation) almost never occurs with benign gastric ulcer. *(Ref. 2, p. 1371)*

299. **(C)** The defect extends beyond the projected wall of the stomach in both, but it is smooth and oval when benign. *(Ref. 2, p. 1372)*

300. **(C)** Both benign and malignant gastric ulcers are most often antral and are usually single and on the lesser curvature. *(Ref. 2, pp. 1371–1372)*

301. **(A)** Benign ulcers should reduce by 50% in two to three weeks at repeat examination, and they often heal completely in four to six weeks. *(Ref. 2, p. 1372)*

302. **(D)** Acute pancreatitis most commonly follows alcoholism or biliary tract disease and can be related to metabolic disorders, drugs, and anatomic

defects. Multiple endocrine neoplasia syndromes are associated with pancreatic tumors, not pancreatitis. *(Ref. 2, p. 1521)*

303. **(B)** Verapamil is a calcium channel blocker and not effective in ulcer therapy. Cimetidine or ranitidine is preferred by many, primarily because of convenience. Cimetidine and ranitidine block histamines-2 (H-2) receptors. The most potent inhibitors of acid production are the proton pump inhibitors (e.g., omeprazole). *(Ref. 2, pp. 1368–1371)*

304. **(A)** Pancreozymin and cholecystokinin possess the same terminal tetrapeptide as gastrin and may explain extragastric effects of gastrin. Gastrin is the most potent known stimulant of gastric acid secretion. It is released from the cytoplasmic secretory granules of gastrin cells (G cells) located in the gastric antrum. *(Ref. 2, pp. 1363–1364)*

305. **(B)** Laboratory tests alone may not permit differentiation of intrahepatic from extrahepatic cholestasis. Ultrasound and CT scan can determine extrahepatic obstruction with good sensitivity and specificity, providing there has been no prior hepatobiliary surgery. *(Ref. 2, p. 231)*

306. **(E)** Intravenous administration of ^{125}I-labelled albumin may show up to a 40% loss in the GI tract in protein-losing enteropathy. Treatment of protein-losing enteropathy is usually directed at the underlying condition. *(Ref. 2, p. 1402)*

307. **(D)** Joint involvement in inflammatory bowel disease may involve sacroiliitis or specific large joint peripheral arthritis. The latter type of arthritis parallels the course of the bowel disease. The sacroiliitis (spondylitic) variety follows an independent course. *(Ref. 2, p. 1413)*

308. **(D)** Hepatitis C is a DNA virus that can now be detected in serum through antibody screening tests. A carrier state may develop and chronic hepatitis may follow acute infection. *(Ref. 2, p. 1463)*

309. **(C)** Acute necrotizing enterocolitis occurs in patients prepared for GI surgery with antibiotics or in liver disease patients on neomycin. In neutropenic patients, *Pseudomonas* can be the cause, but generally *Clostridium difficile* is the organism. *(Ref. 2, pp. 668, 1411)*

310. **(C)** Medium chain triglycerides composed of fatty acids with 6 to 10 carbons are effective when given as a 10% fat emulsion in dextrose and water. *(Ref. 2, p. 468)*

311. **(E)** The patient is typically a middle-aged woman with itching, jaundice, steatorrhea, marked hepatomegaly, and elevated serum lipids. The cause of primary biliary cirrhosis is unknown, but a disordered immune response may be involved. A positive antimitochondrial antibody test is found in over 90% of symptomatic patients. *(Ref. 2, pp. 1487–1488)*

312. **(B)** Postgastrectomy steatorrhea does not result from mucosal abnormality. The mucosa is also normal in pancreatic steatorrhea. Postgastrectomy maldigestion and malabsorption is caused by rapid gastric emptying, reduced dispersion of food in the stomach, reduced luminal levels of bile, rapid transit of food, and impaired pancreatic secretory response. *(Ref. 2, p. 1375)*

313. **(A)** In addition to the string sign, abnormal puddling of barium, and fistulous tracts are other helpful x-ray signs of ileitis. Other radiologic findings in Crohn's disease include skip lesions, rectal sparing, small ulcerations, and fistulas. *(Ref. 2, p. 1409)*

314. **(D)** Fixation of the bowel wall by tumor may produce volvulus, most frequently in the sigmoid colon. Sigmoidoscopy may be therapeutic in cases of sigmoid volvulus. Barium should never be given by mouth to a patient with a possible large bowel obstruction. *(Ref. 2, p. 1431)*

315. **(C)** Most people with *H. pylori* colonization never develop ulceration. However, of those with duodenal ulcer, 90 to 95% are colonized and of those with gastric ulcer 60 to 70% are colonized. For those under 30 years of age, the colonization rate is 10%, but for those over 60 years of age, the colonization rate approximates their age. Low socioeconomic status and institutionalization both increase the colonization rate. *(Ref. 2, p. 1367)*

316. **(A)** Severe weight loss out of proportion to the degree of dysphagia suggests carcinoma of the esophagus. *(Ref. 2, p. 207)*

317. **(C)** Hoarseness following the onset of dysphagia can be caused by an esophageal cancer extending to involve the recurrent laryngeal nerve or because of laryngitis secondary to gastroesophageal reflux. *(Ref. 2, p. 207)*

318. **(A)** Episodic dysphagia to solids of several years' duration suggests a benign disease and is characteristic of a lower esophageal ring. *(Ref. 2, p. 206)*

319. **(C)** Motor dysphagia presents with dysphagia to solids and liquids. Dysphagia due to obstruc-

tion starts with solids and can progress to liquids as well. *(Ref. 2, p. 206)*

320. **(A)** A prolonged history of heartburn and reflux preceding dysphagia indicates a peptic stricture. *(Ref. 2, p. 207)*

321. **(D)** Biliary colic is characterized by pain, not jaundice. *(Ref. 2, p. 62)*

322. **(C)** Sepsis causes conjugated hyperbilirubinemia as well as predominantly unconjugated hyperbilirubinemia (due to decreased hepatic uptake). *(Ref. 2, pp. 230–231)*

323. **(C)** Hereditary disorders of hepatitic glucuronosyl transferase activity such as Gilbert syndrome and Crigler–Najjar types I and II result in unconjugated hyperbilirubinemia. Intrahepatic disorders such as Dubin–Johnson syndrome and Rotor syndrome cause predominantly conjugated hyperbilirubinemia. *(Ref. 2, pp. 230–231)*

324. **(A)** Breast milk jaundice is caused by reversible hepatic glucuronosyl transferase deficiency and results in predominantly unconjugated hyperbilirubinemia. *(Ref. 2, pp. 230–231)*

325. **(A)** Prolonged fasting impairs hepatic uptake of bilirubin, resulting in predominantly unconjugated hyperbilirubinemia. *(Ref. 2, pp. 230–231)*

326. **(B)** Chlorpromazine, oral contraceptives, and androgens cause a cholestatic picture with predominantly conjugated hyperbilirubinemia. Some drugs, e.g., chloramphenicol can inhibit hepatic glucuronosyl transferase activity and cause predominantly unconjugated hyperbilirubinemia. *(Ref. 2, pp. 230–231)*

327. **(G)** Acute erosive gastritis is most commonly seen in critically ill hospitalized patients. Ischemia of the gastric mucosa is a key factor in the syndrome. *(Ref. 2, p. 1378)*

328. **(B)** Type B chronic gastritis is the more common cause of chronic gastritis. It becomes more common with advancing age and is uniformly associated with *H. pylori* infection. Eradication of *H. pylori* produces histologic improvement. *(Ref. 2, p. 1381)*

329. **(A)** Type A chronic gastritis may lead to pernicious anemia. Antibodies to parietal cells and to intrinsic factor are frequently seen in the sera, suggesting an immune or autoimmune pathogenesis. *(Ref. 2, p. 1380)*

330. **(C)** Ménétrier's disease is not a true gastritis as inflammation is not present on histologic examination. It is characterized by large tortuous gastric mucosal folds and usually presents with abdominal pain. Protein-losing enteropathy often develops, resulting in hypoalbuminemia and edema. *(Ref. 2, p. 1381)*

331. **(F)** Gastric surgery seems to accelerate the development of asymptomatic gastritis with progressive parietal cell loss. However, some patients develop bile reflux gastritis with symptoms of pain, nausea, and vomiting. *(Ref. 2, p. 1382)*

332. **(B)** Crohn's disease is characterized by transmural involvement. It is rare in ulcerative colitis. *(Ref. 2, p. 1407)*

333. **(B)** Ulcerative colitis never involves lymph nodes or mesenteric fat, whereas Crohn's disease frequently does. *(Ref. 2, p. 1407)*

334. **(C)** Ulcerative colitis involves the rectum 95% of the time. Crohn's disease results in rectal involvement 50% of the time. *(Ref. 2, p. 1407)*

335. **(B)** Malignancy, although reported in Crohn's is rare in comparison with ulcerative colitis. *(Ref. 2, pp. 1407–1408)*

336. **(D)** Although any joint can be involved, inflammatory bowel disease usually affects knees, ankles, or wrists or else causes a spondylitic syndrome. *(Ref. 2, p. 1413)*

CHAPTER 5

Hematology
Questions

DISEASES OF THE BLOOD

DIRECTIONS (Questions 337 through 361): Each of the questions or incomplete statements below is followed by five suggested answers or completions. Select the ONE that is best in each case.

337. Cryoglobulinemia may be found in association with all of the following EXCEPT

    (A) multiple myeloma
    (B) lymphosarcoma
    (C) systemic lupus
    (D) infectious mononucleosis
    (E) thalassemia

338. Acute myeloblastic leukemia (AML) is characterized by

    (A) peak incidence in childhood
    (B) high leukocyte alkaline phosphatase
    (C) Philadelphia chromosome
    (D) Auer bodies in blast cells
    (E) response to vincristine and prednisone

339. All of the following are generally associated with secondary polycythemia EXCEPT

    (A) Cushing syndrome
    (B) uterine myomata
    (C) hypernephroma
    (D) gastric malignancy
    (E) cerebellar hemangiomas

340. The cytogenetic abnormality in chronic myelogenous leukemia includes

    (A) deletion of 14
    (B) reciprocal translocation of 9 and 22
    (C) translocation of the RAS oncogene
    (D) trisomy 21
    (E) translocation of 8 to 14

341. Infectious mononucleosis is characterized by all of the following EXCEPT

    (A) antibodies to Epstein–Barr virus
    (B) heterophil antibodies
    (C) antinuclear antibodies
    (D) anti-I antibodies
    (E) antibodies to sheep red cells

342. A patient with aplastic anemia receives a bone marrow transplant from an HLA-matched sister. The most likely complication will be

    (A) graft versus host disease
    (B) graft failure
    (C) radiation sickness
    (D) development of leukemia
    (E) secondary skin cancer

343. Hemophilia A can be characterized by

    (A) normal immunoreactive factor VIII
    (B) normal functional factor VIII
    (C) decreased immunoreactive factor VIII
    (D) prolonged bleeding time
    (E) platelet function abnormality

344. Patients homozygous for hemoglobin C may manifest all of the following EXCEPT

    (A) increased target cells
    (B) increased spleen size
    (C) intracellular crystals
    (D) increased osmotic fragility
    (E) marrow hyperplasia

345. Multiple myeloma is often associated with all of the following EXCEPT

    (A) bone pain
    (B) osteoblastic bone lesions
    (C) Bence Jones proteinuria
    (D) occurrence after age 40 in most cases
    (E) myeloma cells in bone marrow

346. Children with homozygous beta-thalassemia who receive a high transfusion regimen should also receive

(A) oral calcium supplements
(B) fresh frozen plasma
(C) desferrioxamine
(D) penicillamine
(E) cryoprecipitate

347. Thrombocythemia can be distinguished from reactive thrombocytosis by

(A) increased megakaryocyte number
(B) increased total platelet mass
(C) increased platelet turnover
(D) normal platelet survival
(E) thromboembolism and hemorrhage

348. Eosinophilia is frequently seen with all of the following EXCEPT

(A) allergic disorders
(B) parasitic infestations
(C) Löffler syndrome
(D) following irradiation
(E) ACTH administration

349. Washed, frozen-thawed, packed red blood cells are used to reduce the transfusion of

(A) non-A, non-B hepatitis
(B) AIDS
(C) malaria
(D) leukocytes
(E) reticulocytes

350. Sickle cell anemia is usually associated with all of the following EXCEPT

(A) hemoglobin S
(B) small- or normal-sized spleen
(C) normal reticulocyte count
(D) shortened erythrocyte life span
(E) normal hemoglobin concentration in the red blood cell

351. A man with a prosthetic aortic valve is most likely to have hemolysis from

(A) thermal injury
(B) isoantibodies
(C) autoantibodies
(D) red cell fragmentation
(E) hemoglobinopathy

352. A decrease in plasma levels of antithrombin III has been responsible for

(A) aspirin sensitivity
(B) heparin resistance
(C) coumadin resistance
(D) platelet dysfunction
(E) disseminated intravascular coagulation

353. Iron deficiency in infancy may be due to all of the following EXCEPT

(A) low birth weight
(B) hemolysis
(C) early clamping of cord
(D) inadequate diet
(E) blood loss

354. The presence of increased levels of 2, 3-DPG in the red cell is associated with

(A) hemolytic anemia due to sulfa drugs
(B) increased oxygen affinity
(C) decreased oxygen affinity
(D) loss of red cell energy
(E) multiple congenital abnormalities

355. All of the following statements are true EXCEPT

(A) people with group AB red blood cells have anti-A and anti-B sera
(B) group O, Rh negative red blood cells are "universal donors"
(C) the red blood cells of 85% of whites are agglutinated by anti-Rh serum
(D) the genotype for group B red blood cells may be BB or BO
(E) the genotype for group O red blood cells is only OO

356. Hemolytic anemias are usually associated with all of the following EXCEPT

(A) erythroid hypoplasia of the marrow
(B) decreased red cell survival
(C) increased numbers of reticulocytes
(D) increased fecal urobilinogen
(E) increased urine urobilinogen

357. Hypochromic microcytic anemia is seen in all of the following EXCEPT

(A) chronic blood loss
(B) thalassemia
(C) thiamine deficiency
(D) pyridoxine deficiency
(E) iron deficiency

358. Elevated platelet counts may be found in all of the following EXCEPT

(A) splenectomized patients
(B) acute hemorrhage
(C) the postoperative period
(D) chronic granulocytic leukemia
(E) penicillin allergy

359. Figure 5.1 (a) and (b) are the x-rays of a 60-year-old white man with pain in the right chest. What is your diagnosis?

(A) aneurysmal bone cyst
(B) multiple myeloma
(C) lymphosarcoma
(D) prostatic metastases
(E) hyperparathyroidism

360. Figure 5.2 is the x-ray of a 30-year-old black woman with recurrent abdominal pain and pallor. What is your diagnosis?

(A) sickle cell anemia
(B) hemangioma
(C) spondylitis deformans
(D) ankylosing spondylitis
(E) multiple myeloma

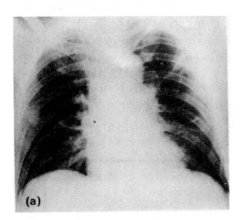

Figure 5.1a

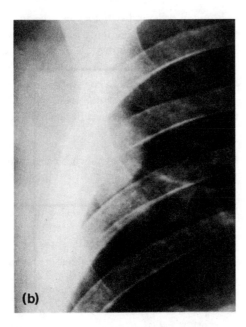

Figure 5.1b

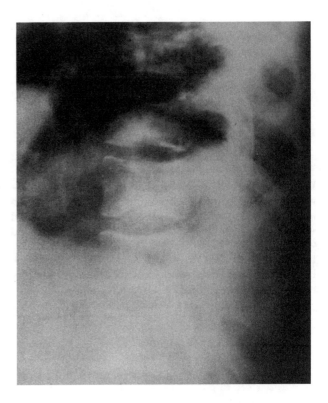

Figure 5.2

TABLE 5.1 CASE WORK-UP

Blood film	Polychromatophilia, some spherocytes
Bilirubin	2.0 mg/100 mL total
	0.3 mg/100 mL direct
Haptoglobin	10 mg/100 mL
Lactate dehydrogenase	200 IU/L
Urine bilirubin	Negative
Antiglobulin test	Positive direct
	Negative indirect

361. The case work-up shown in Table 5.1 is of a 30-year-old woman presenting with a hemoglobin of 6.0 gm/100 mL. The most likely diagnosis is

(A) iron deficiency
(B) congenital spherocytosis
(C) liver failure and hemolysis
(D) splenomegaly and hemolysis
(E) autoimmune hemolytic anemia

DIRECTIONS (Questions 362 through 366): The group of questions below consists of a list of lettered headings followed by a list of numbered words, phrases, or statements. For each numbered word, phrase, or statement, select the ONE lettered heading that is most closely associated with it. Each lettered heading may be selected once, more than once, or not at all.

(A) beta-thalassemia major
(B) hemoglobin H disease
(C) sickle cell disease
(D) hemoglobin C disease
(E) hemoglobin M disease

362. Forms tactoids or liquid crystals when hypoxic

363. A mild hemolytic anemia with intra-erythrocytic crystals seen on fixed blood smears

364. May result from defect in processing of globin messenger RNA

365. Decreased alpha chain production leads to four-beta tetramer formation

366. Bone infarction can occur that may be difficult to distinguish from osteomyelitis

DIRECTIONS (Questions 367 through 378): Each of the questions or incomplete statements below is followed by five suggested answers or completions. Select the ONE that is best in each case.

367. Patients with lymphoma receiving long-term therapy with vincristine may develop all of the following EXCEPT

(A) loss of the Achilles tendon reflex
(B) muscle pains
(C) cardiac arrhythmias
(D) paraesthesia
(E) diplopia

368. Which of the following is NOT involved in prenatal diagnosis of beta-thalassemia?

(A) amniotic fluid analysis
(B) restriction fragment polymorphism
(C) trophoblast biopsy
(D) buccal mucosal cytology
(E) molecular genetic probes

369. The sickle cell trait may include all of the following EXCEPT

(A) vascular occlusive phenomena under stress
(B) renal concentration defect
(C) positive sickle preparation
(D) increased hemoglobin H
(E) hematuria

370. Which of the following statements does NOT describe the macrocytic anemia of pregnancy?

(A) helmet cells and schistocytes are common
(B) it occurs most commonly in the third trimester of pregnancy
(C) it responds to folic acid
(D) the anemia disappears spontaneously on interruption or termination of the pregnancy
(E) splenomegaly is present in about one-third of cases

371. Hemolytic disease of the newborn (erythroblastosis fetalis) due to Rh incompatibility is usually associated with

(A) a positive direct Coombs' test using the mother's red blood cells
(B) toxemia of pregnancy
(C) a negative direct Coombs' test using the baby's red blood cells
(D) simultaneous ABO incompatibility
(E) a positive indirect Coombs' test using the mother's serum

372. Hairy cell leukemia probably responds best to treatment with

    (A) cytosine arabinoside
    (B) ifosfamide
    (C) deoxycoformycin
    (D) interleukin 3
    (E) retinoic acid

373. All of the following are frequently associated with hemolytic anemia due to intravascular red cell destruction EXCEPT

    (A) paroxysmal nocturnal hemoglobinuria
    (B) cold agglutinin disease
    (C) ABO isoantibodies and transfusion
    (D) clostridial sepsis
    (E) glucose-6-phosphate dehydrogenase deficiency and drugs

374. Hereditary persistence of hemoglobin F can best be characterized as

    (A) a cause of sickling red cells
    (B) a disease of infants only
    (C) a variant of thalassemia major
    (D) an anemia exacerbated by Fava beans
    (E) a benign genetic abnormality

375. Which of the following is most typical of peripheral blood films from patients with splenectomy?

    (A) increase in macrophages
    (B) leukopenia
    (C) polycythemia
    (D) Pappenheimer bodies
    (E) nucleated red cells

376. Although type O blood is considered to be the "universal donor," a possible danger in this practice may be

    (A) type O donors have a higher incidence of hepatitis C virus
    (B) type O donors have a shorter survival time when transfused than do other cell types
    (C) at times, type B blood may be mistyped as type O
    (D) type O donors have high titers of anti-A and anti-B in their plasma
    (E) conversion of the recipient to type O blood

377. All of the following are important prognostic factors in acute lymphoblastic leukemia EXCEPT

    (A) age
    (B) total white count
    (C) mediastinal lymphadenopathy

    (D) total platelet count
    (E) response to induction therapy

378. Which of the following drugs does NOT interfere with platelet function?

    (A) dipyridamole
    (B) aspirin
    (C) co-trimoxazole
    (D) sulfinpyrazone
    (E) enteric-coated aspirin

379. All of the following statements concerning sideroblastic anemia are correct EXCEPT

    (A) isoniazid can disrupt heme metabolism and cause sideroblastic anemia
    (B) it can be an inherited condition
    (C) idiopathic cases generally respond to pharmacologic doses of pyridoxine
    (D) can result in acute myelogenous leukemia
    (E) can affect neutrophils and platelets

DIRECTIONS (Questions 380 through 394): This section consists of clinical situations, each followed by a series of questions. Study each situation, and select the ONE best answer to each question following it.

Questions 380 through 384: A 50-year-old white woman presents with a three-week history of tiredness and pallor. A family member has noted some yellowness of her eyes, but she denies darkening of the urine. Physical examination reveals only slight jaundice. Laboratory data include an Hb of 9 gm, reticulocyte count of 12%, a bilirubin in the serum of 2 mg/dL indirect reacting, and some microspherocytes on peripheral smear.

380. The most likely cause of this woman's anemia is

    (A) blood loss externally
    (B) decreased red cell production
    (C) ineffective erythropoiesis
    (D) intravascular hemolysis
    (E) extravascular hemolysis

381. Spherocytosis may be associated with all of the following EXCEPT

    (A) burns
    (B) hereditary spherocytosis
    (C) Coombs'-positive hemolytic anemia
    (D) glucose-6-phosphate dehydrogenase deficiency
    (E) splenomegaly

382. All of the following may be expected in this case EXCEPT

(A) depressed haptoglobin level

(B) increased bilirubin in the urine

(C) increased urobilinogen in the stool

(D) increased methemalbumin in the blood

(E) decreased hemopexin in the blood

383. Bone narrow examination is most likely to show

(A) megaloblastic changes

(B) giant metamyelocytes

(C) increased erythroid to myeloid ratio

(D) increased lymphocytes

(E) shift to left of the myeloid series

384. Other changes in a peripheral blood smear might include all of the following EXCEPT

(A) large polychromatophilic cells

(B) normoblasts

(C) leukocytosis

(D) basophilic stippling

(E) hypochromia

Questions 385 through 389: A 57-year-old man with a history of chronic alcohol ingestion is admitted to the hospital with acute alcoholic intoxication and lobar pneumonia. Physical examination reveals pallor; a large, tender liver; and consolidation of the right lower lobe. Laboratory data include an Hb of 7 gm, WBC of 4000, and platelet count of 85,000.

385. Likely causes for anemia in this man include all of the following EXCEPT

(A) hemorrhagic diathesis

(B) gastrointestinal bleeding

(C) nutritional deficiency

(D) toxic marrow suppression

(E) hemoglobinopathy

386. The most likely vitamin deficiency related to the pancytopenia is

(A) B_{12}

(B) folate

(C) pyridoxine

(D) thiamine

(E) riboflavin

387. Toxic marrow suppression is most likely to affect

(A) developing erythrocytes and myelocytes

(B) mature polymorphonuclear leukocytes

(C) mature red cells

(D) mature platelets

(E) eosinophils

388. Examination of the peripheral smear might show all of the following EXCEPT

(A) target cells

(B) macrocytosis

(C) spur cells

(D) increased platelet adhesiveness

(E) increased segmentation of white cells

389. A deficiency of coagulation factors in this patient would most likely include factors

(A) V and VIII

(B) VIII, IX, XI, and XII

(C) XIII

(D) II, V, VII, X

(E) I, V, VIII

Questions 390 through 394: An 18-year-old man of Italian extraction is found to have a hypochromic microcytic anemia of 10% gm. In addition, there is a fair degree of anisocytosis, poikilocytosis, and targeting on smear. The white blood count is 9500, the platelet count is 240,000, and the reticulocyte count is 7%. The spleen is palpated 5 cm below the left costal margin.

390. The most likely diagnosis is

(A) sickle cell trait

(B) thalassemia minor

(C) hemoglobin S-C disease

(D) iron-deficiency anemia

(E) hereditary spherocytosis

391. Which of the following would be most helpful in distinguishing this case from one of pure iron deficiency anemia?

(A) peripheral blood smear

(B) osmotic fragility test

(C) Ham test

(D) hemoglobin electrophoresis on paper

(E) serum iron determination

392. One would expect to find which of the following in thalassemia minor?

(A) an increased amount of fetal or A_2 hemoglobin

(B) increased osmotic fragility of the red cells

(C) absent bone marrow iron

(D) increased macroglobulins in the serum

(E) small amounts of S hemoglobin

393. The present treatment of choice for thalassemia minor is

(A) splenectomy
(B) removal of the abnormal hemoglobin pigment
(C) purely supportive
(D) plasmapheresis
(E) intramuscular iron

394. Which of the following abnormal hemoglobins characteristically produces targeting in the peripheral blood?

(A) hemoglobin M
(B) hemoglobin S
(C) hemoglobin Zurich
(D) hemoglobin C
(E) hemoglobin Barts

The group of questions below consists of a list of lettered phrases followed by a list of numbered phrases. For each numbered phrase select the ONE lettered heading that is most closely associated with it. Each lettered heading may be selected once, more than once, or not at all.

Questions 395 through 399

(A) iron-deficiency anemia
(B) beta-thalassemia trait
(C) anemia of chronic disease
(D) sideroblastic anemia

395. Serum iron increased, total iron-binding capacity (TIBC) normal, ferritin increased

396. Serum iron normal, TIBC normal, ferritin normal

397. Serum iron decreased, TIBC increased, ferritin decreased, Hb A2 decreased

398. Serum iron decreased, TIBC decreased, serum ferritin increased

399. Generally requires a bone marrow for definitive diagnosis

Questions 400 and 401

(A) spherocytes
(B) schistocytes
(C) sickle cells
(D) acanthocytes
(E) agglutinated cells
(F) Heinz bodies

400. Found in severe liver disease

401. Represent precipitated hemoglobin

402. Caused by loss of red cell membrane

403. Caused by polymerization of an abnormal hemoglobin

404. Caused by trauma to red cell membranes

DIRECTIONS (Questions 405 and 406): Each of the questions or incomplete statements below is followed by five suggested answers or completions. Select the ONE that is best in each case.

405. All the following statements concerning von Willebrand's disease are true EXCEPT

(A) it is a rare disorder
(B) it facilitates platelet adhesion
(C) it is the plasma carrier for coagulation factor VIII
(D) severe forms cause more joint bleeding than hemophilia
(E) it can be treated with a vasopressin analogue

406. All the following statements concerning circulating anticoagulants are correct EXCEPT

(A) they can be IgG antibodies which react to specific coagulation factors
(B) nonspecific circulating anticoagulants cause severe hemorrhage
(C) some circulating anticoagulants may cause thromboembolic disease
(D) may be implicated in spontaneous abortions
(E) abnormal coagulation tests are not corrected by addition of normal plasma

Hematology
Answers and Explanations

337. **(E)** Cryoglobulinemia may be found in association with the first four conditions cited. An association with thalassemia would be unusual. Cryoglobulins are serum proteins that undergo reversible precipitation at low temperatures. Hyperviscosity syndromes may result. *(Ref. 4, p. 1110)*

338. **(D)** Auer bodies are slender, pink, staining rods containing lysozyme and are exclusively seen in AML. Although similar to normal azurophilic granules in content and staining properties, they are distinguished by their gigantic size. Special stains can enhance the detection of Auer bodies. *(Ref. 4, p. 766)*

339. **(D)** Gastric malignancy is not associated with secondary polycythemia. The other tumors listed generally are thought to produce endogenous erythropoietin and are distinguished from primary polycythemia by high levels of erythropoietin. *(Ref. 4, p. 705)*

340. **(B)** The reciprocal translocation involves the long arms of 22 and 9, and results in translocation of the c-abl oncogene. The resultant abnormal chromosome 22 is known as the Philadelphia (Ph[1]) chromosome. *(Ref. 4, p. 203)*

341. **(C)** Antinuclear antibodies are not characteristic of infectious mononucleosis. Heterophil antibodies react against sheep red cells and are not absorbed out by guinea pig kidney. Examination of the blood film reveals a lymphocytosis with atypical lymphocytes. *(Ref. 4, p. 955)*

342. **(A)** Graft versus host disease is a frequent complication of allogeneic marrow transplant. It is caused by a reaction of lymphoid donor cells against host tissue. It can be acute or chronic. Numerous treatment regimes involving methotrexate, glucocorticoids, cyclosporine, and other drugs are used in treatment. *(Ref. 4, p. 1674)*

343. **(A)** Antibodies to factor VIII detect normal quantities in hemophilia A, but function of the molecule is abnormal. The activated partial thromboplastin time (APTT) is prolonged and the prothrombin consumption test is abnormal. The prothrombin time, thrombin clotting time, and bleeding time are usually normal. *(Ref. 4, p. 1461)*

344. **(D)** Homozygous C red cells are often target-shaped with "extra" membrane to make them more resistant to osmotic fragility. However, cells containing principally hemoglobin C are more rigid than normal and their fragmentation in the circulation may result in microspherocytes. The intracellular crystals are simply oxygenated HbC. The spleen is invariably enlarged. *(Ref. 4, p. 626)*

345. **(B)** Bone lesions in myeloma are destructive, but the alkaline phosphatase is usually normal, indicating little blastic activity. Osteolysis, when combined with immobilization can lead to hypercalcemia. It is usually mediated by osteoclast-activating factor from neoplastic myeloma cells in the adjacent marrow. *(Ref. 4, pp. 1115–1116)*

346. **(C)** Iron chelation with desferrioxamine will reduce the toxicity from iron overload if given regularly in high doses. The most lethal toxicity of iron load is iron infiltration of the myocardium with resultant dysfunction and death. *(Ref. 4, p. 534)*

347. **(E)** Reactive thrombocytosis is usually transitory, without thromboembolism, hemorrhage, splenomegaly, or leukocytosis. Causes of secondary thrombocytosis include chronic inflammatory disorders (e.g., rheumatoid arthritis), acute inflammatory disease, acute or chronic blood loss, and malignancy. Recovery from thrombocytopenia ("rebound") can also result in very high platelets. A common cause is withdrawal of alcohol. *(Ref. 4, p. 1403)*

348. (E) Steroids cause decreased numbers of eosinophils to circulate, so that eosinophilia may be seen in Addison's disease, for example. Beta blockers may cause eosinophilia by blocking beta adrenergic eosinopenia. Löffler syndrome is a transient eosinophilia associated with pulmonary infiltrate. *(Ref. 4, p. 845)*

349. (D) Febrile reactions to leukocytes may be severe and cause hypotension, especially in repeatedly transfused patients. Antibodies to platelets can also develop. *(Ref. 4, p. 1614)*

350. (C) Since sickle cell anemia is a chronic hemolytic anemia, the reticulocyte is chronically elevated except in aplastic crises. Infection is the most common precipitant of an aplastic crisis, particularly those caused by parvoviruses. *(Ref. 4, p. 618)*

351. (D) Most valves associated with hemolysis have been aortic, but mitral prostheses or unsuccessful mitral valvuloplasty have caused red cell fragmentation. The reticulocyte count, serum LDH, and plasma hemoglobin levels may be elevated. Haptoglobin concentration is diminished and hemosiderinuria is present. Mild cases can be managed with iron and folic acid supplementation, but on occasion valve replacement is required. *(Ref. 4, p. 654)*

352. (B) Heparin appears to act as catalyst in the inactivation of thrombin by antithrombin III. The heparin-AT III complex is an immediate, potent inhibitor of activated coagulation proteases. *(Ref. 4, p. 1569)*

353. (B) Iron deficiency in infancy is not due to hemolysis. Sixty percent of body iron concentration at birth is contained in circulating hemoglobin. Milk is a poor source of iron, so the most common cause of iron deficiency in infancy is prolonged breast or bottle feeding. Cereals are high in iron content. *(Ref. 4, p. 482)*

354. (C) The 2, 3-DGP binds to the central cavity of the heme molecule and changes the configuration in favor of oxygen release. The other common factors that affect oxygen affinity are temperature and pH. The oxygen affinity of hemoglobin is easily characterized by the P_{50}; the oxygen tension at which hemoglobin is half saturated. *(Ref. 4, p. 380)*

355. (A) Group AB has neither anti-A nor anti-B, as both A and B antigens are on the red cells. It is a rare blood group (only 2 to 3% of population) and if large amounts of blood are required in an AB individual A type blood can be used, as anti-B in the donor plasma rarely destroys AB cells. It

would still be preferable to remove the plasma and use packed red cells. If donor O blood is used, significant hemolysis can occur unless donor plasma is removed. *(Ref. 4, p. 1596)*

356. (A) Hemolytic anemias are not associated with erythroid hypoplasia of the marrow. Erythroid hyperplasia is present except during infections or insults that lead to aregenerative crises. *(Ref. 4, p. 426)*

357. (C) Microcytic hypochromic anemias are caused by disorders of iron, globin, heme, or porphyrin metabolism and are not seen in thiamine deficiency. Thiamine has been implicated in a rare megaloblastic anemia in children. The biochemistry is not understood. *(Ref. 4, p. 1616)*

358. (E) Elevated platelet counts may be found in the first four conditions listed. Penicillin allergy may lower platelet counts. Reactive thrombocytosis is rarely associated with thromboembolic or hemorrhagic phenomena. *(Ref. 4, p. 1463)*

359. (B) There is lytic destruction of the sixth rib with a pathologic fracture and an extrapleural mass. The most common manifestation of multiple myeloma is multiple, "punched-out" lesions in the flat and tubular bones. Some may appear as a discrete lytic lesion and remain as a solitary lesion. *(Ref. 4, p. 1114)*

360. (A) The diagnosis is sickle cell anemia. There is a biconcave appearance or configuration of the vertebral bodies, giving rise to a "fish mouth" appearance. Some sclerotic changes are seen. *(Ref. 4, p. 614)*

361. (E) Autoimmune hemolytic anemia is the most likely diagnosis. Spherocytosis is seen as well in burn victims, in microangiopathic hemolysis, and in congenital spherocytosis. *(Ref. 4, p. 666)*

362. (C) A number of factors influence the rate and degree of hemoglobin S aggregation including concentration of S in the cell, cellular dehydration, and the length of time in deoxy conformation. *(Ref. 4, p. 614)*

363. (D) The patients with homozygous hemoglobin C disease have mild hemolysis, splenomegaly, target cells, and hemoglobin C crystals. Unlike sickle cell disease, the prognosis is favorable. *(Ref. 4, p. 626)*

364. (A) In one class of beta-thalassemia (beta-plus), there is a mutation that affects processing of the beta-globin messenger RNA precursor. *(Ref. 4, p. 525)*

365. (B) A moderately severe decrease in alpha-chain production leads to the formation of very unstable four-beta-chain tetrameres that are useless in oxygen transport. *(Ref. 4, p. 530)*

366. (C) If the bone infarction occurs in proximity to a joint, an effusion can develop. The underlying pathology is a vaso-occlusive phenomenon. *(Ref. 4, p. 614)*

367. (C) In addition to the four symptoms cited, other neurologic symptoms include motor weakness, muscle atrophy, ptosis, facial palsy, and ileus. Neurologic toxicity is usually the result of a cumulative dose and usually begins when the total dose exceeds 6 mg/m². Parasthesia of fingers and feet and loss of deep tendon reflexes are the usual initial manifestation. *(Ref. 4, p. 283)*

368. (D) Lengthening or shortening of DNA fragments following restriction enzyme treatment may help to identify an affected fetus. It is possible to identify about 80% of cases with prenatal diagnosis. *(Ref. 4, p. 533)*

369. (D) The renal concentrating defect and positive sickle prep are constant, but occlusive phenomena and hematuria may occur under stress. In sickle cell trait more than half the hemoglobin is hemoglobin A. Thus the cells are resistant to sickling until an oxygen tension of about 15 mm Hg. *(Ref. 4, p. 625)*

370. (A) The megaloblastic anemia of pregnancy is the most common of all folate deficient states. Dilutional anemia and iron deficiency also occur in pregnancy. In pregnancy a low hemoglobin concentration may simply be due to a disproportionate increase in plasma volume, rather than a true anemia. The exact hormonal mechanism is unknown. *(Ref. 4, pp. 426, 446)*

371. (E) This condition is usually associated with a positive Coombs' test using the baby's red blood cells and a positive indirect Coombs' test using the mother's serum. Prevention of Rh immunization by the administration of Rh antibody (via Rh immune globulin) has been an effective preventive measure for this disorder. *(Ref. 4, p. 687)*

372. (C) Deoxycoformycin produces complete remissions in hairy cell leukemia. Recombinant alpha-interferon may also be effective. The disease is characterized by "hairy" cells in blood and bone marrow, splenomegaly, and pancytopenia. *(Ref. 4, p. 1025)*

373. (B) Other categories of intravascular red cell destruction include erythrocyte fragmentation, autoimmune hemolytic anemias, and thermal in-juries. Cold agglutinins agglutinate human red cells at temperatures below body temperature. Red cell destruction is usually extravascular. It can be secondary to mycoplasma pneumonia infection, but despite the presence of cold agglutinins, hemolysis in this infection is unusual. *(Ref. 4, p. 485)*

374. (E) Hemoglobin F is evenly distributed among red cells, unlike the increased F in other conditions. It is a heterogeneous condition, and can be classified into deletion and nondeletion forms. *(Ref. 4, p. 510)*

375. (E) The spleen normally functions to pit nuclei and their fragments from red cells. The spleen has immune functions and filter functions. It also enhances iron re-utilization and acts as a reservoir and blood volume regulator. In disease states it can be a site of extramedullary hematopoiesis. *(Ref. 4, p. 59)*

376. (D) There is a danger that type A₂ may be mistyped as O. Anti-A and anti-B in the plasma are usually absorbed in the recipient's tissues. *(Ref. 4, p. 1596)*

377. (D) Age under two or over ten years, white count over 100,000, and presence of a mediastinal mass are all adverse prognostic indicators. It is the most common malignancy in children under age 15 in the United States. In white children only, there is a sharp peak of incidence between age 3 and 7. *(Ref. 4, p. 994)*

378. (C) Aspirin in usual clinical dosage inhibits platelet aggregation and prolongs the bleeding time. Aspirin inhibits platelet function by acetylating and irreversibly inactivating the enzymes cyclo-oxygenase. Penicillins and cephalosporins can also impair both platelet adhesion and activation. Co-trimoxazole can inhibit marrow production of platelets, but not their function. *(Ref. 4, p. 1426)*

379. (C) A trial of pyridoxine at 200 mg/day for 2 to 3 months should be attempted, but the response rate is low. Many toxic agents (e.g., alcohol, alkylating agents, isoniazid, lead, chloramphenicol) can cause sideroblastic anemia. The inherited form is an X-linked disorder and is quite rare. About 10% of cases will develop acute myelogenous leukemia; this might be higher if the anemia is associated with alkylating agents. Neutropenia and thrombocytopenia occur frequently. *(Ref. 2, p. 1725)*

380. (E) Extravascular hemolysis usually occurs in the liver, spleen, or other RE sites and liberates bilirubin unconjugated. Intrinsic causes of hemolytic anemia are usually inherited and are a result of abnormalities of membranes, red cell enzymes, globins, or heme. Extrinsic hemolysis is a result of mechanical forces, chemicals or microorganisms, antibodies, or sequestration in the monocyte–macrophage system. *(Ref. 4, p. 426)*

381.   **(D)**   Spherocytosis is not associated with glucose-6-phosphate dehydrogenase deficiency. Spherocytes are characterized by normocytic hyperchromic indices with MCHC between 37% and 40%. The typical changes in G-6-PD deficiency include the presence of Heinz bodies. The cell morphology is not usually changed unless hemolysis is very severe. *(Ref. 4, pp. 565, 599)*

382.   **(B)**   All mechanisms listed help to clear hemoglobin or heme from the plasma. Unconjugated bilirubin is not cleared by the kidney because it is tightly bound to plasma proteins. *(Ref. 4, p. 426)*

383.   **(C)**   Bone marrow examination is most likely to show increased erythroid to myeloid ratio. Erythroid hyperplasia is common to all hemolytic anemias and may develop megaloblastic features unless folate is supplied. *(Ref. 4, p. 426)*

384.   **(E)**   Hypochromia would not be a change in the peripheral blood smear. Reticulocytes are large polychromatophilic cells that may have basophilic stippling. Normoblasts are released in brisk hemolysis. Hypochromia is seen in disturbances of hemoglobin synthesis. Examples include iron deficiency, and the various thalassemia. *(Ref. 4, p. 426)*

385.   **(E)**   Hemoglobinopathy is not a likely cause of anemia in this patient. Gastrointestinal bleeding from a duodenal ulcer, gastritis, or bleeding varices with iron deficiency are the more common causes. *(Ref. 4, p. 456)*

386.   **(B)**   Folate deficiency results from decreased intake and malabsorption. Body folate stores are meager, and therefore easily depleted when intake is poor. Alcohol itself can depress folate levels acutely and also can cause pancytopenia directly. *(Ref. 4, p. 456)*

387.   **(A)**   Alcohol is directly toxic to dividing and maturing cells but may also affect neutrophil function. The hematologic effects of alcohol may be direct, or indirect, via diet, infection, liver disease, and gastrointestinal disease. The resulting hematologic abnormalities may be profound. *(Ref. 4, p. 1588)*

388.   **(D)**   The peripheral smear would not show increased platelet adhesiveness. The red cell changes may result from folate deficiency, associated liver disease, or plasma lipid concentration changes. *(Ref. 4, p. 456)*

389.   **(D)**   Coagulation factors II, V, VII, and X would most likely be deficient. These are some of the factors that are synthesized in the liver, but V is not dependent on vitamin K. *(Ref. 4, p. 1285)*

390.   **(B)**   Thalassemia minor usually represents a heterozygous state and is often asymptomatic. Symptoms may develop during periods of stress such as pregnancy or severe infection. Hemoglobin values are usually in the 9 to 11 g/dL range. The red cells are small and poorly hemoglobinized. *(Ref. 4, p. 510)*

391.   **(E)**   A serum iron determination would be most helpful. Iron stores in thalassemia are greatly increased, as in most chronic hemolytic anemias. *(Ref. 4, p. 510)*

392.   **(A)**   An increased amount of fetal A_2 hemoglobin would be expected. As beta chains are decreased, the alpha chains combine with gamma and delta chains to make F and A_2. *(Ref. 4, p. 510)*

393.   **(C)**   The present treatment of choice is purely supportive. Care is taken to watch for anemia during intercurrent illness, due to aregenerative crises. *(Ref. 4, p. 510)*

394.   **(D)**   Hemoglobin C characteristically produces targeting in the peripheral blood. Targeting is also seen in liver disease and may represent redundant membrane. *(Ref. 4, p. 626)*

395.   **(D)**   Sideroblastic anemia is associated with an increased serum iron and ferritin. TIBC is generally normal. Hb A_2 is usually decreased. *(Ref. 2, pp. 1724–1725)*

396.   **(B)**   Beta thalassemia trait is characterized by normal iron studies and an elevated Hb A_2. *(Ref. 2, p. 1724)*

397.   **(A)**   Iron deficiency is characterized by low serum iron and ferritin and an increase in TIBC. Hb A_2 is low. *(Ref. 2, p. 1724)*

398.   **(C)**   Anemia of chronic disease is characterized by decreased serum iron and TIBC, an elevated ferritin and normal Hb A_2. *(Ref. 2, p. 1724)*

399.   **(D)**   Beta thalassemia trait is diagnosed by demonstrating an elevated HB A_2, iron deficiency by iron studies and ferritin levels, and anemia of chronic disease by demonstrating a chronic disease. Sideroblastic anemia generally

requires a bone marrow revealing ringed sidero-blasts for diagnosis. *(Ref. 2, p. 1724)*

400. (D) Acanthocytes are found in severe liver disease and might result from abnormal membrane lipids. *(Ref. 2, p. 1744)*

401. (F) Heinz bodies, precipitated hemoglobin, are found in disorders with unstable hemoglobin or after oxidant stress. *(Ref. 2, p. 1744)*

402. (A) Spherocytes are caused by loss of membrane, as in hereditary spherocytosis or autoimmune hemolytic anemia. *(Ref. 2, p. 1744)*

403. (C) Sickle cell disease results in polymerization of HbS and the characteristic sickle cells. *(Ref. 2, p. 1744)*

404. (B) Schistocytes are caused by traumatic disruption of the red cell membrane, e.g., microangiopathic syndromes. *(Ref. 2, p. 1744)*

405. (A) Von Willebrand's disease is the most common inherited bleeding disorder, occurring in up to 1 in 800 to 1,000 individuals. The von Willebrand factor facilitates platelet adhesion by linking platelet membrane receptors to vascular subendothelium and also serves as the plasma carrier for factor VIII. The rare severe form (type III) can occasionally cause hemarthrosis similar to mild hemophilia. The usual treatment, when required, is cryoprecipitate or factor VIII concentrates. However, milder forms often respond to DDAVP, a vasopressin analogue. *(Ref. 2, p. 1801)*

406. (B) Nonspecific circulating anticoagulants prolong coagulation tests by binding to phospholipids, and may be measured by their ability to bind to the complex phospholipid cardiolipin. They are associated with thromboembolic disease and spontaneous midtrimester abortions, not hemorrhage. Specific inhibitors are generally IgG antibodies to factor VIII, and are most common in multiply transfused hemophiliacs. Circulating anticoagulants are diagnosed by the failure of normal plasma to correct abnormal coagulation tests. *(Ref. 2, pp. 1808–1809)*

CHAPTER 6

Oncology
Questions

DIRECTIONS (Questions 407 through 432): Each of the questions or imcomplete statements below is followed by five suggested answers or completions. Select the ONE that is best in each case.

407. All of the following statements about the pattern of cancer occurrence in the United States are true EXCEPT

    (A) cancer is the second most common cause of death

    (B) cancer is the most common cause of death in middle-aged women

    (C) incidence rates for cancer are generally higher in men than women

    (D) colon and rectum cancers have the highest mortality rate when considering both men and women

    (E) about 75 to 80% of all cancers in the United States are due to environmental factors

408. All of the following hereditary pre-neoplastic syndromes are inherited in an autosomal dominant pattern EXCEPT

    (A) neurofibromatosis

    (B) tuberous sclerosis

    (C) ataxia–telangiectasia

    (D) von Hippel–Lindau syndrome

    (E) Peutz–Jeghers syndrome

409. Which of the following statements concerning the epidemiology of hepatitis B virus (HBV), and hepatocellular carcinoma (HCC) is correct?

    (A) previous HBV infection dramatically increases the risk of hepatocellular carcinoma

    (B) HCC only occurs in the setting of cirrhosis

    (C) age of infection is not relevant to likelihood of HCC

    (D) cirrhosis and HCC are the most common causes of death for those with HB_sAg chronic carrier state in Taiwan

    (E) the chronic carrier state of HB_sAg increases the relative risk of HCC by 10-fold in endemic areas such as Taiwan

410. Which of the following statements concerning ionizing radiation and malignancy is correct?

    (A) malignancies occur within ten years of exposure

    (B) leukemia has the shortest latency period of all malignancies

    (C) large exposure is required to develop the most serious malignancies

    (D) risk increases with advancing age at time of exposure

    (E) therapeutic radiation therapy given without chemotherapy does not increase the risk of a second malignancy

411. Appropriate cancer screening for a 25-year-old woman would include

    (A) mammography every five years

    (B) Pap smear at least every three years

    (C) stool for occult blood

    (D) chest x-ray every three years

    (E) physical examination of the breast by a physician

412. A 25-year-old woman presents with intermittent double vision. A CXR reveals an anterior mediastinal mass. Further evaluation will include

    (A) measurement of serum calcium

    (B) MRI scan of the brain

    (C) evaluation of T cell function

    (D) measurement of serum gamma globulins

    (E) assessment of glucose tolerance

413. A 40-year-old nonsmoking woman with a history of moderate alcohol use presents with a four-month history of weight loss and dysphagia. An important finding on physical examination related to this presentation would be

    (A) pigmentation of the lips

    (B) telangiectasia of oropharynx

    (C) lichen planus

    (D) hyperkeratosis of palms

    (E) psoriasis vulgaris

414. All the following statements concerning Barrett's esophagus are correct EXCEPT

(A) it is a major risk factor for squamous cell cancer of the esophagus

(B) it can be found in up to 20% of patients undergoing esophagoscopy for esophagitis

(C) the histological changes include development of a columnar cell-lined esophagus

(D) medical control of reflux will not affect likelihood of malignant changes

(E) up to half of patients with Barrett's esophagus may develop malignancy

415. Which of the following is a risk factor for carcinoma of the stomach?

(A) high fat diet

(B) high socioeconomic status

(C) high protein diet

(D) high alcohol consumption

(E) low dietary vitamin A

416. Methotrexate exerts its antitumor effect by

(A) preventing absorption of folic acid

(B) inhibiting dihydrofolate reductase

(C) preventing formation of messenger RNA

(D) forming a cytotoxic metabolite

(E) preventing proper functioning of membrane ATPase

417. Which of the following statements concerning cancer of the pancreas is correct?

(A) tumors of the pancreas are divided almost equally between those arising from the exocrine portion and those arising from the endocrine portion

(B) most endocrine tumors of the pancreas are malignant

(C) the body of the pancreas is the most common site of malignancy

(D) ductal adenocarcinoma is the most common pancreatic cancer

(E) extension is through local invasion; metastases are a late manifestation

418. Which of the following statements concerning physical examination of a patient with suspected hepatocellular carcinoma (HCC) is correct?

(A) hepatomegaly is rarely present

(B) the majority have hepatic bruits

(C) ascites is usually caused by malignant peritoneal spread

(D) Virchow nodes in the supraclavicular region are as common as with gastric cancer

(E) acute splenomegaly is usually caused by the tumor

419. All of the following statements concerning cancer of the biliary system are correct EXCEPT

(A) liver flukes are the most common predisposing factor for biliary cancer

(B) it is rare in patients with ulcerative colitis

(C) peripheral (intrahepatic) cholangiocarcinomas have the highest frequency of jaundice

(D) hepatolithiasis is a predisposing factor

(E) a third of cases of sclerosing cholangitis may have cholangiocarcinoma as well

420. Which of the following statements concerning small bowel tumors is correct?

(A) carcinoid tumors frequently present with flushing, watery diarrhea, and asthma

(B) malignant adenocarcinoma most frequently occur in the duodenum

(C) malignant tumors bleed more frequently than benign tumors

(D) Peutz–Jeghers syndrome is characterized only by benign hamartoma

(E) most primary gastrointestinal lymphomas are located in the ileum

421. Which of the following factors improves the prognosis for carcinoma of the colon?

(A) age under 40

(B) male gender

(C) rectal bleeding

(D) small tumor size

(E) location in the rectum

422. Which of the following statements is correct for both carcinoma of the uterine cervix and carcinoma of the uterine endometrium?

(A) associated with diabetes mellitus and obesity

(B) most common in middle age

(C) associated with nulliparity

(D) common in Jews and Muslims

(E) associated with herpes virus type 2 (HSV-2) infection

423. The risk of breast cancer is increased by

(A) early onset of menopause

(B) early onset of menarche

(C) late-life radiation exposure

(D) multiparity

(E) early full-term pregnancy

424. All of the following statements provide a rationale for systemic adjuvant therapy in breast cancer EXCEPT

(A) size of the local tumor at presentation does not correlate with "cure" rate

(B) there is no orderly pattern of tumor cell dissemination

(C) a clinically detectable breast cancer is already advanced (about 30 doublings) and has had ample opportunity to establish distant micrometastases

(D) tumor growth fraction is inversely related to population size

(E) the optimal kinetic conditions to achieve cure exist if microscopic foci of disease are present after curative surgery and/or radiation therapy

425. The following statements about malignant pleural mesothelioma are all true EXCEPT

(A) up to half of the cases have no known asbestos exposure

(B) most have bilateral involvement at the time of diagnosis

(C) pleural plaques or interstitial fibrosis are apparent in only 20% of plain radiographs

(D) pain is a frequent presenting symptom

(E) therapeutic irradiation can be a predisposing factor

426. Which of the following statements about sarcomas of bone is correct?

(A) most dissemination is blood-borne

(B) lung metastases are a late sign

(C) local lymph node involvement is very common

(D) articular cartilage is a common plane for tumor spread

(E) skip metastases within the same bone are common and unrelated to prognosis

427. All of the following concerning the epidemiology and natural history of malignant melanoma are true EXCEPT

(A) the incidence and mortality in white populations are rising throughout the world

(B) there is a shift in the United States to less localized disease on presentation, resulting in a higher mortality

(C) most melanomas occur in relatively young persons who have not had years of constant exposure to sunlight

(D) for most cases lymph node involvement is not the most important prognostic factor

(E) incidence rates are higher in persons residing closer to the equator

428. The following statements concerning staging of Hodgkin's disease are all true EXCEPT

(A) over half of patients have advanced (III or IV) disease after all staging procedures

(B) B symptoms occur in about one quarter of those with Hodgkin's disease

(C) if B symptoms are present, chemotherapy, with or without radiation therapy, is a mandatory part of treatment

(D) lymphocyte predominant and nodular sclerosing forms of Hodgkin's disease are more commonly diagnosed in stages I and II

(E) increasing use of effective chemotherapy regimes has meant that staging laparotomy is less commonly performed

429. Which of the following statements comparing Hodgkin's disease and lymphocytic lymphoma is correct?

(A) lymphocytic lymphoma is more likely to be localized than Hodgkin's disease at time of diagnosis

(B) involvement of Waldeyer's ring and epitrochlear nodes is similar in both conditions

(C) the spleen is more frequently involved in Hodgkin's disease

(D) both spread by hematogenous and noncontiguous nodal spread

(E) marrow involvement is common in both diseases

430. A 68-year-old man presents with left axillary adenopathy that on biopsy reveals a low-grade lymphocytic lymphoma. Which of the following statements is correct?

(A) staging in this type of disorder is not relevant

(B) if disease is widespread, early aggressive chemotherapy will result in an improved prognosis for survival

(C) the disease is likely to be widespread at time of diagnosis

(D) untreated, the prognosis is measured in months

(E) his age is not a relevant factor in treatment

431. All of the following statements concerning aggressive lymphocytic lymphoma are true EXCEPT

    (A) untreated, survival is measured in months
    (B) localized disease is effectively treated with radiation therapy.
    (C) cure is more likely than with low-grade (indolent) lymphomas
    (D) surgical treatment of gastric lymphoma alone is inadequate
    (E) elderly patients should be treated similarly to younger patients

432. All the following statements concerning cutaneous lymphomas are true EXCEPT

    (A) they can be associated with leukemic cells
    (B) are of T cell origin
    (C) have a geographic distribution
    (D) have a high cure rate
    (E) can be related to viral infection

DIRECTIONS (Questions 433 through 465): The group of questions below consists of a list of lettered headings followed by a list of numbered words, phrases, or statements. For each numbered word, phrase, or statement, select the ONE lettered heading that is most closely associated with it. Each lettered heading may be selected once, more than once, or not at all.

Questions 433 through 439

    (A) Hispanic Americans
    (B) White Americans
    (C) Black Americans
    (D) Native Americans
    (E) Chinese Americans
    (F) Japanese Americans
    (G) Filipino Americans

433. Have the lowest cancer rates for both sexes

434. Have very high rates of melanoma

435. Have the highest rates for breast, corpus uteri, and ovarian cancer

436. Have especially high rates for cervix cancer

437. Have elevated rates for nasopharynx and liver cancer

438. Have high rates for stomach cancer

439. Have high cancer rates at least partially due to socioeconomic factors

Questions 440 through 444

    (A) aflatoxin
    (B) alcoholic beverages
    (C) alkylating agents
    (D) anabolic steroids
    (E) arsenic
    (F) asbestos
    (G) benzene
    (H) chewing tobacco
    (I) tobacco smoke
    (J) ultraviolet radiation
    (K) virus, Epstein–Barr
    (L) virus, hepatitis B
    (M) virus, human papillomavirus
    (N) vinyl chloride

440. Associated with cancer of the mouth and liver

441. Increases risk of lung cancer two-fold and cancer of peritoneum 100-fold

442. Can cause different cancers, some secondary to intermittent severe exposure, others due to cumulative dose

443. Is linked to cancer of the cervix, vulva, and penis

444. Is linked to cancer even with indirect exposure

Questions 445 through 449

    (A) cancer metastatic to the lung
    (B) squamous cell cancer of the lung
    (C) adenocarcinoma of the lung
    (D) small cell cancer of the lung
    (E) large cell cancer of the lung

445. The most common type of lung cancer in the United States

446. Has the best prognosis of all malignant lung cancers

447. Likeliest to cause nonmetastatic hypercalcemia

448. Associated with syndrome of inappropriate antidiuretic hormone (SIADH)

449. Associated with myasthenic syndrome (Eaton–Lambert syndrome)

Questions 450 through 454

(A) methotrexate

(B) cytarabine

(C) 5-Fluorouracil

(D) bleomycin

(E) doxorubicin

(F) mithramycin

(G) cisplatin

(H) busulfan

(I) cyclophosphamide

(J) vincristine

450. Can cause profound hypocalcemia

451. Can cause hepatic fibrosis

452. Can cause erythema, induration, thickening, and eventual peeling of the skin on the fingers, palms, and extremity joints.

453. Can cause acute cardiac failure

454. Frequently causes hemorrhagic cystitis

Questions 455 through 457

(A) anaplastic thyroid cancer

(B) follicular cancer of the thyroid

(C) lymphoma of the thyroid

(D) papillary cancer of the thyroid

(E) medullary thyroid cancer

455. Has the best prognosis of all thyroid malignancies

456. Is more common in areas of iodine deficiency

457. Is associated with the most specific marker available in clinical oncology

Questions 458 through 461

(A) lymphocyte predominant Hodgkin's disease

(B) nodular sclerosing Hodgkin's disease

(C) mixed cellularity Hodgkin's disease

(D) lymphocyte depleted Hodgkin's disease, reticular type

(E) lymphocyte depleted Hodgkin's disease, diffuse fibrosis type

(F) all variants of Hodgkin's disease

458. The only form of Hodgkin's disease more common in women

459. Reed–Sternberg cells can be difficult to locate in this variant

460. This variant has a particularly good outcome

461. Can be accompanied by a non-necrotizing epithelioid granulomatous reaction

Questions 462 through 465: The following questions refer to the relief of pain in patients with metastatic cancer.

(A) nonsteroidal anti-inflammatory drugs (NSAIDs)

(B) opioids

(C) amphetamines

(D) anticonvulsants

(E) phenothiazines

(F) butyrophenones

(G) steroids

462. This group of medications is particularly useful for pain from bony metastases

463. Leukopenia and thrombocytopenia can limit the use of the most widely used drug in this category

464. Can be particularly useful for headaches

465. Can be useful in controlling opioid-induced sedation

DIRECTIONS (Questions 466 through 469): This section consists of clinical situations, each followed by a question or a series of questions. Study each situation, and select the ONE best answer to each question following it.

Question 466: A 65-year-old man with a 45 pack/year history of smoking presents with hematuria. His hemoglobin is 18.5 gm and his liver enzymes are twice normal. He has lost 15 pounds in weight. Which of the following statements is correct?

(A) his hemoglobin level represents stress polycythemia

(B) the elevated hemoglobin indicates a poor prognosis

(C) his tumor is nonresectable

(D) a chest x-ray is a useful test

(E) a palpable abdominal mass is very unlikely

Question 467: A 53-year-old woman presents with a 0.5-cm invasive carcinoma of the breast detected on mammography. The appropriate local therapy for the tumor would be

    (A) simple mastectomy with axillary dissection

    (B) radiation therapy to breast and axilla

    (C) local excision plus radiation therapy

    (D) local excision and axillary dissection followed by radiation therapy

    (E) local excision and axillary sampling

Question 468: An asymptomatic 74-year-old gentleman has a high ESR noted on routine blood work done with a yearly physical examination. A follow-up protein electrophoresis reveals a monoclonal IgG spike. All of the following will help differentiate a monoclonal gammopathy of unknown significance (MGUS) from multiple myeloma EXCEPT

    (A) M-component level of 7 g/dL

    (B) absence of bone lesions

    (C) Bence Jones (BJ) protein < 1.0 g/24 hour

    (D) bone marrow plasma cells less then 10%

    (E) normal hemoglobin level

Question 469: A 68-year-old woman presents to her attending physician feeling unwell and having lost 10 pounds in weight. Physical examination reveals left axillary lymphadenopathy. Biopsy reveals well-differentiated adenocarcinoma. Liver scan and bone scan suggest widespread metastases. Which statement concerning her further management is correct?

    (A) the response rate for metastatic adenocarcinoma (well-differentiated) of unknown primary site is so poor that no investigation or treatment is indicated

    (B) the pancreas is a common site for origin of this tumor

    (C) extensive work-up, including colonoscopy, abdominal CAT scan, and mammography will define subsets which benefit from treatment

    (D) special studies of the excised lymph node are not useful in determining the site of origin

    (E) metastatic breast cancer is the most common cause of adenocarcinoma of unknown primary site in women

Oncology

Answers and Explanations

407. **(D)** Lung cancer is still number one in mortality when both sexes are considered. Although number two behind CVS mortality, among women 35 to 74, cancer is the leading cause of death. Only breast, gallbladder, and thyroid cancers are more common in women than men. The environmental contribution to cancer is calculated by comparing US rates of specific cancers to the rates for the country with the lowest risk. *(Ref. 10, p. 154)*

408. **(C)** Ataxia–telangiectasia is inherited in an autosomal recessive manner. It is associated with nonHodgkin's lymphoma, acute lymphocytic leukemia, and stomach cancer. *(Ref. 10, p. 178)*

409. **(D)** Only the chronic carrier state increases HCC risk, not previous infection. The majority, but not all, of HCC associated with HBV occurs in the setting of cirrhosis (60 to 90%). Because the latency period is 35 years of HBV infection before HCC supervenes, early life infection is strongly correlated with HCC. The chronic carrier state of HB_sAg in endemic areas such as Taiwan is associated with a relative risk of 217 for the development of HCC. Over half the chronic carriers of HB_sAg in such a population will die of cirrhosis or HCC. *(Ref. 10, p. 187)*

410. **(B)** Radiation-induced malignancies tend to occur at the age where that particular malignancy would normally occur. Therefore the latency period can be forty years or more. The latency period tends to be shortest (5 to 7 years) for leukemia. The risk for most malignancies is greatest with early-life radiation, and evidence suggests that therapeutic radiation confers excess risk as well. The amount of exposure determines the likelihood of developing malignancy, not its severity. *(Ref. 10, pp. 215–218)*

411. **(B)** There is universal agreement on the need for regular Pap smears in young women. There is no need to screen for colon cancer (fecal occult blood) or lung tumors (CXR). Mammography, if indicated for screening, would only be for older women. More authorities recommend breast self-examination rather than physical examination by a physician. *(Ref. 10, p. 565)*

412. **(D)** An anterior mediastinal mass with ocular muscular weakness suggests the association of a thymoma with myasthenia gravis. About 5 to 10% of patients with thymoma will also have hypogammaglobulinemia. *(Ref. 10, p. 767)*

413. **(D)** The history of weight loss and dysphagia suggests carcinoma of the esophagus, a disease most common in older men who drink and smoke heavily. Tylosis, a disease characterized by hyperkeratosis of the palms and soles and papillomata of the esophagus is inherited in an autosomal-dominant manner. Affected individuals have a high likelihood of developing squamous cell cancer of the esophagus. *(Ref. 10, pp. 776, 780)*

414. **(A)** Barrett's esophagus, characterized by a columnar cell-lined esophageal mucosa, is a major risk factor for adenocarcinoma of the esophagus. Although acid reflux may be a predisposing factor, there is no evidence that either medical or surgical antireflux measures alter the outcome. *(Ref. 10, pp. 793–794)*

415. **(E)** Low dietary vitamin A and C, low fat and protein consumption, and low socioeconomic status predispose to gastric cancer, as do ingestion of nitrates and smoked foods. Smoking is a risk factor, but alcohol is not. *(Ref. 10, p. 820)*

416. **(B)** The likeliest mode of action of methotrexate is by tightly binding dihydrofolate reductase (DHFR). DHFR maintains the intracellular folate pool in its fully reduced form as tetrahydrofolates. These compounds are required in the de novo synthesis of pyrimidines and purines. *(Ref. 10, pp. 358–359)*

417. (D) Ductal adenocarcinoma comprises 80% of all cancers of the pancreas. The proximal pancreas is the most common site, with only 20% occurring in the body and 5 to 10% in the tail. About 95% of the tumors arise from the exocrine portion of the gland, and these are usually malignant. Most of the endocrine tumors are benign. Early development of metastases are characteristic of pancreatic adenocarcinoma. *(Ref. 10, pp. 851–852)*

418. (E) Chronic splenomegaly and ascites in patients with HCC is usually due to the underlying liver disease. Acute splenomegaly may be due to portal vein occlusion by the tumor. Virchow nodes are extremely rare in HCC, but have been reported. The majority have hepatomegaly (50 to 90%), but less than a quarter have an abdominal bruit. *(Ref. 10, pp. 894–895)*

419. (C) Hilar tumors (Klatskin tumors) are almost three times more likely to cause jaundice than intrahepatic tumors. Liver flukes such as *Clonorchis sinensis* are the most common predisposing factors world-wide. Up to 10% of people with liver stones may develop biliary cancer, but it is much rarer in those with ulcerative colitis (less than 1%). At autopsy of patients with sclerosing cholangitis, 33 to 42% have cholangiocarcinoma as well. *(Ref. 10, p. 900)*

420. (B) Adenocarcinoma, the most common malignancy of the small bowel is most common proximally, particularly in the duodenum. Small bowel lymphomas are most common in the ileum, but the stomach is the most common site of gastrointestinal lymphoma. Carcinoids usually present with local symptoms. Carcinoid syndrome is present only with hepatic metastases. Benign tumors bleed more frequently than malignant ones. Malignant adenocarcinomas can occur in Peutz–Jeghers syndrome. *(Ref. 10, pp. 917–923)*

421. (C) Rectal bleeding is a good prognostic sign, perhaps because surface erosion manifests early. Young age, male gender, and location in the rectum all indicate a poorer prognosis. Unlike most tumors, no correlation with tumor size and prognosis has been established for colon cancer. *(Ref. 10, pp. 940–942)*

422. (B) The peak age for carcinoma of the cervix is between 48 to 55 years. For endometrial cancer the peak is from ages 55 to 60. Endometrial cancer is associated with nulliparity, diabetes mellitus, and obesity. Cervical cancer is associated with HSV-2 infections, and is less common in Jews and Muslims, perhaps because of circumcision among male partners. *(Ref. 10, pp. 1168–1169, 1195–1196)*

423. (B) Breast cancer risk is reduced by 20% for each year that menarche is delayed. Early menopause, natural or surgical, also decreases risk. Early (age 18 or 19) full-term pregnancy and multiparity decrease the risk. Radiation exposure is a risk factor primarily in adolescence, and is marginal after the age of 40. *(Ref. 10, pp. 1266–1267)*

424. (A) Clinical evidence and experiments with tumor transplantation in mice suggest that the volume of the initial tumor is an important prognostic factor. Thus, in tumors of similar biological nature a larger volume suggests greater likelihood of metastatic disease. *(Ref. 10, pp. 1301–1302)*

425. (B) Only 5% have bilateral involvement at the time of presentation. In 30 to 50%, no history of asbestos exposure is apparent. Among the other postulated causes are therapeutic irradiation. The most common presenting symptoms are dyspnea and nonpleuritic chest pain. *(Ref. 10, p. 1491)*

426. (A) Bones lack a lymphatic system, and most dissemination is blood-borne. As a result, lung metastases are an early sign of hematogenous spread. Lymph nodes are uncommonly involved, and indicate a poor prognosis. Articular cartilage is thought to be a natural barrier to direct articular extension by tumor. Skip metastases, tumor nodules in the same bone, but not in continuity with the main tumor, are rare (< 1%) and connote a poor prognosis. *(Ref. 10, p. 1513)*

427. (B) There has been a steady increase to presentation with localized disease (81% by 1990) in the United States. As a result, thickness of the tumor is the most important prognostic factor in the majority of cases. The increasing mortality in the United States is caused by the increasing incidence of disease. Although cumulative sun exposure is a major factor in melanoma (e.g., more frequent near the equator) it cannot explain such things as the more common occurrence of some types in relatively young people. It is possible that brief, intense exposure to sunlight may contribute to or initiate carcinogenic events. *(Ref. 10, p. 1616)*

428. (C) Stage IB Hodgkin's disease is effectively treated with radiation therapy alone. Some reports suggest that stage IIB can be similarly treated. Although physical exam and CXR will initially suggest that 90% of patients with Hodgkin's disease have localized disease, by the end of staging, 60% will be stage III or IV. The purpose of staging laparotomy is to determine whether radiation alone will be used for treatment. As chemotherapy usage increases, the necessity for staging laparotomy decreases. *(Ref. 10, pp. 1826–1831)*

429. **(C)** The spleen is commonly involved in Hodgkin's disease but not lymphocytic lymphoma. Hodgkin's disease is more likely to be localized and spreads via contiguous nodes, not by the hematogenous or noncontiguous nodal spread characteristic of lymphocytic lymphoma. Marrow, CNS, and other non-nodal sites are more commonly involved in lymphocytic lymphoma. As well, Waldeyer's ring and epitrochlear nodes, occasionally involved in lymphocytic lymphoma, are almost never involved in Hodgkin's disease. *(Ref. 10, p. 1882)*

430. **(C)** About 85% of low-grade lymphocytic lymphomas are widespread at the time of diagnosis. However, staging is still important as radiation therapy can be curative for localized (stage I, II) disease. Because the prognosis for this malignancy is measured in years, it has been difficult to demonstrate a survival benefit for aggressive chemotherapy. The poor prognosis for lymphoma in older patients might be a result of less aggressive therapy. *(Ref. 10, pp. 1892–1899)*

431. **(B)** Even if disease seems to be localized, systemic chemotherapy is always required in aggressive lymphocytic lymphomas. Although untreated survival is dismal, the chances of a cure with current chemotherapy are about 60%, much better than in low-grade lymphomas. The poor prognosis of elderly patients might be secondary to lower doses of chemotherapy. Treatment should be based on toxicities actually experienced rather than making excessive anticipatory dose reductions for the elderly. *(Ref. 10, pp. 1904–1913)*

432. **(D)** Cutaneous lymphomas are of T-cell origin and are more common in other parts of the world, such as Japan. Patients with adult T-cell lymphoma–leukemia (ATLL), have acute fulminant courses characterized by skin invasion and leukemic cells. This syndrome is clearly related to human T-cell lymphotropic virus-1 (HTLV-1) and there is a possibility that HTLV-5 might be the agent for mycosis fungoides and the Sezary syndrome. ATLL responds poorly to treatment, and therapy for the low-grade malignancies controls symptoms but does not result in cure. *(Ref. 10, pp. 1928–1934)*

433. **(D)** Native Americans of both sexes have low cancer rates, but cancer rates (for women) for stomach, biliary tract, cervix, and kidney are surprisingly high. *(Ref. 10, pp. 162–164)*

434. **(B)** Whites have high rates for melanoma, lymphoma, leukemia, and lip cancer. *(Ref. 10, p. 162)*

435. **(B)** Whites have high cancer rates for breast, corpus uteri, testis, bladder, brain, colon, and rectum. *(Ref. 10, p. 162)*

436. **(A)** Although Hispanic Americans have relatively low cancer rates (66% of that for White Americans and 54% of that for Black Americans), they do have high rates for cancer of the cervix. *(Ref. 10, pp. 162–163)*

437. **(E)** Chinese Americans have a rate of nasopharyngeal cancer 23 times greater than White Americans and liver cancer rates 7 times greater than White Americans. *(Ref. 10, pp. 162–163)*

438. **(F)** Japanese Americans have a three-fold increase in stomach cancer rate compared to White Americans, but this is lower than rates in Japan. *(Ref. 10, pp. 155, 162–164)*

439. **(C)** The excess risk of cancers of the stomach, esophagus, lung, and cervix among Black Americans is diminished when socioeconomic variations are factored in. *(Ref. 10, p. 165)*

440. **(B)** Alcoholic beverages combine with tobacco smoking to increase cancer of the mouth, and by causing cirrhosis can lead to liver cancer. *(Ref. 10, p. 170)*

441. **(F)** Asbestos exposure causes more deaths from lung cancer (two-fold increase) than from mesothelioma (100-fold increase) because the latter tumor is so rare. *(Ref. 10, p. 172)*

442. **(J)** Sun exposure severe enough to cause sunburn is associated with increased risk of melanoma, whereas other skin cancers are more related to cumulative exposure. *(Ref. 10, p. 173)*

443. **(M)** Although causation is not definite, a high proportion of cervical cancers reveal HPV-16 and HPV-18 on biopsy. HPV has also been isolated from vulvar, penile, and anal cancers. *(Ref. 10, p. 176)*

444. **(I)** Tobacco smoke constituents and metabolites can be detected in the body fluids of exposed nonsmokers. Evidence suggests that nonsmoking women married to smokers have a 30% excess risk for lung cancer. *(Ref. 10, p. 170)*

445. **(C)** Adenocarcinoma is now the most common form of lung cancer, accounting for 40% of the total cases. *(Ref. 10, p. 677)*

446. (B) Because of its tendency for early exfoliation and obstruction, squamous cell cancer is often detected at an earlier stage. Even correcting for this, there is some suggestion that its prognosis is still better, perhaps because of its slow growth rate. *(Ref. 10, p. 677)*

447. (B) Nonmetastatic hypercalcemia occurs in up to 15% of all squamous cell cancers. *(Ref. 10, p. 2029)*

448. (D) SIADH occurs in up to 9% of all small cell cancers of the lung. *(Ref. 10, p. 2029)*

449. (D) Eaton–Lambert syndrome is unusual, but can occur in up to 6% of small cell lung cancer. *(Ref. 10, p. 2046)*

450. (F) Mithramycin is often used therapeutically for malignant hypercalcemia. In higher antitumor doses it is too toxic for routine use. *(Ref. 10, p. 383)*

451. (A) Liver toxicity is most common when methotrexate is used on a daily basis, such as for psoriasis. Myelosuppression and GI mucositis are the most common side effects in cancer therapy. *(Ref 10, p. 361)*

452. (D) Although lung injury is the most serious complication of bleomycin, this unusual skin reaction is more frequent, occurring in almost 50% of patients. *(Ref. 10, p. 376)*

453. (E) Doxorubicin can cause a cumulative, dose-dependent cardiomyopathy that can result in congestive heart failure. However an acute, non-dose-related, myocarditis–pericarditis, can also occur. It can cause arrhythmias, heart failure, or pericardial effusions. *(Ref. 10, p. 379)*

454. (I) Cyclophosphamide causes hemorrhagic cystitis in up to 10% of patients because active metabolites are excreted. Adequate hydration and frequent urination can decrease the frequency of this complication. *(Ref. 10, p. 404)*

455. (D) Papillary cancer has the best prognosis of all thyroid cancers. Although it is seven times more common than follicular cancer, fewer people die from it. In common with other thyroid cancers, age seems to be an independent risk factor for poor prognosis. *(Ref. 10, pp. 1333–1335)*

456. (B) Follicular cancer is more common in areas of iodine deficiency such as Switzerland, perhaps related to the prolonged stimulatory effect of TSH. In contrast, papillary carcinoma is more common in areas with a high-iodine diet (Swe-

den) or areas with iodination of salt (United States). *(Ref. 10, pp. 1337–1338)*

457. (E) Serum calcitonin elevation is specific for medullary thyroid cancer and is the most specific tumor marker now available. When combined with provocative agents (e.g., calcium, pentagrastin) it is also the most sensitive tumor marker available. *(Ref. 10, p. 1339)*

458. (B) Nodular sclerosing Hodgkin's disease is more common in women, and is particularly common in younger age groups. *(Ref. 10, p. 1822)*

459. (A) In lymphocyte predominant Hodgkin's disease multiple sections often have to be examined to find Reed–Sternberg cells. Some authorities question whether such cells are necessary for diagnosis of this form. *(Ref. 10, p. 1821)*

460. (A) Most patients with lymphocyte predominant Hodgkin's disease have clinically localized disease and are asymptomatic; the prognosis is usually favorable. *(Ref. 10, p. 1821)*

461. (F) This is a frequent accompaniment of Hodgkin's disease and can be found in involved lymph nodes and may be extensive enough to obscure the presence of Hodgkin's disease. Rather than evidence of occult involvement, the presence of granulomas implies, stage for stage, a better prognosis than those without this reaction. *(Ref. 10, p. 1823)*

462. (A) Prostaglandins play a role in bone resorption in metastatic disease, perhaps explaining the effectiveness of NSAIDs for this type of pain. Aspirin has been shown to have an antitumor effect in an animal bone tumor model. *(Ref. 10, p. 2428)*

463. (D) Carbamazepine is an anticonvulsant used widely as an adjuvant analgesic for neuralgic pain caused by either tumor infiltration or surgical nerve injury. Because cancer patients commonly have compromised hematologic reserve, the leukopenia and thrombocytopenia caused by carbamazepine may limit its use. *(Ref. 10, p. 2435)*

464. (G) Steroids are useful for controlling pain in patients with leptomeningeal metastases or headache from increased intracranial pressure. *(Ref. 10, p. 2436)*

465. (C) Usually sedation can be controlled by altering opioid dosage, or switching to a drug with a shorter half-life, as well as stopping other sedating medications. If this fails, amphetamine, methylphenidate, and caffeine can be used to counteract the sedative effect. *(Ref. 10, p. 2433)*

466. **(D)** The age, history of smoking, and polycythemia in a patient with hematuria strongly suggests a renal cell carcinoma. The elevated hemoglobin represents increased erythropoietin production and is not related to prognosis. Elevated liver enzymes and weight loss can represent nonmetastatic effects of malignancy and can reverse with resection. Almost half of patients will have a palpable abdominal mass on presentation. The chest x-ray is a useful test as three-quarters of those with metastatic disease will have lung metastases. *(Ref. 10, p. 1026)*

467. **(D)** Breast-conserving surgery is now recommended for small tumors. Radiation therapy will decrease local recurrence rates. For tumors less than 1 cm, adjuvant therapy is indicated only if axillary nodes are positive. Therefore in this case an axillary dissection will provide important therapeutic information. *(Ref. 10, pp. 1283–1287)*

468. **(A)** IgG spikes greater than 5g/dL strongly suggest myeloma rather than MGUS, where the spike is less than 3.5 g/dL, the marrow has fewer than 10% plasma cells, and the BJ proteinuria is less than 1.0 g/24 hours. Depressed hemoglobin levels, elevated calcium levels, progressive bone lesions, and impaired renal function suggest more advanced stages of multiple myeloma. *(Ref. 10, pp. 1994–1995)*

469. **(B)** At autopsy, lung and pancreas are the most common primaries identified (about 40%). Generally the prognosis is poor, but some subsets in whom effective treatment is available can be identified by clinical criteria with only moderate investigations. These include peritoneal carcinomatosis in women (responds to treatment for ovarian cancer), predominant skeletal metastases in men (can reflect prostatic cancer), and women with axillary lymphadenopathy (can reflect breast cancer). In the latter scenario, studies for estrogen and progesterone receptors are very useful in guiding therapy. *(Ref. 10, pp. 2074–2076)*

CHAPTER 7

Diseases of the Nervous System
Questions

DIRECTIONS (Questions 470 through 499): Each of the questions or incomplete statements below is followed by five suggested answers or completions. Select the ONE that is best in each case.

470. Alzheimer's disease (presenile dementia) is associated with

    (A) atrophy of the frontal and temporal poles
    (B) atrophy of the entire frontal and temporal lobes
    (C) cranial nerve palsies
    (D) transient episodes of hemiplegia
    (E) hemianesthesia

471. Chronic progressive chorea (Huntington's) is characterized by all of the following EXCEPT

    (A) hereditary disorder
    (B) childhood onset
    (C) mental deterioration
    (D) atrophy of the cortex
    (E) enlargement of the ventricles on pneumoencephalogram

472. Migraine headaches may be associated with all of the following focal neurologic signs EXCEPT

    (A) diplopia
    (B) dysphasia
    (C) paresthesia
    (D) weakness
    (E) seizure

473. The diagnosis in an infant with convulsions, chorioretinitis, and x-ray evidence of calcification of the brain is most likely to be

    (A) Tay–Sachs disease
    (B) hydrocephalus
    (C) kernicterus
    (D) toxoplasmosis
    (E) congenital neurosyphilis

474. Occlusion of the right posterior cerebral artery is most likely to cause

    (A) homonymous hemianopia
    (B) total blindness
    (C) sudden death
    (D) infarction of the right brain stem
    (E) a right-sided hemiplegia

475. In amyotrophic lateral sclerosis, one finds

    (A) a long history of remissions and exacerbations
    (B) sensory loss in the distribution of peripheral nerves
    (C) focal seizures
    (D) signs of ventral horn and lateral column involvement
    (E) cogwheel rigidity

476. Transient episodes of vertigo, slurred speech, diplopia, and paresthesias suggest

    (A) basilar artery insufficiency
    (B) anterior communicating artery aneurysm
    (C) hypertensive encephalopathy
    (D) pseudobulbar palsy
    (E) occlusion of the middle cerebral artery

477. A right homonymous hemianopia is due to a lesion of the

    (A) right optic nerve
    (B) chiasm
    (C) right optic radiations
    (D) right occipital lobe
    (E) left optic radiations

478. Café-au-lait spots are seen in association with

(A) atrophy of the proximal musculature

(B) optic atrophy

(C) multiple subcutaneous nodules

(D) congenital nystagmus

(E) mental retardation

479. A lesion of the oculomotor nerve can result in

(A) paralysis of the lateral gaze

(B) ptosis of the eyelid

(C) widening of the palpebral fissure

(D) inability to turn the eye downward and outward

(E) deviation of the eye inward

480. Injury to the ulnar nerve results in

(A) atrophy of the muscles of the thenar eminence

(B) wrist drop

(C) inability to oppose the thumb

(D) sensory loss of the palmar surface of the thumb, index, and middle fingers

(E) impaired adduction and abduction of the fingers

481. The syndrome of familial periodic paralysis may be associated with all of the following EXCEPT

(A) hyperkalemia

(B) hypokalemia

(C) normokalemia

(D) hypercalcemia

(E) epinephrine sensitivity

482. The combination of polyneuritis and confusion, disorientation, loss of memory, and tendency to confabulate is most likely due to

(A) pernicious anemia

(B) alcoholism

(C) cerebrovascular disease of the carotid system

(D) Charcot–Marie–Tooth disease

(E) dermatomyositis

483. Signs and symptoms of involvement of the peripheral nerves in the form of pains, paresthesias, motor weakness, and reflex loss develop in a fairly large percentage of patients with

(A) heart disease

(B) dermatomyositis

(C) hypothyroidism

(D) diabetes mellitus

(E) adrenal insufficiency

484. A subdural hematoma

(A) is practically always of venous origin

(B) is rarely seen in infancy

(C) is due to injury to the middle meningeal artery

(D) is always chronic

(E) does not usually occur in the absence of trauma

485. An acoustic neuroma is most likely to lead to a palsy of the

(A) fourth cranial nerve

(B) sixth cranial nerve

(C) eighth cranial nerve

(D) tenth cranial nerve

(E) eleventh cranial nerve

486. Figure 7.1 (a) shows a plaque of demyelination in the optic nerve as compared to a normal sample in Figure 7.1 (b). What is the most likely cause of this phenomenon?

(A) diabetic microvascular disease

(B) arteriosclerosis

(C) trauma

(D) multiple sclerosis

(E) Creutzfeldt–Jakob disease

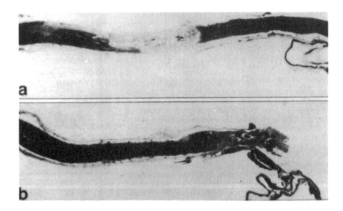

Figure 7.1

487. The LEAST common presenting symptom in the disease illustrated above is

(A) leg weakness

(B) paresthesias

(C) visual loss

(D) sphincter impairment

(E) incoordination

488. In tuberous sclerosis, all of the following may be found EXCEPT

(A) facial nevi

(B) mental retardation

(C) renal tumors

(D) pituitary atrophy

(E) convulsions

489. Muscular wasting and/or atrophy can commonly occur in all of the following EXCEPT

(A) syringomyelia

(B) vincristine neuropathy

(C) Cushing syndrome

(D) amyotrophic lateral sclerosis

(E) myasthenia gravis

490. A patient complaining of persistent drowsiness associated with narcolepsy will show all of the following specific signs EXCEPT

(A) automatic behavior

(B) cataplexy

(C) hypnagogic hallucinations

(D) parasthesias

(E) sleep paralysis

491. Tremors are seen in

(A) hypopituitarism

(B) marijuana use

(C) hyperthyroidism

(D) myxedema

(E) iron overdose

492. The pathologic changes in Friedreich's ataxia are found in the

(A) spinal cord tracts

(B) basal ganglia

(C) cerebral cortex

(D) peripheral autonomic nerves

(E) peripheral motor nerves

493. In hepatolenticular degeneration (Wilson's disease), there is usually

(A) a reduction of copper excretion in the urine

(B) an increase of the serum ceruloplasmin content

(C) no renal involvement

(D) retention of normal neurologic movements

(E) a peculiar greenish-brown pigmentation of the cornea

494. Ophthalmoplegia may be found in

(A) optic atrophy

(B) ophthalmic zoster

(C) paralysis agitans

(D) Horner syndrome

(E) myasthenia gravis

495. Involvement of the optic chiasm with defects in the visual fields can occur in

(A) a pituitary adenoma

(B) a falx meningioma

(C) a craniopharyngioma

(D) an aneurysm of the internal carotid artery

(E) a glioblastoma

496. Fasciculations can be found in

(A) amyotrophic lateral sclerosis

(B) myotonic muscular dystrophy

(C) amyotonia congenita

(D) tabes dorsalis

(E) migraine

497. The cardinal features of Parkinson's disease (paralysis agitans) include

(A) constant fine tremor

(B) muscle atrophy

(C) akinesia

(D) pupillary constriction

(E) spontaneous remission

498. Hydrocephalus may result from all of the following EXCEPT

(A) aqueductal stenosis

(B) absence of the foramina of Luschka

(C) adhesions in the meningeal space in the basal cisterns

(D) agenesis of the corpus callosum

(E) glioblastoma

499. Demyelinization within the central nervous system may be a common feature in all of the following processes EXCEPT

(A) vascular lesions

(B) malignancy

(C) infectious processes

(D) nutritional deficiencies

(E) postvaccinial

500. Seizures after head injury

(A) are inevitable

(B) are more often generalized than focal

(C) always indicate a brain abscess

(D) usually occur immediately

(E) are usually on the dominant side

501. Magnetic resonance imaging (MRI) of the brain is superior to computed tomography (CT) in all of the following circumstances EXCEPT

(A) demonstrating Chiari malformation

(B) imaging demyelinating diseases (e.g., multiple sclerosis)

(C) imaging small lacunes

(D) diagnosing an acute hemorrhage

(E) searching for metastatic disease

502. Which of the following statements concerning the lateral medullary syndrome is correct?

(A) invariably caused by occlusion of the posterior–inferior cerebellar artery

(B) causes contralateral sensory impairment

(C) causes contralateral ataxia

(D) causes ipsilateral paralysis of tongue

(E) causes ipsilateral paralysis of arm and leg

503. Which of the following statements concerning hypertensive hemorrhage in the pons is correct?

(A) evolves over several hours

(B) coma can occur, but is uncommon

(C) the prognosis is relatively good

(D) pupils are small and reactive

(E) it is the most common form of hypertensive hemorrhage

504. Tropical spastic paraparesis (TSP)

(A) is ruled out by evidence of cerebellar signs

(B) is associated with a definite sensory level

(C) can be spread by sexual activity

(D) rarely involves the bladder

(E) is characterized by rapid progression once symptoms and signs develop

DIRECTIONS (Questions 505 through 508): This section consists of a clinical situation, followed by a series of questions. Study the situation, and select the ONE best answer to each question following it.

Questions 505 and 506

505. A 40-year-old woman complains of episodes of severe unilateral facial pain of a stabbing quality that is intermittent for several hours, then disappears for several days. Physical examination is entirely normal. The most likely diagnosis is

(A) trigeminal neuralgia

(B) herpes zoster

(C) acoustic neuroma

(D) Bell's palsy

(E) diabetic neuropathy

506. The most effective therapy for the condition described in the preceding case history is

(A) morphine

(B) indomethacin

(C) cimetidine

(D) carbamazepine

(E) xylocaine gel

Question 507: A 63-year-old man suddenly becomes acutely ill and has a fever of 102.4°F. There is pain in the eye and the orbits are painful to pressure. There is edema and chemosis of the conjunctivas and eyelids. The bulbs are proptosed. There is diplopia and ptosis, and the pupils are slow in reacting. The most likely diagnosis is

(A) cavernous sinus thrombosis

(B) chorioretinitis

(C) subarachnoid hemorrhage

(D) brain abscess

(E) none of these

Question 508: A 20-year-old woman presents with a history of rapid loss of vision in one eye. Examination reveals pain on movement of the eyeball. The pupillary reactions are normal, as is the appearance of the fundi. Perimetry shows a large central scotoma. The most likely diagnosis is

(A) optic atrophy

(B) papilledema

(C) retrobulbar neuritis

(D) amblyopia ex anopsia

(E) hysteria

Question 509: A 67-year-old man has episodes lasting up to five minutes, which consist of numbness of the left side of his body with impaired vision in his right eye. The most likely diagnosis is

(A) posterior cerebral artery insufficiency

(B) parietal lobe neoplasm

(C) parasagittal meningioma

(D) AV malformation

(E) internal carotid artery insufficiency

Questions 510 and 511

510. An 18-year-old man develops fever, headache, and generalized seizures. CSF shows mononuclear cell pleocytosis and increased protein. The EEG shows bilateral periodic discharges from the temporal leads and slow-wave complexes at regular intervals of 2 to 3 per second. A CT scan shows bilateral, small, low-density temporal lobe lesions. The best diagnostic procedure in this setting is

(A) angiography

(B) cerebral biopsy

(C) radionuclide scan

(D) acute viral titers

(E) CSF culture

511. The patient in the preceding case history is most likely to respond to treatment with

(A) penicillin or tetracycline

(B) chloramphenicol

(C) vidarabine or acyclovir

(D) erythromycin or tetracycline

(E) steroids

Question 512: A 24-year-old woman develops bilateral foot drop, progressing over one week to paralysis of both legs and lower trunk. There are no constitutional symptoms or signs. The CSF protein is very high. The most likely diagnosis is

(A) diabetic neuropathy

(B) alcoholic neuropathy

(C) Guillain-Barré syndrome

(D) cyanide poisoning

(E) poliomyelitis

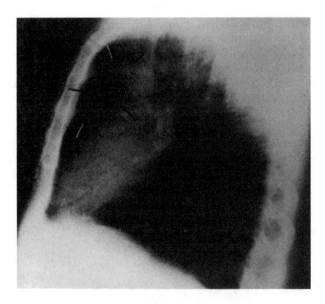

Figure 7.2

Questions 513 through 515: A 37-year-old woman complains of drooping eyelids at the end of the day. Further history reveals difficulty in chewing food and some weakness in climbing stairs. On examination, there is weakness of eyelids, masticatory muscles, and thigh flexors. There is no sensory abnormality and reflexes are normal. The chest x-ray is shown in Figure 7.2.

513. What does the chest x-ray show?

(A) bronchogenic carcinoma

(B) Hodgkin's disease

(C) teratoma

(D) thyroid tumor with retrosternal extension

(E) thymoma

514. The cause of the patient's symptoms is

(A) hypercalcemia

(B) myasthenia gravis

(C) multiple sclerosis

(D) thyroid storm

(E) meningeal lymphoma

515. All of the following treatments may be used in this patient EXCEPT

(A) adrenergic drugs

(B) surgery

(C) plasmapheresis

(D) cholinergic drugs

(E) steroids

DIRECTIONS (Questions 516 through 540): The group of questions below consists of lettered headings followed by a list of numbered phrases. For each numbered phrase, select the ONE lettered heading that is most closely associated with it. Each lettered heading may be selected once, more than once, or not at all.

Questions 516 through 520

(A) simple partial seizure

(B) complex partial seizures

(C) tonic–clonic (grand mal) seizures

(D) absence (petit mal) seizures

(E) myoclonic seizures

(F) status epilepticus

516. Seen in Creutzfeldt–Jakob disease

517. Temporal lobe most common site of origin

518. A generalized seizure without convulsive muscular activity

519. Can result in "Jacksonian march"

520. Almost always starts in childhood

Questions 521 through 525

(A) phenytoin

(B) carbamazepine

(C) phenobarbital

(D) primidone

(E) sodium valproate (valproic acid)

(F) ethosuximide

(G) clonazepam

(H) trimethadione

521. Used for absence attacks, it can cause ataxia, tremor, bone marrow suppression, and hepatotoxicity

522. Is the drug of choice for myoclonic seizures

523. Can be used for tonic–clonic (grand mal) and partial seizures and can cause gum hyperplasia and lymphadenopathy

524. Used for tonic–clonic and partial seizures, it can increase metabolism of other drugs

525. Useful in myoclonic seizures and absence attacks, but development of tolerance can limit its effectiveness

Questions 526 through 530

(A) associated with peripheral (labyrinthine) vertigo but not central (brain stem or cerebellum) vertigo

(B) associated with central vertigo but not peripheral vertigo

(C) associated with *both* central and peripheral vertigo

(D) associated with *neither* central nor peripheral vertigo

526. Tinnitus often present

527. Visual fixation inhibits symptoms

528. Symptoms chronically present

529. Pure horizontal nystagmus without torsional component

530. Can by caused by ischemia

Questions 531 through 535

(A) essential anisocoria

(B) Horner syndrome

(C) tonic pupil (Holmes–Adie syndrome)

(D) Argyll–Robertson pupil

(E) midbrain pupils

(F) atropinized pupils

(G) oculomotor palsy

531. A unilateral small, round pupil with brisk response to light and near stimuli; associated with ptosis

532. Results in the largest pupils

533. Small, irregular, bilateral; responds to near stimuli but poorly to light

534. Can be caused by a parasympathetic lesion at the ciliary ganglion

535. Commonly caused by an infection

Questions 536 through 540

    (A) anterior horn cell
    (B) peripheral nerve
    (C) neuromuscular junction
    (D) muscle

536. Reflexes are decreased out of proportion to weakness

537. Diurnal fluctuations are common

538. Atrophy is early and marked

539. Most likely to cause distal weakness

540. Characteristic facial features

Diseases of the Nervous System

Answers and Explanations

470. (B) Alzheimer's disease is associated with atrophy of the entire frontal and temporal lobes. Microscopically, there is diffuse loss of cells in all layers, secondary gliosis, and neurofibrillar degeneration. The typical senile plaques are enlarged degenerating axonal endings surrounding a core primarily composed of extracellular amyloid. *(Ref. 6, p. 637)*

471. (B) The most common onset is the appearance of abnormal movements, but it may include psychotic episodes or frank mental deterioration. Huntington's chorea is not characterized by onset in childhood. Despite being a genetic disorder (linked to a gene on short arm of chromosome 4), the typical age of onset is about 35 to 40 years of age. The range of age of onset is quite wide however. *(Ref. 6, p. 647)*

472. (E) Migraine headaches are not associated with seizure. Because migraine is a functional disorder, it is rare for the symptoms to occur in the same location at every attack. The pathophysiology of migraine is likely vasoconstriction in the pre-headache phase, with subsequent increased flow. The aura of classic migraine likely is caused by ischemia. *(Ref. 6, p. 773)*

473. (D) Toxoplasmosis is the most likely diagnosis. The infection has a predilection for the central nervous system and the eye and produces encephalitis in utero. Symptoms are usually evident in the first few days of life. Other manifestations of congenital toxoplasmosis include inanition, microcephaly, mental retardation, spasticity, and microphthalmus. *(Ref. 6, p. 171)*

474. (A) Occlusion of the right posterior cerebral artery is most likely to cause homonymous hemianopia. This artery conveys blood to the inferior and medial portion of the posterior temporal and occipital lobes and to the optic thalamus. *(Ref. 6, p. 212)*

475. (D) Signs of ventral horn and lateral column involvement are found in amyotrophic lateral sclerosis. The most severe changes are in the region of the corticospinal tract as well as in the anterior roots and the peripheral nerves. The disease is one of constant progression rather than remissions and exacerbations and death usually occurs within five years. There is no sensory loss, no seizure diathesis, as only the motor system is involved. There can be signs of hyperreflexia and spasticity depending on the balance of upper and lower motor neuron damage, but not cogwheel rigidity. *(Ref. 6, p. 683)*

476. (A) Basilar artery insufficiency is suggested by the transient episodes. The basilar artery is formed by the two vertebral arteries and supplies the pons, the midbrain, and the cerebellum. With vertebrobasilar transient ischemic attacks (TIAs), tinnitus, vertigo, diplopia, ataxia, hemiparesis, and bilateral visual impairment are common findings. *(Ref. 6, p. 226)*

477. (E) The hemianopia is due to a lesion of the left optic radiations. The posterior cerebral artery arises from the basilar artery but is sometimes a branch of the internal carotid. With posterior cerebral artery lesions affecting the occipital cortex, it is possible for the hemianopia to be an isolated finding. *(Ref. 6, p. 208)*

478. (C) Café-au-lait spots are seen in association with multiple subcutaneous nodules. Neurofibromatosis is an inherited disorder with multiple tumors of the spinal or cranial nerves, tumors of the skin, and cutaneous pigmentation. *(Ref. 6, p. 364)*

479. (B) The lesion can result in ptosis of the eyelid. There is also loss of the ability to open the eye, and the eyeball is deviated outward and slightly downward. With complete lesions, the pupil is dilated, does not react to light, and loses the power of accommodation. *(Ref. 6, p. 418)*

480. (E) Injury to the ulnar nerve results in impaired adduction and abduction of the fingers. The fibers arise from the eighth cervical and the first thoracic segments. The ulnar is a mixed nerve with sensory supply to the medial hand. *(Ref. 6, p. 431)*

481. (D) The familial periodic paralysis syndrome is usually associated with low potassium, but normal or high levels may occur. It is characterized by recurrent attacks of weakness or paralysis of the somatic musculature, with loss of the deep tendon reflexes and may be aggravated by epinephrine. *(Ref. 6, p. 720)*

482. (B) The combination of symptoms is typical of chronic alcohol abuse. The mental symptoms are suggestive of Korsakoff syndrome. A distal limb sensory-motor neuropathy is also typical of alcoholism. The confusion and disorientation are typical for acute alcohol intoxication. *(Ref. 6, pp. 901–903)*

483. (D) These signs and symptoms develop in a fairly large percentage of patients with diabetes mellitus. Loss of proprioceptive sensation together with absent reflexes superficially resembles tabes dorsalis. If sensory loss is severe, Charcot joints can develop. *(Ref. 6, p. 614)*

484. (A) A subdural hematoma is practically always of venous origin. It is almost always secondary to a minor or severe injury to the head but may occur in blood dyscrasias or cachexia in the absence of trauma. Acute subdural hematomas commonly present with a fluctuating level of consciousness and hemiplegia (spastic type). Chronic subdurals may also present with seizures or papilledema. *(Ref. 6, p. 384)*

485. (C) An acoustic neuroma is most likely to lead to a palsy of the eighth cranial nerve. Deafness, headache, ataxia, tinnitus, and diplopia are seen, as well as facial paresthesias. Acoustic neuromas represent 5% to 10% of all intracranial tumors. They develop from Schwann cells and generally grow very slowly. They may be very large before symptoms develop. *(Ref. 6, p. 288)*

486. (D) Visual loss in multiple sclerosis varies from slight blurring to no light perception. Other eye symptoms include diplopia and pain. The classic syndrome of optic or retrobulbar neuritis occurs in 50% of cases at some point in the disease, and it may be the presenting symptom. *(Ref. 6, p. 417)*

487. (D) Weakness, especially of the legs, is the major presenting symptom of multiple sclerosis. Both sphincter impairment and vertigo occur at

presentation in about 6% of the cases. When the presenting symptoms relate to cerebellar or corticospinal dysfunction, the prognosis tends to be worse than a presentation with sensory symptoms. *(Ref. 6, p. 757)*

488. (D) Tuberous sclerosis is an autosomal-dominant disease with a wide variety of clinical phenotypes. Lesions occur in the nervous system, skin, bones, retina, kidney, and elsewhere. The skin lesions include facial nevi (fibroma molluscum) and patches of skin fibrosis. Hard nodules are found throughout the brain. Seizures and mental retardation can occur. *(Ref. 6, p. 591)*

489. (E) While muscle wasting can occur in myasthenia gravis it is not a direct cause of the disease. Rather, it is not focal but diffuse, and is encountered in patients with malnutrition secondary to severe dysphagia. This nonspecific wasting occurs in about 10% of cases. The other syndromes mentioned characteristically have muscle wasting. *(Ref. 6, p. 700)*

490. (D) Hypnagogic hallucinations are almost always visual. They occur most frequently at the onset of sleep, either during the day or at night. They are generally very vivid. Cataplexy is a brief loss of muscle power without loss of consciousness. The patient is fully aware of what is going on. The paralysis may be complete or partial. A similar set of symptoms can occur when falling asleep or awakening, and is called sleep paralysis. Automatic behavior can be confused with complex partial seizures. Parasthesias are not part of the narcolepsy syndrome. *(Ref. 6, pp. 815–816)*

491. (C) In hyperthyroidism, neurologic symptoms include tremors of the hands, exophthalmos, lid lag, stare, and muscle weakness. The muscle weakness of hyperthyroidism affects the pelvic girdle and to a lesser extent, the shoulder girdle. Reflexes are normal or increased and sensation is normal. It must be differentiated from myasthenia gravis, which may also accompany thyrotoxicosis. *(Ref. 6, p. 831)*

492. (A) The pathologic changes are found in the spinal cord tracts. Degeneration is seen in the posterior funiculi, the lateral corticospinal tract, and the spino-cerebellar tracts. The disease is usually inherited as an autosomal recessive. Ataxia, sensory loss, nystagmus, reflex changes, clubfeet, and kyphoscoliosis are the characteristic findings. The heart is frequently involved and cardiac disease is a common cause of death. *(Ref. 6, p. 629)*

493. **(E)** In Wilson's disease, there is usually a reduction of the serum ceruloplasmin content. Signs and symptoms of injury to the basal ganglia are accompanied by cirrhosis of the liver. Renal involvement is characterized by persistent aminoaciduria. The most common neurologic finding is tremor. The corneal pigmentation (Kayser–Fleischer ring) is the most important diagnostic finding on physical examination. If it is absent any neurological findings cannot be ascribed to Wilson's disease. *(Ref. 6, p. 541)*

494. **(E)** In myasthenia gravis, weakness of the facial and levator palpebrae muscles produces a characteristic expressionless facies with drooping of the eyelids. Weakness of the ocular muscles may cause paralysis or weakness of individual muscles, paralysis of conjugate gaze, ophthalmoplegia, or a pattern similar to internuclear ophthalmoplegia. *(Ref. 6, p. 701)*

495. **(A)** Adenomas of the pituitary gland constitute approximately 15% of intracranial tumors, with the chromophobic type most common. With macroadenomas, some degree of pituitary insufficiency is common. With microadenomas the other pituitary functions may be completely normal. *(Ref. 6, p. 823)*

496. **(A)** In approximately two-thirds of the patients with amyotrophic lateral sclerosis, the initial symptom of the disease is weakness and wasting of the extremities. The fasciculations can be a very prominent part of the disease. This is rare in other neurologic disorders. *(Ref. 6, p. 683)*

497. **(C)** The characteristic triad in Parkinson's disease (tremor, rigidity, akinesia) has been expanded to include postural instability. This forms the mnemonic TRAP. Autonomic instability is also common. Findings on exam also include mask-like facies, dysarthria, stooped posture, and abnormal gait. *(Ref. 6, p. 658)*

498. **(D)** Adults may develop hydrocephalus as a result of occlusion of CSF pathways by tumors in the third ventricle, brain stem, or posterior fossa. In adults the symptoms of obstructive hydrocephalus include headache, lethargy, malaise, incoordination, and weakness. Seizures do not usually occur. Dementia, altered consciousness, ocular nerve palsies, papilledema, ataxia, or corticospinal tract signs may be present. *(Ref. 6, p. 253)*

499. **(B)** Myelin is a complex protein lipid carbohydrate structure, which forms part of the cell membrane of the oligodendroglia. Vascular lesions cause demyelination because of ischemia. Papovaviruses can cause progressive multifocal leukoencephalopathy in patients with HIV infection, or less commonly, malignancy. Acute disseminated encephalomyelitis has been described after smallpox or rabies vaccination. Nutritional deficiencies can also cause demyelination (e.g., pernicious anemia with B_{12} deficiency). *(Ref. 6, pp. 122, 124, 564, 692)*

500. **(B)** In the majority of cases, seizures do not develop until several months after the injury, six to eighteen months being the most common interval. The more severe the injury, the greater the likelihood of seizures. For severe injuries with penetration of the dura, some authorities recommend prophylactic anticonvulsants for 1 to 2 years. There is no firm evidence for this however. *(Ref. 6, pp. 388–389)*

501. **(D)** CT scan is still superior to MRI in certain circumstances, particularly in the emergency setting for diagnosing hemorrhage and fractures of the face, temporal bone, and base of the skull. It also demonstrates calcification within lesions of the brain better than MRI. *(Ref. 2, p. 2212)*

502. **(B)** The lateral medullary syndrome causes ipsilateral numbness but also contralateral involvement of pain and thermal sense by affecting the spinothalamic tract. It can be caused by occlusion of the vertebral, posterior–inferior cerebellar, and superior, middle, or inferior medullary arteries. Ipsilateral ataxia and falling to the side of the lesion are common. Ipsilateral paralysis of the tongue is characteristic of medial medullary syndrome which also causes contralateral paralysis of arm and leg. Paralysis of the body is not characteristic of lateral medullary syndrome, but ipsilateral paralysis of palate and vocal cord does occur. Ipsilateral Horner syndrome, nystagmus, diplopia, vertigo, nausea, and vomiting are characteristic. *(Ref. 2, p. 2244)*

503. **(D)** Pontine hemorrhage is associated with impaired oculocephalic reflexes and small reactive pupils. It generally evolves over a few minutes, usually with coma and quadriplegia. The prognosis is poor and death often occurs within hours. Putamenal hemorrhage is the most common form of hypertensive hemorrhage. *(Ref. 2, pp. 2251–2252)*

504. **(C)** TSP is frequently associated with a retroviral (HTLV-1) infection that can be spread through blood transfusion, sexual contact, intravenous drug use, and vertical transmission from mother to child. It is slowly progressive, and bladder involvement is characteristic. Sensory symptoms are usually mild and a true sensory level is almost never found. On occasion cranial nerve findings, frontal release signs, and cerebellar signs (tremor, dysmetria) are present. *(Ref. 2, pp. 2317–2318)*

505. **(A)** The cause of trigeminal neuralgia (tic douloureux) is unknown, although some cases may be caused by compression of the trigeminal nerve by arteries or veins of the posterior fossa. The pain occurs in paroxysms and is strictly limited to one or more branches of the fifth cranial nerve. Paroxysms may be brief or last up to 15 minutes. There is no objective sensory loss, but the patient may complain of hyperesthesia of the face. Watering of the eye on the involved side may occur during an attack. *(Ref. 6, pp. 419–420)*

506. **(D)** This anticonvulsant drug is given in doses varying from 400 to 800 mg/day. Phenytoin has also been used. The two drugs can also be used in combination. Operative procedures include alcohol injection of the nerve or ganglion, partial section of the nerve in the middle or posterior fossa, decompression of the root and medullary tractotomy. Percutaneous thermal destruction of the affected branch extracranially is also possible. *(Ref. 6, pp. 421, 800)*

507. **(A)** Cavernous sinus thrombosis is usually secondary to suppurative processes in the orbit, the nasal sinuses, or the upper half of the face. The optic discs are swollen, and there may be numerous surrounding small or large hemorrhages if the orbital veins are occluded. Visual acuity is normal or moderately impaired. *(Ref. 6, p. 244)*

508. **(C)** In the vast majority of cases, retrobulbar neuritis occurs as an episode in a demyelinating disease such as multiple sclerosis. It is the first manifestation of multiple sclerosis in 15% of cases, and occurs at some point in 50% of all patients with the disease. The course of the disease is that of gradual spontaneous improvement. *(Ref. 6, p. 417)*

509. **(E)** Internal carotid artery insufficiency is the most likely diagnosis. Abnormalities are found in the extracranial arteries in more than one-half of the patients with symptomatic cerebral infarction. Current treatment is carotid endarterectomy for severe stenosis, and aspirin therapy for lesser degrees of stenosis. *(Ref. 6, p. 211)*

510. **(B)** The patient's findings strongly suggest herpes simplex encephalitis. This is generally caused by HSV-1. When the disease is suspected appropriate antiviral therapy (acyclovir) should be started immediately. CT scan is not helpful in diagnosis, but MRI scans may be diagnostic. Brain biopsy, once the diagnostic test of choice, is rarely performed. *(Ref. 6, p. 114)*

511. **(C)** Vidarabine is relatively nontoxic, but does produce immunosuppression and has some degree of neurotoxicity. Acyclovir selectively inhibits viral DNA polymerase. Acyclovir is currently the treatment of choice. Because it is relatively nontoxic, therapy can be started even if the diagnosis is only presumptive. *(Ref. 6, p. 114)*

512. **(C)** Guillain–Barré syndrome often appears days to weeks after a viral upper respiratory or gastrointestinal infection. The initial symptoms are due to symmetric limb weakness. Parasthesias may be present. Unlike most other neuropathies, proximal muscles may be affected more than distal muscles early in the disease. Tendon reflexes are usually lost within a few days. Protein content of the CSF is usually high with a few days of onset. *(Ref. 6, p. 611)*

513. **(E)** The thymus tissue is often abnormal, with encapsulated tumors occurring in about 15% of cases. Almost all thymomas occur in patients over age 30. Even without thymoma, thymectomy can result in remission in patients with generalized myasthenia. Its benefit is delayed for months or more, so it is not an emergency treatment for myasthenia. *(Ref. 6, p. 697)*

514. **(B)** The most common presenting symptoms relate to weakness of eye muscles causing ptosis or diplopia. Difficulty in chewing, dysarthria, and dysphagia are also common. The differential diagnosis includes all diseases that cause weakness of oropharyngeal or limb muscles. These include the muscular dystrophies, amyotrophic lateral sclerosis, and progressive bulbar palsies among others. Most other conditions do not improve after injection of edrophonium or neostigmine. *(Ref. 6, p. 701)*

515. **(A)** Cholinergic drugs are largely inhibitors of cholinesterase. Prednisone may improve as many as 80% of patients. Thymectomy helps patients with no thymoma, but thymoma patients don't do as well. Plasmapheresis benefits most patients but needs to be repeated at intervals. *(Ref. 6, p. 701)*

516. **(E)** Myoclonic seizures are sudden, brief, single, or repetitive muscle contractions involving one body part or the entire body. Loss of consciousness does not occur unless other types of seizures co-exist. These seizures can be idiopathic or associated with Creutzfeldt–Jakob disease, uremia, hepatic failure, subacute leukoencephalopathies, and some hereditary disorders. *(Ref. 2, pp. 2223–2226)*

517. (B) Complex partial seizures were once classified as temporal lobe epilepsy. Although the temporal lobe (especially the hippocampus or amygdala) is the most common site of origin, some seizures have been shown to originate from mesial parasagittal or orbital frontal regions. *(Ref. 2, p. 2224)*

518. (D) Pure absence seizures consist of the sudden cessation of ongoing conscious activity without convulsive muscular activity or loss of postural control. They can be so brief as to be inapparent, but can last several minutes. There is usually no period of postictal confusion. *(Ref. 2, p. 2225)*

519. (A) Simple partial seizures can occur with motor, sensory, autonomic, or psychic symptoms. When a partial motor seizure spreads to adjacent neurons a "Jacksonian march" can occur, e.g., right thumb to right hand and right arm to right side of face. *(Ref. 2, p. 2224)*

520. (D) Absence seizures almost always begin in young children (age 6 to 14). They may first present as learning difficulties in school. The EEG is diagnostic, revealing brief 3 Herz spike and wave discharges occurring synchronously throughout all the leads. *(Ref. 2, p. 2225)*.

521. (E) Valproic acid can be used for typical and atypical seizures, myoclonic seizures and tonic–clonic seizures. It causes little sedation, and does not impair cognition. However, the blood count and liver tests must be monitored for a time after initiation of therapy to ensure the safety in an individual patient. *(Ref. 2, pp. 2230–2231)*

522. (E) Valproic acid is the drug of choice for atypical absence seizures and myoclonic seizures. *(Ref. 2, p. 2231)*

523. (A) Phenytoin can cause gum hyperplasia and hirsutism, which are particularly unpleasant side effects in young women. As well lymphadenopathy, ataxia, incoordination, confusion, and cerebellar toxicity can occur. *(Ref. 2, pp. 2230–2231)*

524. (C) Phenobarbital is effective for tonic–clonic and partial seizures. It has few if any systemic side effects, but can cause sedation and dulling of intellect. It induces liver enzymes, which can enhance the metabolism of other drugs. *(Ref. 2, pp. 2230–2231)*

525. (G) Clonazepam is used in the treatment of typical and atypical absence seizures as well as myoclonic seizures. It causes drowsiness and irritability but few systemic symptoms. Unfortunately the development of tolerance can limit its effectiveness. *(Ref. 2, pp. 2230–2231)*

526. (A) Tinnitus and/or deafness are commonly present in peripheral vertigo, but usually absent in central vertigo. *(Ref. 2, p. 97)*

527. (A) Visual fixation may inhibit both nystagmus and vertigo in peripheral vertigo. There is no inhibition in central vertigo. *(Ref. 2, p. 97)*

528. (B) Peripheral vertigo is episodic and finite, although the episodes may be prolonged. It is often recurrent. Central vertigo may be present all the time. It is often milder than peripheral vertigo. *(Ref. 2, p. 97)*

529. (B) Pure horizontal nystagmus is common in central vertigo but not peripheral, where a torsional component is usually present. Pure vertical or pure torsional nystagmus only occurs in central vertigo. *(Ref. 2, pp. 97–98)*

530. (C) Both central and peripheral vertigo can be caused by ischemia. *(Ref. 2, p. 97)*

531. (B) Horner syndrome results in a small, round pupil on one side. Light and near reaction is brisk and response to mydriatics and miotics is normal. The affected pupil will not dilate in the dark, so darkness accentuates the anisocoria. *(Ref. 2, pp. 101–102)*

532. (F) Atropinized pupils can reach a diameter of 8 to 9 m. This does not occur in other syndromes. *(Ref. 2, p. 102)*

533. (D) Argyll–Robertson pupils are small, irregular, and often bilateral. The response to light is impaired, but the response to near vision is preserved. *(Ref. 2, p. 102)*

534. (C) The tonic pupil (Holmes–Adie syndrome) is caused by a parasympathetic lesion at or distal to the ciliary ganglion. The pupil is large, usually unilateral, with absent response to light. A bright room, by causing constriction of the normal pupil, accentuates the anisocoria. *(Ref. 2, pp. 101–102)*

535. (D) The Argyll–Robertson pupil is a manifestation of syphilis, a treponemal infection. *(Ref. 2, p. 102)*

536. (B) Peripheral nerve lesions result in reflex loss greater than the degree of weakness. Reflex loss is variable in anterior horn cell disease, and decreased proportionately in muscle disease. In neuromuscular junction disorders reflexes are characteristically normal. *(Ref. 2, p. 2361)*

537. **(C)** Diurnal fluctuations, and pathologic fatigue, are common in disorders of neuromuscular transmission (e.g., myasthenia gravis). *(Ref 2, p. 2360)*

538. **(A)** In diseases of the anterior horn cell atrophy is marked and early. Muscle disease can result in marked atrophy, but much later in the course of the disease. Atrophy is generally moderate in peripheral nerve disease and absent in disorders of the neuromuscular junction. *(Ref. 2, pp. 2360–2361)*

539. **(B)** Peripheral nerve disease is the most likely to cause distal weakness, and is the only one of the four to also cause sensory symptoms. *(Ref. 2, pp. 2360–2361)*

540. **(D)** Certain muscle diseases such as myotonic dystrophy and facioscapulohumeral dystrophy have virtually pathognomonic facial features. *(Ref. 2, p. 2361)*

CHAPTER 8

Kidneys
Questions

DISEASES OF THE KIDNEYS: FLUIDS AND ELECTROLYTES

DIRECTIONS (Questions 541 through 578): Each of the questions or incomplete statements below is followed by five suggested answers or completions. Select the ONE that is best in each case.

541. All of the following substances are added to the urine by means of tubular secretion EXCEPT

(A) potassium
(B) hydrogen ion
(C) penicillin
(D) urea
(E) creatinine

542. Ten days after a kidney transplant, the patient develops allograft enlargement, fever, oliguria, and hypertension. The most likely cause is

(A) steroid hyperglycemia
(B) erythrocytosis
(C) hyperacute rejection
(D) acute rejection
(E) renal artery stenosis

543. The most characteristic urinary finding of acute glomerulonephritis is

(A) proteinuria
(B) microhematuria
(C) granular casts
(D) erythrocyte casts
(E) hyaline casts

544. Electron microscopy of glomerular lesions in poststreptococcal glomerulonephritis will show

(A) diffuse mesangial deposits
(B) no deposits
(C) electron-dense endothelial deposits
(D) closed capillary lumen
(E) subepithelial humps

545. In the diuresis following relief of urinary obstruction, the urine is

(A) dilute and alkaline
(B) low in sodium
(C) concentrated
(D) acidic
(E) none of the above

546. Chronic phenacetin ingestion may lead to

(A) glomerulosclerosis
(B) papillary necrosis
(C) cortical necrosis
(D) tubular necrosis
(E) nephrolithiasis

547. Acute glomerulonephritis may be mimicked by all of the following EXCEPT

(A) periarteritis nodosa
(B) allergic purpura
(C) subacute bacterial endocarditis
(D) pyelonephritis
(E) lupus erythematosus

548. The nephrotic syndrome is characterized by all of the following signs EXCEPT

(A) edema
(B) proteinuria
(C) hypoalbuminemia
(D) hyperlipemia
(E) hypertension

549. Metabolic alkalosis is likely to be caused by

(A) extracellular fluid volume expansion
(B) hyperkalemia
(C) mineralocorticoid excess
(D) decreased distal salt delivery
(E) bicarbonate deprivation

550. The kidney in sickle cell anemia is characterized by

(A) an inability to acidify the urine

(B) a decrease in glomerular filtration

(C) an inability to concentrate the urine

(D) pyuria

(E) a salt-losing state

551. In patients with gout, renal disease is often manifested by all of the following EXCEPT

(A) glomerulonephritis

(B) pyelonephritis

(C) urate crystals

(D) vascular sclerosis

(E) proteinuria

552. Intravenous pyelography (IVP) must be performed with special caution in patients with

(A) hyperparathyroidism

(B) pyelonephritis

(C) nephrolithiasis

(D) hypernephroma

(E) multiple myeloma

553. Amyloidosis of the kidneys may be associated with all of the following EXCEPT

(A) leprosy

(B) hypertension

(C) retinitis

(D) ulcerative colitis

(E) hematuria

554. Renal involvement in multiple myeloma is characterized by

(A) nitrogen retention

(B) hypertension

(C) retinitis

(D) edema

(E) hematuria

555. A patient with a mass in the lung develops hyponatremia, increased effective circulating volume, and high urine osmolality. He most likely has

(A) nephrotic syndrome

(B) inappropriate ADH production

(C) renal metastases from lung cancer

(D) lung metastases from hypernephroma

(E) renal tubular acidosis

556. Hematuria presenting as initial bleeding only, may be due to

(A) kidney tumor

(B) ureteral stone

(C) severe bladder hemorrhage

(D) urethral lesions

(E) none of the above

557. Papillary necrosis is prone to occur in

(A) diabetes mellitus

(B) glomerulonephritis

(C) pyelonephritis

(D) hypertension

(E) cortical necrosis

558. Magnesium deficiency may be seen in all of the following EXCEPT

(A) cerebellar hemangioma

(B) malabsorption syndromes

(C) chronic alcoholism

(D) long-term parenteral therapy

(E) diabetic acidosis

559. All of the following are true of orthostatic proteinuria EXCEPT

(A) it is more pronounced in lordosis

(B) it is aggravated by prolonged standing

(C) it manifests protein-free early-morning urine

(D) it only occurs with renal parenchymal disease

(E) that up to 3 gm/L is seen

560. Hypernephroma has been associated with all of the following EXCEPT

(A) polycythemia

(B) fever

(C) hematuria

(D) renal vein thrombosis

(E) high incidence of hypertension

561. Blood levels of all of the following rise in acute renal failure EXCEPT

(A) creatinine

(B) sodium

(C) potassium

(D) uric acid

(E) urea

562. Hypernatremia includes all of the following responses EXCEPT

(A) thirst

(B) decreased secretion of ADH

(C) movement of water out of cells

(D) decreased rate of sweating

(E) concentration of urine

563. The nephropathy of potassium depletion is most strikingly characterized by

(A) inability to concentrate urine

(B) inability to dilute urine

(C) erythrocyte casts

(D) granular casts

(E) renal potassium wasting

564. Inappropriate secretion of antidiuretic hormone may be associated with

(A) massive edema

(B) hypernatremia

(C) dehydration

(D) urine osmolality that is inappropriately low

(E) benign intrathoracic lesions

565. The largest volume of water is reabsorbed in the nephron at the

(A) collecting ducts

(B) proximal convolution

(C) distal convolution

(D) ascending loop of Henle

(E) descending loop of Henle

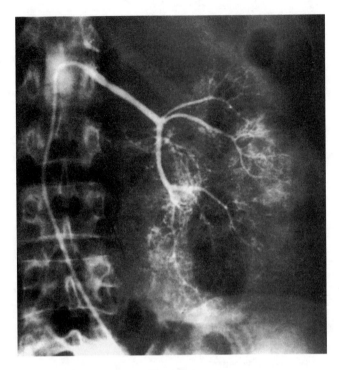

Figure 8.1

566. Figure 8.1 is a selective renal arteriogram done on a 64-year-old man who was admitted for hematuria after slipping on an icy pavement. What is your diagnosis?

(A) renal cell carcinoma

(B) kidney contusion and laceration

(C) transitional cell carcinoma

(D) renal hamartoma

(E) renal hemangioma

567. Which of the following conditions is commonly associated with urinary tract infection?

(A) anemia

(B) exercise

(C) diabetes mellitus

(D) influenza

(E) aspergillus

568. Which of the following is NOT associated with rapidly progressive (subacute) glomerulonephritis?

(A) pernicious anemia

(B) bacterial endocarditis

(C) Goodpasture syndrome

(D) lupus erythematosus

(E) poststreptococcal disease

569. Most likely to be associated with the nephrotic syndrome is

(A) sickle cell diseases
(B) medullary sponge kidney
(C) radiation nephritis
(D) staphylococcal infection
(E) amyloid disease

570. In acute renal failure, peritoneal dialysis is preferred over hemodialysis in

(A) cerebral trauma
(B) hypercatabolic states
(C) severe lung disease
(D) atrial premature beats
(E) drug overdose

571. Polyuria is commonly seen in all of the following EXCEPT

(A) hyperkalemia
(B) hypercalcemia
(C) glycosuria
(D) hypokalemia
(E) polydipsia

572. Most commonly associated with toxemia of pregnancy is

(A) second pregnancies
(B) third pregnancies
(C) twin pregnancies
(D) extremes of reproductive age
(E) sickle cell anemia

573. Which of the following statements is most likely to be true of polycystic kidney disease?

(A) it frequently affects only one kidney
(B) pregnancy aggravates the disease
(C) episodic oliguria is common
(D) other organs do not contain cysts
(E) renal transplantation is often indicated

574. Which of the following is NOT usually associated with renal lithiasis?

(A) cystinuria
(B) thalassemia
(C) hereditary glycinuria
(D) primary hyperoxaluria
(E) sarcoidosis

575. Late medical complications of transplantation with a renal allograft include all of the following EXCEPT

(A) atherosclerotic disease
(B) opportunistic infection
(C) aseptic necrosis of the hip
(D) an increase in lung cancer
(E) an increase in lymphoma

576. Which of the following agents requires a major dose reduction in the face of chronic renal failure?

(A) erythromycin
(B) doxycycline
(C) tobramycin
(D) isoniazid
(E) vincristine

577. Sudden deterioration of renal function in a diabetic should lead one to the diagnosis of

(A) papillary necrosis
(B) acute pyelonephritis
(C) chronic pyelonephritis
(D) renal calculi
(E) polyposis of the bladder

578. Isolated hematuria (i.e., only red blood cells present, no pathological proteinuria, casts or other abnormalities on urinalysis and normal renal function) is a common finding in all the following EXCEPT

(A) urinary tract stones
(B) primary renal disease
(C) trauma
(D) malignant renal tumors
(E) benign renal tumors

DIRECTIONS (Questions 579 through 589): The group of questions below consists of a list of lettered headings followed by a list of numbered words, phrases, or statements. For each numbered word, phrase, or statement, select the ONE lettered heading that is most closely associated with it. Each lettered heading may be selected once, more than once, or not at all.

Questions 579 through 583

    (A) metabolic acidosis
    (B) metabolic alkalosis
    (C) respiratory acidosis
    (D) respiratory alkalosis

579. Diarrhea leads to significant bicarbonate loss with a normal anion gap

580. Acute onset leads to somnolence, confusion, and ultimately CO_2 narcosis

581. Can result from primary hyperaldosteronism because of renal bicarbonate generation

582. May be associated with isoniazid toxicity in which oxygen utilization by tissues is thought to be impaired

583. May occur acutely as a result of anxiety or salicylism

Questions 584 through 589

    (A) nephrogenic diabetes insipidus
    (B) central diabetes insipidus
    (C) primary polydipsia
    (D) solute diuresis
    (E) natriuretic syndrome

584. May occur during course of acute tubular necrosis

585. Causes the greatest amount of medullary washout

586. Can be caused by hypokalemia

587. Can be caused by major tranquilizers

588. After fluid deprivation test little or no response to vasopressin

589. Can be caused by high protein tube feeds

DIRECTIONS (Questions 590 through 595): A 75-year-old man is referred from a local nursing home because of a serum sodium of 120. Each lettered heading gives a possible cause of his hyponatremia. Each numbered statement gives a description of clinical findings. For each numbered phrase select the ONE lettered heading that is most closely associated with it. Each lettered heading may be selected once, more than once, or not at all.

    (A) congestive heart failure
    (B) extra-renal fluid losses
    (C) syndrome of inappropriate ADH (SIADH)
    (D) polydipsia
    (E) essential hyponatremia
    (F) renal failure
    (G) endocrine cause of hyponatremia
    (H) renal fluid losses
    (I) artifactual
    (J) osmotic
    (K) impaired diuresis

590. Blood pressure 100/50, neck veins not visible, urine sodium 30 mmol/liter

591. Left hemiplegia

592. Depression being treated with amitriptyline

593. Postural drop in blood pressure, urine sodium 5 mmol/liter

594. Pitting edema

595. Uric acid low, urinary sodium 40 mmol/liter

DIRECTIONS (Questions 596 through 600): A 30-year-old woman comes to medical attention because of a low potassium. The group of questions below concerns the possible causes for her hypokalemia. Each lettered heading gives a possible cause of hypokalemia. Each numbered statement gives a description of clinical findings. For each numbered phrase select the ONE lettered heading that is most closely associated with it. Each lettered heading may be selected once, more than once, or not at all.

(A) lower gastrointestinal losses
(B) prior use of diuretics
(C) renal tubular acidosis (RTA)
(D) current use of diuretics
(E) malignant hypertension
(F) primary hyperaldosteronism
(G) glucocorticoid excess

596. Normal blood pressure, urine K^+ 15 mmol/L, bicarbonate above normal

597. Hypertension, low plasma renin, low plasma aldosterone

598. Normal blood pressure, urine K^+ 40 mmol/L, low serum bicarbonate

599. Hypertension, low plasma renin, high plasma aldosterone

600. Normal blood pressure, urine K^+ 15 mmol/L, bicarbonate low

DIRECTIONS (Questions 601 through 610): For each numbered phrase select the ONE lettered heading that is most closely associated with it. Each lettered heading may be selected once, more than once, or not at all.

(A) associated with prerenal azotemia but *not* intrinsic renal azotemia
(B) associated with intrinsic renal azotemia but *not* prerenal azotemia
(C) associated with *both* prerenal and intrinsic renal azotemia
(D) associated with *neither* prerenal nor intrinsic renal azotemia

601. Oliguria is helpful in determining the cause

602. Urine sodium concentration < 10 mmol/L

603. Urine specific gravity < 1.012

604. Fractional excretion of sodium is a sensitive test

605. Plasma BUN/creatinine ratio (mg/dL) < 10

DIRECTIONS (Questions 606 through 610): Each lettered heading below describes a mixed acid–base disorder. Each numbered phrase gives a cause of a mixed acid–base disorder. For each numbered phrase select the ONE lettered heading that is most closely associated with it. Each lettered heading may be selected once, more than once, or not at all.

(A) metabolic acidosis and respiratory acidosis
(B) metabolic acidosis and respiratory alkalosis
(C) metabolic alkalosis and respiratory acidosis
(D) metabolic alkalosis and respiratory alkalosis
(E) metabolic alkalosis and metabolic acidosis

606. Salicylate overdose

607. Sepsis

608. Chronic pulmonary disease on steroids

609. Renal failure with vomiting

610. Hepatic cirrhosis complicated by acute renal failure

Kidneys

Answers and Explanations

541. (D) Urea is filtered at the glomerulus and thereafter any movement in or out of tubules is a passive process depending on gradients, not secretion. Reabsorption of urea in the distal tubule and collecting duct when urine flow is reduced results in the disproportionate elevation of urea nitrogen over creatinine in prerenal azotemia. *(Ref. 1, p. 486)*

542. (D) Renal scans initially show a reduction in excretion with cortical retention. This is the most common type of rejection. Most acute rejections will respond to immunosuppressive agents if diagnosed early. In contrast, immediate nonfunction of a graft can be caused by damage to the kidney during procurement and storage. Such problems are becoming less frequent. Obstruction, vascular compression, and ureteral compression are other causes of primary nonfunction of a renal graft. *(Ref. 1, p. 549)*

543. (D) Granular and erythrocyte casts are both present, but the latter indicate bleeding from the glomerulus and are most characteristically seen. Red cells reach the urine probably via capillary wall "gaps," and form casts as they become embedded in concentrated tubular fluid with a high protein content. Proteinuria is invariably present, but is not as specific. *(Ref. 1, p. 552)*

544. (E) These humps are discrete, electron-dense nodules that persist for about eight weeks and are highly characteristic of the disease. Light microscopy reveals diffuse proliferation, and immunofluorescence reveals granular IgG and C3. About 95% will resolve spontaneously. *(Ref. 1, p. 552)*

545. (A) The urine is dilute and alkaline and contains much sodium. The large volume is due in part to osmotic diuresis following urea accumulation. Careful attention to fluid and electrolytes is important to prevent hypokalemia, hypomagnesemia, hyponatremia or hypernatremia, and volume depletion. *(Ref. 1, p. 583)*

546. (B) Chronic phenacetin ingestion may lead to papillar necrosis. Satisfactory understanding of the pathogenesis is lacking, but sensitivity reactions or industrial contaminants have been suggested. Depletion of reducing equivalents such as glutathione may also play a role. *(Ref. 1, p. 573)*

547. (D) Pyelonephritis does not mimic acute glomerulonephritis. The characteristic elevation and subsequent fall of the antistreptolysin O titer is excellent evidence for a preceding strep infection. *(Ref. 1, p. 552)*

548. (E) The blood pressure is often normal, and the heart is not enlarged. Unlike glomerulonephritis, the onset of nephrotic syndrome is often insidious. Gross hematuria and red cell casts are infrequent. Renal function is often normal at time of presentation. *(Ref. 1, pp. 559–560)*

549. (C) Mineralocorticoid excess leads to metabolic alkalosis, primarily because of renal bicarbonate generation. Other major mechanisms for metabolic alkalosis include ECF volume contraction, potassium depletion, and increased distal salt delivery. Less common causes are Liddle syndrome, bicarbonate loading (posthypercapneic alkalosis) and delayed conversion of administered organic acids. *(Ref. 1, p. 526)*

550. (C) In sickle cell anemia the kidney is characterized by an inability to concentrate the urine. Papillary necrosis may also occur in patients with homozygous sickle cell disease or sickle cell trait. *(Ref. 1, p. 585)*

551. (A) In patients with gout, renal disease is not manifested by glomerulonephritis. Twenty percent to forty percent of patients show albuminuria, which is rarely heavy in quantity and usually intermittent. *(Ref. 1, p. 1110)*

552. (E) Danger of acute renal failure after IVP has led to caution, especially in patients with multiple myeloma. The patient should not be dehydrated if the IVP is necessary. *(Ref. 1, pp. 496, 529)*

553. **(E)** Amyloidosis of the kidneys does not cause hematuria. Amyloidosis is commonly encountered as a complication of chronic suppuration and causes of amyloidosis include osteomyelitis and tuberculosis. *(Ref. 1, pp. 494, 1141–1145)*

554. **(A)** Nitrogen retention is characteristic of renal involvement in multiple myeloma. Hypercalcemia may produce transient or irreversible renal damage as do amyloid and myeloma cell infiltrates. *(Ref. 1, pp. 572, 974)*

555. **(B)** The urine osmolality in patients with SIADH need not be hypertonic to plasma, but only inappropriately high compared with serum. The major characteristics of SIADH include hyponatremia, volume expansion without edema, natriuresis, hypouricemia, normal or reduced serum creatinine level, with normal thyroid and adrenal function. *(Ref. 1, p. 511)*

556. **(D)** Urethral lesions may cause hematuria that presents as initial bleeding only. Investigation of hematuria includes urinalysis, hematologic evaluation, radiologic evaluation, cystoscopy, and renal biopsy. *(Ref. 1, pp. 493–494)*

557. **(A)** Papillary necrosis is prone to occur in diabetes mellitus. It is also seen in sickle cell disease, chronic alcoholism, vascular disease, and analgesic abuse. Radiologic findings of papillary necrosis include caliceal clubbing, papillary cavities, and caliceal filling defects (secondary to a sloughed papilla, the ring sign). *(Ref. 1, p. 572)*

558. **(A)** Magnesium deficiency is usually accompanied by hypocalcemia, and it is not seen in cerebellar hemangioma. Symptoms include lethargy, weakness, and irritability. Tetany, with positive Chvostek's and Trousseau's sign, may result from the accompanying hypocalcemia. *(Ref. 1, pp. 535, 1138–1139)*

559. **(D)** Orthostatic proteinuria occurs in many conditions and not only with renal parenchymal disease. Perhaps three-quarters of adolescents and young adults have proteinuria on prolonged standing or strenuous exercise. *(Ref. 1, p. 553)*

560. **(E)** Hypernephroma is not associated with a high incidence of hypertension. Hematuria, flank pain, and abdominal mass is the classical presentation, but metastases may be the first sign. *(Ref. 1, p. 616)*

561. **(B)** Blood levels of sodium do not rise in acute renal failure. Patients with acute tubular necro-

sis do spontaneously excrete a moderately high percentage of filtered water and filtered sodium. *(Ref. 1, pp. 529–530)*

562. **(B)** Decreased secretion of ADH is not a response in hypernatremia. Hypernatremia is the chemical expression of water deficit, and the adjustments in physiology retain or acquire water. *(Ref. 2, p. 248)*

563. **(A)** Inability to concentrate urine persists with dehydration; however, diluting ability is usually well preserved. The urine samples are not usually profoundly hypotonic in hypokalemic nephropathy, because it is relative vasopressin resistance, not complete resistance, that occurs. *(Ref. 1, pp. 513, 1243)*

564. **(E)** Intrathoracic lesions may be benign or malignant, and the latter may secrete a substance similar to lysine vasopressin. Nevertheless, bronchogenic carcinoma is the most common intrathoracic lesion causing SIADH. *(Ref. 1, p. 509)*

565. **(B)** The largest volume of water is reabsorbed in the nephron at the proximal convolution. Maximally concentrated urine depends on ADH, which allows distal convoluted tubes and collecting ducts to become permeable to water. *(Ref. 1, p. 485)*

566. **(A)** The diagnosis is renal cell carcinoma. There is marked hypervascularity of the left kidney. The arteries are irregular and tortuous, following a random distribution. There are small vessels within the renal vein that indicate the blood supply of the neoplastic thrombosis involving the renal vein. The kidney is enlarged and abnormally bulbous in the lower pole. *(Ref. 1, p. 497)*

567. **(C)** Urinary tract infections are increased in diabetes mellitus as well as pregnancy, hypertension, primary renal diseases, and urinary obstruction. *(Ref. 1, pp. 590, 595)*

568. **(A)** Abrupt onset and rapid progression are the rule with blood in the urine, anemia, oliguria, and azotemia. Pernicious anemia is primarily a disorder of vitamin B_{12} absorption secondary to an autoimmune disorder. The kidneys are not primarily involved. *(Ref. 1, pp. 557–559)*

569. **(E)** In addition to amyloid disease, other conditions associated with the nephrotic syndrome are secondary syphilis, malaria, and treatment with gold salts. Minimal change nephrotic syndrome, focal glomerular sclerosis, membranous nephropathy, and membranoproliferative glomeru-

lonephritis are the primary renal diseases that present as nephrotic syndrome. *(Ref. 1, p. 560)*

570. (A) Peritoneal dialysis is preferred with cerebral trauma and also myocardial infarction because of risk of hemorrhage or hypotension with hemodialysis. *(Ref. 1, p. 544)*

571. (A) Diabetes insipidus from hormonal or nephrogenic causes also produce polyuria. Central diabetes insipidus can be caused by trauma, tumor, or granulomatous disease, but is idiopathic in 30% to 40% of cases. Nephrogenic DI can be familial or acquired. Drugs, hypokalemia, and hypercalcemia are common acquired causes of nephrogenic DI. *(Ref. 1, pp. 568, 1242–1243)*

572. (D) Hydatidiform moles, first pregnancies, and extremes of reproductive age are associated with toxemia. The clinical manifestations of severe toxemia include headache, epigastric pain, visual disturbances, and hypertension. *(Ref. 1, p. 600)*

573. (E) Renal transplantation is utilized in end-stage renal failure. The transplanted kidney cannot be affected by the disease. Hepatic and pancreatic cysts are also common in autosomal-dominant polycystic kidney disease. Intracranial aneurysms are also more frequent. *(Ref. 1, p. 611)*

574. (B) Cystinuria is a congenital disorder associated with decreased tubular resorption of cystine, arginine, ornithine, and lysine. Thalassemia is not associated with kidney stones. *(Ref. 1, p. 604)*

575. (D) Increase in neoplasms in renal transplant recipients include cervical carcinoma, lymphoma, and cutaneous malignancies. Osteoporosis and persistent hyperparathyroidism are other bony complications. Risk of infection is related to degree of immunosuppression. *(Ref. 1, p. 550)*

576. (C) Tetracyclines should also have their dose reduced in chronic failure because of their hepatotoxicity with increased blood levels. Newer antibiotics are often used instead of aminoglycosides to reduce risk of renal damage. *(Ref. 1, p. 574)*

577. (A) Severe infection of the renal pyramids in association with vascular disease or obstruction leads to papillary necrosis. *(Ref. 1, p. 597)*

578. (B) Primary renal diseases rarely present with isolated hematuria. Benign recurrent hematuria or IgA nephrology usually have red blood cell casts present as well. Analgesic nephropathy usually causes modest proteinuria as well as hematuria. The hematuria of papillary necrosis is usually associated with some proteinuria. In contrast, urinary tract stones, trauma, benign and malignant tumors, tuberculosis, and prostate disease frequently present with isolated hematuria. *(Ref. 2, p. 238)*

579. (A) The anion gap is calculated as the sodium concentration minus the chloride plus the bicarbonate concentration. Other causes of bicarbonate loss with normal anion gap include proximal renal tubular acidosis and primary hyperparathyroidism. *(Ref. 1, pp. 522–523)*

580. (C) Causes of acute respiratory acidosis include narcotic overdose, myasthenia gravis, airway obstruction, and trauma to the chest. Acute increases in $Paco_2$ result in carbon dioxide narcosis. This starts with somnolence and confusion and can lead to coma. Asterixis may be present. Cerebral vasodilation may result in frank papilledema. *(Ref. 1, pp. 527–528)*

581. (B) The disorder can occur in volume-expanded patients in which the alkalosis is unresponsive to sodium chloride loading, as in primary hyperaldosteronism or volume contraction with secondary hyperaldosteronism. *(Ref. 1, pp. 525–527)*

582. (A) Impaired oxygen utilization leads to lactic acidosis, accumulation of lactate, and increased anion gap. *(Ref. 1, pp. 523–525)*

583. (D) During acute hyperventilation, plasma bicarbonate concentrations fall by approximately 3 mEq/L when the arterial pressure of CO_2 falls to about 25 mm Hg. *(Ref. 1, p. 528)*

584. (E) The diuretic phase of acute tubular necrosis is characterized by large losses of sodium and water. *(Ref. 2, p. 239)*

585. (C) Primary polydipsia can cause greater medullary wash-out than either nephrogenic or central diabetes insipidus because primary polydipsia tends to cause expansion of the extracellular fluid volume. This tends to increase total delivery of NaCl and water to the inner medulla. It also increases renal blood flow, and increased flow through the vasa recta reduces ability to trap solutes in the medulla. *(Ref. 2, p. 239)*

586. (A) Nephrogenic diabetes insipidus can be caused by hypokalemia as well as hypercalcemia. *(Ref. 2, p. 239)*

587. (C) Both thioridazine and chlorpromazine have been associated with primary polydipsia. *(Ref. 2, p. 239)*

588. **(C)** There is little or no response to vasopressin after fluid deprivation in primary polydipsia, because of medullary wash-out, not vasopressin deficiency. Complete nephrogenic diabetes insipidus also will not respond; however, incomplete nephrogenic diabetes insipidus will show some response. *(Ref. 2, p. 239)*

589. **(D)** High protein tube feeds may cause a solute diuresis because of excessive excretion of urea. Other causes of solute diuresis include glucosuria, mannitol, radiographic contrast media, and chronic renal failure. *(Ref. 2, p. 234)*

590. **(H)** The combination of extracellular fluid (ECF) volume contraction with a high urinary sodium (> 20 mmol/L) suggests renal fluid loss. This is commonly caused by diuretics or glucosuria. *(Ref. 2, pp. 244–247)*

591. **(C)** SIADH is associated with many CNS diseases including meningitis, encephalitis, tumors, trauma, stroke, and acute porphyria. It is assumed that ADH in these patients is secreted in response to direct stimulation of the hypothalamic osmoreceptors. *(Ref. 2, p. 245)*

592. **(C)** Amitriptyline is one of the psychoactive drugs that cause SIADH. Others include haloperidol, thioridazine, and carbamazepine. Oral hypoglycemics (chlorpropamide, tolbutamide) and antineoplastic drugs (vincristine, vinblastine, cyclophosphamide) are also associated with SIADH. *(Ref. 2, p. 246)*

593. **(B)** The combination of ECF volume contraction and a low urinary sodium (< 10 mmol/L) suggests extra-renal sodium loss. Common causes are vomiting, diarrhea, or excessive sweating. *(Ref. 2, p. 244)*

594. **(A)** The hyponatremia associated with nephrotic syndrome, cirrhosis, or congestive heart failure is characterized by edema. It is felt that the hyponatremia is caused by a decrease in "effective" circulating volume secondary to decreased cardiac output or sequestration of fluid. *(Ref. 2, p. 245)*

595. **(C)** SIADH is characterized by a low uric acid and a urine sodium greater than 20 mmol/L. *(Ref. 2, pp. 245–247)*

596. **(B)** In patients who have prior diuretic use resulting in hypokalemia at the time of evaluation, the bicarbonate tends to be elevated and the urine K+ low (< 25 mmol/L). *(Ref. 2, pp. 250–251)*

597. **(G)** Glucocorticoid and licorice ingestion, can result in hypertension with low plasma renin and aldosterone levels. *(Ref. 2, pp. 250–251)*

598. **(C)** Type I and II RTA cause hypokalemia with high K+ excretion (> 25 mmol/L), and a low bicarbonate in the absence of hypertension. Diabetic ketoacidosis can also result in this constellation of findings. *(Ref. 2, pp. 250–251)*

599. **(F)** Primary hyperaldosteronism is characterized by hypertension with high plasma aldosterone and low plasma renin. *(Ref. 2, pp. 250–251)*

600. **(A)** In lower GI loss (diarrhea) the blood pressure is normal, the urine K+ low (< 25 mmol/L) and the bicarbonate is either normal or low. *(Ref. 2, pp. 250–251)*

601. **(D)** Oliguria does not help in determining the cause of acute renal failure. Complete anuria suggests, but does not prove, that obstruction is present. *(Ref. 2, p. 1270)*

602. **(A)** The kidney tries to conserve sodium in prerenal azotemia and the result is a low urine Na+ concentration (< 10 mmol/L). *(Ref. 2, pp. 1269–1271)*

603. **(B)** The urine osmolality approximates plasma in intrinsic renal azotemia and is usually below 1.012. *(Ref. 2, p. 1270)*

604. **(C)** The fractional excretion of sodium relates sodium clearance to creatinine clearance and is more sensitive than direct measurements of Na+ excretion. In prerenal azotemia, sodium is avidly resorbed from glomerular filtrate, but not in intrinsic renal azotemia, because of tubular epithelial cell injury. Creatinine is resorbed less efficiently in both conditions. Therefore the fractional excretion of sodium is less than 1% in prerenal azotemia (often much less) while it is greater than 1% in intrinsic renal azotemia.

$$\text{Fractional excretion of sodium \%} = \frac{U_{Na} \, P_{Cr}}{P_{Na} \, U_{Cr}} \times 100$$

(Ref. 2, pp. 270–271)

605. **(B)** The ratio of BUN/creatinine is usually < 10 to 15 in intrinsic renal disease and > 20 in prerenal azotemia. *(Ref. 2, pp. 270–271)*

606. **(B)** Metabolic acidosis and respiratory alkalosis are seen in salicylate overdose. *(Ref. 2, p. 261)*

607. **(B)** Sepsis can cause cardiovascular insufficiency with lactic acidosis, while the fever and endotoxemia stimulate the respiratory center causing respiratory alkalosis. *(Ref. 2, p. 261)*

608. **(C)** Chronic pulmonary disease often causes respiratory acidosis while the steroids frequently used in therapy may cause a metabolic alkalosis. *(Ref. 2, p. 261)*

609. **(E)** Renal failure causes metabolic acidosis, while the loss of H^+ ions in vomiting cause a metabolic alkalosis. *(Ref. 2, p. 261)*

610. **(B)** Hepatic cirrhosis frequently results in chronic respiratory alkalosis. Acute renal failure with metabolic acidosis is common in patients with cirrhosis. *(Ref. 2, p. 261)*

CHAPTER 9

Muscles and Joints
Questions

DISEASES OF THE MUSCULOSKELETAL SYSTEM

DIRECTIONS (Questions 611 through 631): Each of the questions or incomplete statements below is followed by five suggested answers or completions. Select the ONE that is best in each case.

611. Marfan syndrome involves all of the following EXCEPT

    (A) abnormalities of the eye
    (B) marked obesity
    (C) excessively long tubular bones
    (D) kyphoscoliosis
    (E) dissecting aneurysm

612. The function of interleukin-2 is most likely to be

    (A) macrophage activation
    (B) chemotaxis for monocytes
    (C) antiviral activity
    (D) bone resorption
    (E) T lymphocyte replication

613. The basic defect in the genetic mucopolysaccharidosis is

    (A) insulin deficiency
    (B) abnormal elastic tissue
    (C) excess iron in tissue
    (D) homocystinuria
    (E) abnormal lysosomal enzymes

614. The single most useful laboratory test for the diagnosis of systemic lupus erythematosus (LE) is

    (A) LE cells
    (B) fluorescence antinuclear antibody test
    (C) erythrocyte sedimentation rate
    (D) antibodies to native DNA
    (E) antinucleolar antibodies

615. Cardiac manifestations of polyarteritis nodosa may include all of the following EXCEPT

    (A) hypertension
    (B) coronary insufficiency
    (C) pericarditis
    (D) granulomatous myocarditis
    (E) bicuspid aortic valve

616. Juvenile rheumatoid arthritis (Still's disease) is characterized by all of the following EXCEPT

    (A) daily high fevers
    (B) lymphadenopathy
    (C) pleuritis
    (D) cervical spondylitis
    (E) tests for the rheumatoid factor that are usually positive

617. X-ray findings in degenerative joint disease (osteoarthritis) include all of the following EXCEPT

    (A) narrowing of the joint space
    (B) osteoporosis
    (C) marginal lipping
    (D) bony sclerosis
    (E) irregularity of joint surfaces

618. Sjögren syndrome (keratoconjunctivitis sicca) is associated with all of the following EXCEPT

    (A) xerostomia
    (B) inflammation in the salivary glands
    (C) Aschoff nodules
    (D) arthritis
    (E) inflammation in the lacrimal glands

619. A diagnostically helpful ophthalmic finding in lupus erythematosus is

    (A) cytoid bodies
    (B) microaneurysm
    (C) Argyll–Robertson pupil
    (D) macular degeneration
    (E) nystagmus

620. The most common portion of the gastrointestinal tract to become involved in scleroderma is the

(A) esophagus
(B) stomach
(C) duodenum
(D) ileum
(E) colon

621. Raynaud's phenomenon

(A) may lead to gangrene of the fingers
(B) is almost always due to scleroderma
(C) occurs when scleroderma is always well established
(D) causes fingers to turn red in cold water
(E) affects the sexes equally

622. Pseudogout can be distinguished from gout by means of

(A) positive birefringent crystals
(B) acute onset
(C) involvement of single joints
(D) involvement of large joints
(E) association with diabetes

623. A 10-year-old child with recurrent signs and symptoms of palpable purpura on the buttocks, arthralgias, colicky abdominal pain, diarrhea, and microscopic hematuria is most likely to have

(A) influenza
(B) hypersensitivity vasculitis
(C) juvenile rheumatoid arthritis
(D) systemic lupus erythematosus
(E) Wegener's granulomatosis

624. A 75-year-old woman has abrupt onset of soreness and severe stiffness of the shoulders and upper thighs with low-grade fever. Physical examination is entirely normal, but the ESR is over 100 mm/hr. The most likely diagnosis is

(A) dermatomyositis
(B) osteoarthritis
(C) polymyalgia rheumatica
(D) midline granuloma
(E) sarcoidosis

625. The patient in the above case history is most likely to require treatment with

(A) intravenous high-dose steroids
(B) acetylsalicylic acid
(C) indomethacin
(D) low-dose steroids by mouth
(E) topical steroid creams

626. Malignancy is classically associated with

(A) systemic lupus erythematosus
(B) scleroderma
(C) dermatomyositis
(D) polyarteritis
(E) Weber–Christian disease

627. Takayasu syndrome is characterized by

(A) high pressure in the legs and low pressure in the arms
(B) low pressure in the legs and high pressure in the arms
(C) high-pitched diastolic murmur
(D) occurrence in older males
(E) hypertension

628. Figure 9.1 is the x-ray of a 40-year-old white man with symptoms of sinusitis and an incidental finding in the skull. Your diagnosis would be

(A) normal variant
(B) osteomyelitis
(C) Paget's disease
(D) hemangioma
(E) metastatic disease

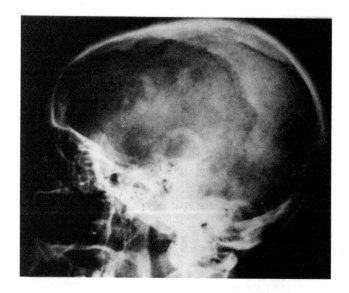

Figure 9.1

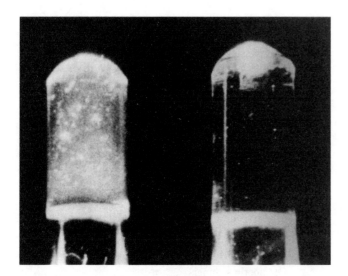

Figure 9.2

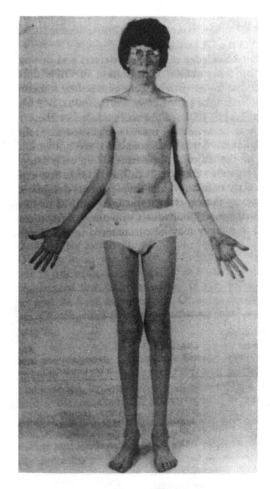

Figure 9.3

629. A mucin clot test is shown in Figure 9.2 with the normal control on the left and the patient's fluid on the right. The patient's most likely diagnosis is

    (A) degenerative joint disease

    (B) traumatic arthritis

    (C) systemic lupus

    (D) scleroderma

    (E) gout

630. Joint fluid aspiration is also analyzed for all of the following EXCEPT

    (A) sodium content

    (B) viscosity

    (C) bacterial culture

    (D) cytology

    (E) inclusions

631. The usual cause of death in the condition pictured in Figure 9.3 is

    (A) ruptured esophageal varices

    (B) berry aneurysm

    (C) aortic aneurysm

    (D) respiratory failure

    (E) sepsis

DIRECTIONS (Questions 632 through 641): For each numbered phrase select the ONE lettered heading that is most closely associated with it. Each lettered heading may be selected once, more than once, or not at all.

Questions 632 through 636

(A) associated with dermatomyositis but *not* temporal arteritis

(B) associated with temporal arteritis but *not* dermatomyositis

(C) associated with *both* dermatomyositis and temporal arteritis

(D) associated with *neither* dermatomyositis nor temporal arteritis

632. Renal disease is common

633. Leukocytosis

634. Intensity of skin manifestations related to exposure to sun

635. Systemic manifestations

636. Optic atrophy

Questions 637 through 641

(A) associated with rheumatoid arthritis but *not* osteoarthritis

(B) associated with osteoarthritis but *not* rheumatoid arthritis

(C) associated with *both* rheumatoid arthritis and osteoarthritis

(D) associated with *neither* rheumatoid arthritis nor osteoarthritis

637. Pain relieved by rest, aggravated by use

638. Prolonged stiffness after rest

639. Cartilaginous and bony enlargement of the terminal interphalangeal joints of the fingers

640. Narrowing of joint spaces on x-ray

641. Lack of correlation between x-ray changes and symptoms

DIRECTIONS (Questions 642 through 653): Each of the questions or incomplete statements below is followed by five suggested answers or completions. Select the ONE that is best in each case.

642. Leukopenia is a common finding in

(A) periarteritis nodosa

(B) systemic lupus erythematosus (SLE)

(C) scleroderma

(D) dermatomyositis

(E) osteoarthritis

643. Hypertrophic osteoarthrophy (HOA) is associated with

(A) rheumatoid factor

(B) aortic stenosis

(C) periosteal inflammation

(D) traumatic fracture

(E) artificial hip replacement

644. Pulmonary manifestations of rheumatoid arthritis include all of the following EXCEPT

(A) pleural effusion

(B) cavitating lesions

(C) intrapulmonary nodules

(D) interstitial fibrosis

(E) diffuse pneumonitis

645. The arthritis accompanying ulcerative colitis is usually associated with

(A) asymmetric involvement of the knees and ankles

(B) coincident regional enteritis

(C) progressive crippling course

(D) symmetrical small joint involvement

(E) sciatic nerve compression

646. Which of the following is NOT characteristic of psoriatic arthritis?

(A) distal interphalangeal joint involvement

(B) association with sacroiliitis

(C) nail lesions

(D) major involvement of the knees

(E) "pencil-in-cup" deformity

647. Lyme disease, the inflammatory arthropathy with regional clustering is characterized by all of the following EXCEPT

(A) tick-borne spirochete infection

(B) circulating immune complexes

(C) clustering in desert areas

(D) neurologic abnormalities

(E) response to penicillin

648. Which of the following is NOT characteristic of Wegener's granulomatosis?

(A) nodular pulmonary lesions

(B) congestive heart failure

(C) intractable rhinitis and sinusitis

(D) terminal uremia

(E) aggressive clinical course

649. The rheumatoid factor

(A) is positive in 10 to 20% of juvenile rheumatoid arthritis

(B) is positive in almost 100% of "classical" rheumatoid arthritis

(C) is seen only in rheumatoid arthritis

(D) has a molecular weight of about 160,000

(E) is frequently present in osteoarthritis

650. Systemic nodular panniculitis (Weber–Christian disease) may be characterized by

(A) rapidly fatal course

(B) increase in hemoglobin

(C) lymphocytosis

(D) inflammatory subcutaneous nodules

(E) infectious etiology

651. The Ehlers–Danlos syndrome is characterized by

(A) thickening of the skin

(B) mental retardation

(C) increased incidence of skin carcinoma

(D) thrombocytopenia

(E) habitual dislocation of joints

652. Synovial fluid characteristics in traumatic arthritis are

(A) clear

(B) poor mucin clot

(C) small fibrin clot

(D) 5,000 to 50,000 WBC/mm$_2$

(E) acellular

653. In dermatomyositis, the course of muscle necrosis can be followed by repeated

(A) serum creatinine kinase (CK)

(B) sedimentation rates

(C) urine transaminase enzymes

(D) electromyography

(E) alkaline phosphatase

654. Which of the following statements concerning renal disease in systemic lupus erythematous (SLE) is correct?

(A) evidence of any pathological change on renal biopsy indicates a poor prognosis

(B) rapidly deteriorating renal function and an active urine sediment require prompt renal biopsy

(C) about 50% of patients with SLE have immunoglobulins in glomeruli

(D) presence of anti-DNA antibodies is associated with active nephritis

(E) mesangial involvement suggests a poor prognosis

655. Which of the following statements concerning the articular manifestations of rheumatoid arthritis (RA) is correct?

(A) wrists are rarely involved

(B) involvement of hands is characteristically asymmetric

(C) fever up to 40°C is common with joint involvement

(D) ulnar deviation at the wrist is common

(E) absence of morning stiffness makes RA an unlikely cause of articular symptoms

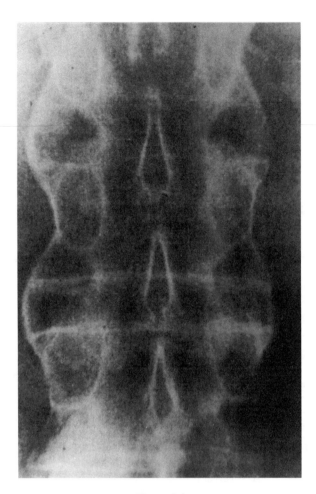

Figure 9.4

DIRECTIONS (Questions 656 through 659): This section consists of a clinical situation, followed by a series of questions. Study the situation, and select the ONE best answer to each question following it. A 22-year-old man has a history of low back pain and stiffness. After several months of mild symptoms, he notes more severe stiffness at night and hip pain. On physical examination, there is paravertebral muscle tenderness and limited flexion of the lumbar spine. A diastolic murmur is heard. Figure 9.4 shows an x-ray of the lumbar spine.

656. The most likely diagnosis is

(A) Reiter syndrome
(B) Marfan syndrome
(C) ankylosing spondylitis
(D) rheumatoid arthritis
(E) pseudogout

657. The diastolic murmur is likely to be

(A) mitral stenosis
(B) tricuspid stenosis
(C) aortic insufficiency
(D) pulmonic insufficiency
(E) tetralogy of Fallot

658. The most likely extra-articular manifestation of this disease is

(A) colitis
(B) iridocyclitis
(C) psoriasis
(D) urethritis
(E) cardiac conduction disturbances

659. All of the following are recommended for therapy of this condition EXCEPT

(A) indomethacin
(B) phenylbutazone
(C) exercise programs
(D) sleep without a pillow
(E) radiotherapy

DIRECTIONS (questions 660 through 684): The lettered phrases below are followed by a list of numbered phrases. For each numbered phrase select the ONE lettered heading that is most closely associated with it. Each lettered heading may be selected once, more than once, or not at all.

Questions 660 through 664

(A) associated with hemolysis
(B) seen in mixed connective tissue disease
(C) most sensitive test for SLE
(D) most sensitive test for drug-induced LE
(E) causes false positive VDRL
(F) relatively disease specific

660. antinuclear antibodies (ANA)

661. anti-ds DNA (ds = double-stranded)

662. anticardiolipin

663. antihistone

664. anti-RNP

Questions 665 through 669

    (A) Felty syndrome

    (B) rheumatoid vasculitis

    (C) episcleritis

    (D) Sjögren syndrome

    (E) rheumatoid nodules

    (F) rheumatoid pleural involvement

    (G) Caplan syndrome

    (H) pericardial disease

    (I) rheumatoid nodules

665. May present as small brown spots in the nail folds

666. Most common form of eye involvement

667. Associated with increased frequency of infections

668. Found in association with occupational lung disease

669. Commonly involves Achilles tendon

Questions 670 through 674

    (A) associated with osteoporosis but *not* osteomalacia and rickets

    (B) associated with osteomalacia and rickets but *not* osteoporosis

    (C) associated with *both* osteoporosis and osteomalacia and rickets

    (D) associated with *neither* osteoporosis nor osteomalacia and rickets

670. Associated with Looser's zones

671. May be associated with vitamin deficiency

672. May be part of an inherited disorder

673. Alkaline phosphatase usually elevated

674. Calcium supplementation is an effective treatment

Questions 675 through 679

    (A) associated with pseudogout but *not* gout

    (B) associated with gout but *not* pseudogout

    (C) associated with *both* gout and pseudogout

    (D) associated with *neither* gout nor pseudogout

675. Caused by more than one kind of crystal

676. Can be treated with steroid injections

677. Increased prevalence with advanced age

678. With effective treatment, progressive arthritis can be prevented

679. May be associated with end-stage renal failure

Questions 680 through 684

    (A) polyarteritis nodosa (PAN)

    (B) Churg–Strauss disease

    (C) Henoch–Schönlein purpura

    (D) vasculitis associated with infectious diseases

    (E) vasculitis associated with connective tissue diseases

    (F) Wegener's granulomatosis

    (G) giant cell arteritis

    (H) Kawasaki disease

    (I) Behçet syndrome

680. Pulmonary involvement and peripheral eosinophilia are common

681. Aneurysms and renal involvement are characteristic

682. Associated with a specific serum test when the disease is active

683. Most common in children and often remits spontaneously after several episodes

684. Characterized by oral and genital ulceration

Muscles and Joints

Answers and Explanations

611. **(B)** In Marfan syndrome, inheritance is autosomal dominant, and the aortic lesion is a cystic medial necrosis with loss of elastic tissue. The syndrome does not include marked obesity. Mitral valve prolapse can also be part of the syndrome. Dislocation of the lens is the most apparent eye abnormality. Severe chest deformities and long limbs are characteristic. High arched palate, high pedal arches, and pes planus are common. *(Ref. 2, p. 2116)*

612. **(E)** Interleukin-2 is a lymphokine that functions as a T cell growth factor. Interleukin-1 stimulates synovial dendritic cells to produce collagenase. In addition, interleukin-2 activates cytotoxic T cells to become active killer cells. *(Ref. 2, p. 1558)*

613. **(E)** Each syndrome in the genetic mucopolysaccharidosis is caused by a mutation-produced deficiency in the activity of a lysosomal enzyme. For example, Tay–Sachs disease is caused by a deficiency of hexosaminidase A, resulting in accumulation of G_{M2} ganglioside. Gaucher's disease is caused by a deficiency of β-glucocerebrosidase resulting in an accumulation of glucosylceramide. *(Ref. 2, p. 2092)*

614. **(D)** Antibodies to a variety of specific antigens can be measured, including native DNA, low molecular weight RNA species, and single-stranded DNA. The preferable test is antibody to double-stranded DNA (anti-dsDNA) which is present in about 70% of cases and relatively disease specific. Antinuclear antibodies (ANA) are present in 95% of cases and are a good screening test. They are not very specific, however. *(Ref. 2, p. 1644)*

615. **(E)** The first four conditions listed may be cardiac manifestations. Heart failure is responsible for, or contributes to, death in one-sixth to one-half of polyarteritis nodosa cases. About three quarters of patients have cardiac involvement at

autopsy. A bicuspid valve is usually a congenital abnormality. *(Ref. 2, pp. 1671–1672)*

616. **(E)** In Still's disease, tests for the rheumatoid factor are not always positive. In about 25% of patients, especially when less than six years old, prominent systemic symptoms occur. *(Ref. 2, pp. 302, 1653)*

617. **(B)** Osteoporosis is not a finding in osteoarthritis. Early pathologic changes occur in the joint cartilage; subsequently, new bone formation develops. There is often not a clear correlation between x-ray findings, symptoms, and functional impairment in osteoarthritis. *(Ref. 2, p. 1696)*

618. **(C)** Sjögren syndrome is not associated with Aschoff nodules. The lack of secretions may also involve the entire respiratory tract, vagina, and skin. The ratio of women to men is 9:1. Close to a third of patients with rheumatoid arthritis, SLE, and scleroderma develop Sjögren syndrome. *(Ref. 2, p. 1663)*

619. **(A)** Cytoid bodies are a diagnostically helpful ophthalmic finding. Other systems involved in LE include skin, cardiopulmonary, neurologic, and lymph node. The most common symptoms of SLE are arthralgias and myalgias. These are almost universal. Cytoid bodies are white exudates in the retina. *(Ref. 2, p. 1646)*

620. **(A)** Esophageal symptoms are present in more than 50% of patients. The pathology consists of a thin mucosa and increase in collagen in the lamina propria, submucosa, and serosa. Muscle atrophy is prominent and ulceration secondary to scleroderma or acid reflux is common. *(Ref. 2, p. 1657)*

621. **(A)** Raynaud's phenomenon may lead to gangrene of the fingers. The soft tissue of the fingertips is lost, and the bone of the terminal phalanges may be resorbed. IgA is the antibody class most often seen in the immune complexes of these patients. The renal involvement is a mild glomerulitis with red blood cell casts. Most patients recover completely, some without any specific therapy (i.e., glucocorticoids). *(Ref. 2, pp. 1139, 1657)*

622. **(A)** Pseudogout is distinguishable from gout by positive birefringent crystals. Calcium pyrophosphate crystals are short, blunt rhomboids, and urate crystals are needle-shaped with negative birefringence. *(Ref. 2, p. 1698)*

623. **(B)** The child most likely has Henoch–Schönlein purpura, a hypersensitivity vasculitis affecting skin, gastrointestinal tract, and renal glomeruli. *(Ref. 2, p. 1674)*

624. **(C)** Difficulty in getting out of bed or rising from a chair may suggest polymyositis, but the muscles are normal. In general, polymyalgia rheumatica causes painful muscles, not weak muscles. However, pain may lead to profound disuse atrophy and apparent muscle weakness. In these cases, the normal CK and nonspecific muscle biopsy still allow accurate differentiation from polymyositis. *(Ref. 2, p. 132)*

625. **(D)** The response of pain and stiffness to 20 mg of prednisone is dramatic. Long-term treatment with 5 mg of prednisone prevents symptoms. Mild cases may respond to nonsteroidal anti-inflammatory medication. *(Ref. 2, p. 132)*

626. **(C)** Most tumors associated with dermatomyositis have been bronchogenic carcinomas, but many others have occurred. About 8% of all cases of myositis are associated with malignancy. The malignancy may antedate or postdate the myositis by up to two years. Age over 60 makes malignancy more likely. *(Ref. 2, p. 2380)*

627. **(A)** High pressure in the legs and low pressure in the arms characterize Takayasu syndrome. Clinical manifestations include easy fatigability of the arms and atrophy of the soft tissues of the face. *(Ref. 2, p. 1677)*

628. **(C)** There is a rarefied area involving the frontal and parietal bones. This is an early stage of Paget's disease where calvarial thickening and foci or radiopacity are not present within the radiolucent area. At this stage of the disease, a cross section through the margin of the lesion reveals a compact inner and outer table in the normal portion, whereas the diploe widens and extends to the outer and inner surfaces of the calvarium without a change in the calvarial thickness in the lesion. *(Ref. 2, p. 2191)*

629. **(E)** When acetic acid is added, a good ropy clot forms in normal joint fluid, but a poor clot forms in severe inflammatory arthritis, including gout and rheumatoid arthritis. *(Ref. 2, p. 1690)*

630. **(A)** Other analyses may include Gram stain, white count and differential, color, crystals, proteins, and rheumatoid factor. *(Ref. 2, p. 1690)*

631. **(C)** The patient has Marfan syndrome. Aortic involvement occurs in about 80%, with degenerative changes predominating. *(Ref. 2, p. 2116)*

632. **(D)** Autopsy has shown renal arteritis, but clinical disease is rare in either condition. *(Ref. 2, pp. 1461, 1677, 2379)*

633. **(C)** In both conditions, leukocytosis is moderate and is largely due to increased neutrophils. *(Ref. 2, pp. 1677, 2379)*

634. **(A)** In dermatomyositis, skin rashes can mimic erythema nodosum, eczema, or exfoliative dermatitis. *(Ref. 2, pp. 1677, 2379)*

635. **(C)** Systemic manifestations in both conditions include fever, weakness, anemia, and leukocytosis. *(Ref. 2, pp. 1677, 2379)*

636. **(B)** In temporal arteritis, sudden onset of blindness may occur in one or both eyes from ophthalmic or vertebral artery disease. *(Ref. 2, pp. 1677, 2379)*

637. **(C)** In both conditions, judicious rest and a mixture of exercise and physiotherapy are used to prevent deformity. *(Ref. 2, pp. 1653, 1697)*

638. **(A)** In rheumatoid arthritis, morning stiffness is an almost invariable feature, and severity varies with the extent of the disease. *(Ref. 2, pp. 1651, 1695)*

639. **(B)** Heberden's nodes are bony protuberances at the dorsal margins of distal interphalangeal joints, which appear in osteoarthritis. *(Ref. 2, pp. 1696)*

640. **(C)** Aside from joint narrowing, osteophyte formation is seen in degenerative joint disease, but radiolucent subchondral cysts are seen in both. *(Ref. 2, pp. 1653, 1696)*

641. **(B)** In osteoarthritis, deformities characterizing Heberden's nodes may be marked but these are not associated with pain or inflammation. *(Ref. 2, p. 1696)*

642. **(B)** Leukopenia occurs in about one-half of the SLE patients, and the differential count is usu-

ally normal. Lymphocytes and platelets can also be reduced. *(Ref. 2, p. 1647)*

643. **(C)** Mononuclear cell infiltration and edema develop in the periosteum, synovial membrane, and joint capsule. Secondary HOA (e.g., lung cancer) is more common than primary HOA. *(Ref. 2, p. 1705)*

644. **(B)** Diffuse interstitial fibrosis and pneumonitis may progress to a honeycomb appearance on x-ray, with bronchiectasis and chronic cough. Pleural involvement is very common at autopsy, but infrequently causes symptoms. If present, pleural fluid is low in glucose and complement levels. *(Ref. 2, p. 1652)*

645. **(A)** Also reported in ulcerative colitis is a more common association with erythema nodosum and uveitis than is found in other types of arthritis. *(Ref. 2, pp. 1702–1703)*

646. **(D)** Resorption of the distal end of the bone produces the "pencil," which projects into a cup-like erosion in the adjacent joint surface. Most patients with psoriatic arthritis also have nail involvement. Only about a quarter actually develop a progressive destructive disease. *(Ref. 2, pp. 1701–1702)*

647. **(C)** The neurologic complications occur in about 15% of patients, and include encephalopathy with memory impairment. Clustering occurs in wooded areas where the tick is found. Response to antibiotics is best in early disease before arthritis and neurological manifestations occur. *(Ref. 2, p. 746)*

648. **(B)** In Wegener's granulomatosis, arteries, arterioles, venules, and capillaries are involved with necrotizing inflammation. Congestive heart failure is not a characteristic feature. An aggressive course with death due to renal involvement is characteristic of untreated Wegener's. Cyclophosphamide has been dramatically successful in treating the disease. Glucocorticosteroids are often used initially as well, but they are relatively ineffective on their own. *(Ref. 2, pp. 1674–1675)*

649. **(A)** The rheumatoid factor is positive in 10 to 20% of juvenile rheumatoid arthritis cases. One-third of patients have monoarticular arthritis, most often in a knee or an ankle. The rheumatoid factor is frequently present in asymptomatic elderly patients and has little diagnostic efficacy in that group. *(Ref. 2, pp. 1689–1690)*

650. **(D)** The disease shows frequent remissions and exacerbations of lesions and is rarely fatal. It is

occasionally associated with lymphoma. Panniculitis may also be secondary to other systemic diseases such as SLE, pancreatic diseases, and α-$_1$-antitrypsin deficiency. *(Ref. 2, p. 2135)*

651. **(E)** In the Ehlers–Danlos syndrome, skin hyperextensibility, fragility, and bruisability are marked, and this condition may create difficulties at operation. Habitual dislocation of joints is also a characteristic of this syndrome. *(Ref. 2, p. 2113)*

652. **(C)** In traumatic arthritis, swellings, ecchymoses, muscular spasms, and tenderness tend to be present, but fractures must be excluded. Synovial fluid is bloody and has a small fibrin clot. *(Ref. 2, p. 1690)*

653. **(A)** The course of muscle necrosis can be best followed by repeated CK determinations. Repeated muscle biopsies are rarely required. *(Ref. 2, p. 2383)*

654. **(D)** Presence of high titer of anti-ds DNA, persistently abnormal urinalysis and low complement increases the risk of severe nephritis. Although most patients have immunoglobulin deposition in the glomeruli, only half develop clinical nephritis. Some patterns of involvement, mesangial or mild focal proliferative nephritis, have a good prognosis. Rapidly deteriorating renal function with an abnormal urine sediment mandates urgent treatment, but not necessarily urgent biopsy. *(Ref. 2, p. 1644)*

655. **(E)** As in most inflammatory arthritides, the patient with RA generally has morning stiffness of greater than one hour. Wrist involvement is nearly universal and is associated with radial deviation (unlike the ulnar deviation of the digits), and carpal tunnel syndrome. Hand involvement characteristically involves the proximal interphalangeal and metacarpophalangeal joints in a symmetrical involvement. High fever ($> 38°C$) even with active synovitis should suggest an intercurrent problem such as infection. *(Ref. 2, p. 1651)*

656. **(C)** The disease is 30 times more prevalent among the relatives of patients than the general population. There is a striking association with the histocompatibility antigen HLA-B$_{27}$. *(Ref. 2, p. 1665)*

657. **(C)** The frequency of aortic insufficiency has been about 4%. Other cardiac valve anomalies are not increased in incidence. *(Ref. 2, p. 1666)*

658. **(B)** Iridocyclitis occurs in about one-quarter of patients. Cardiac conduction disturbances occur in about 10%. Pain, photophobia, and increased lacrimation are the usual symptoms. Attacks are unilateral and tend to recur. *(Ref. 2, p. 1665)*

659. **(E)** Radiotherapy was formerly used to reduce pain and inflammation, but was associated with a 10-fold incidence of leukemia. The most common indication for surgery in ankylosing spondylitis is hip joint surgery. *(Ref. 2, p. 1667)*

660. **(C)** Although not specific, ANA is positive in 95% of patients with SLE. A repeatedly negative test makes SLE unlikely. *(Ref. 2, p. 1644)*

661. **(F)** Anti-ds DNA is relatively disease specific and associated with nephritis and clinical activity. Anti-ss DNA is not very specific. *(Ref. 2, p. 1644)*

662. **(E)** The presence of anticardiolipin antibodies is associated with false-positive VDRL, vascular thrombosis, and spontaneous abortion. *(Ref. 2, p. 1644)*

663. **(D)** Antihistone antibodies are seen in 95% of drug-induced LE and in 70% of those with SLE. *(Ref. 2, p. 1644)*

664. **(B)** Anti-RNP is found in high titer in syndromes with features of polymyositis, scleroderma, lupus, and mixed connective tissue disease. *(Ref. 2, p. 1644)*

665. **(B)** Although widespread vasculitis is rare, limited forms of vasculitis are not, particularly in white patients with high titers of rheumatoid factor. Cutaneous vasculitis usually presents as crops of small brown spots in the nail beds, nail folds, and digital pulp. *(Ref. 2, p. 1652)*

666. **(D)** Direct eye involvement with the rheumatoid process (episcleritis or scleritis) occurs in less than 1% of patients. However, 15% to 20% may develop Sjögren syndrome with attendant keratoconjunctivitis sicca. *(Ref. 2, p. 1652)*

667. **(A)** Felty syndrome consists of chronic RA, splenomegaly, and neutropenia. The increased frequency of infections is due to both decreased number and function of neutrophils. *(Ref. 2, p. 1652)*

668. **(G)** Caplan syndrome is a diffuse nodular fibrotic process which may result when rheumatoid nodules occur in the lungs of patients with pneumoconiosis. *(Ref. 2, p. 1652)*

669. **(E)** Rheumatoid nodules occur in 20% to 30% of patients with RA. Common locations include the olecranon bursa, the proximal ulna, the Achilles tendon and the occiput. *(Ref. 2, p. 1651)*

670. **(B)** The characteristic radiologic signs of osteomalacia are Looser's zones (pseudofractures). They are radiolucent bands perpendicular to the bone's surface and are particularly common in the femur, pelvis, scapula, upper fibula, and metatarsals. They occur at sites where major arteries cross the bones and might be due to the mechanical stress of the vessel's pulsations. The major x-ray finding of osteoporosis is decreased mineral density, at least until fractures supervene. *(Ref. 2, pp. 2173, 2178–2179)*

671. **(C)** The most common cause of osteomalacia is vitamin D deficiency. Scurvy, caused by vitamin C deficiency, is commonly characterized by osteoporosis. *(Ref. 2, pp. 2173, 2177)*

672. **(C)** Osteoporosis is a feature of heritable disorders of connective tissue such as osteogenesis imperfecta, homocystinuria, Ehlers–Danlos syndrome, and Marfan syndrome. Numerous forms of inherited renal disease, as well as inherited disorders of vitamin D metabolism can cause osteomalacia and rickets. *(Ref. 2, pp. 2173, 2177)*

673. **(B)** The alkaline phosphatase is usually, but not invariably, elevated in osteomalacia. It is normal in osteoporosis unless a fracture has occurred. *(Ref. 2, pp. 2174, 2179)*

674. **(D)** Although chronic calcium deficiency may be a factor in its pathogenesis, osteoporosis is rarely effectively treated with calcium alone. The low calcium levels often associated with osteomalacia are treated primarily with vitamin D therapy. *(Ref. 2, pp. 2175–2176, 2179–2182)*

675. **(A)** Pseudogout can be caused by calcium pyrophosphate dihydrate (CPPD), calcium hydroxyapatite (HA), or calcium oxalate (CaOx). *(Ref. 2, p. 1698)*

676. **(C)** Both gout and pseudogout respond to intraarticular steroid injections. *(Ref. 2, pp. 1699, 2085)*

677. **(A)** Pseudogout, particularly CPPD and HA deposition increase in prevalence with advancing age. With CPPD deposition disease over 80% of patients are over age 60. *(Ref. 2, pp. 1698–1699)*

678. **(B)** There is no effective way of removing calcium crystals from joints, so pseudogout is frequently progressive. Effectively lowering serum uric acid levels will result in urate crystals dissolving and even tophi can resolve. Allopurinol is the most common urate lowering medication. *(Ref. 2, pp. 1700, 2085–2086)*

679. **(C)** Both pseudogout (especially HA and CaOx) and gout are more frequent in the setting of end-stage renal disease. Gout can also contribute to renal disease directly by causing nephrolithiasis or urate nephropathy. *(Ref. 2, pp. 1699–1701, 2084–2085)*

680. **(B)** Churg–Strauss can be very similar to polyarteritis nodosa, except renal involvement is less common and less severe. Pulmonary involvement often dominates the clinical presentation and peripheral eosinophilia is common. *(Ref. 2, pp. 1672–1673)*

681. **(A)** PAN is a multisystem, necrotizing vasculitis of small- and medium-sized muscular arteries. Aneurysmal dilations of the arteries are characteristic. Nonspecific signs and symptoms are the usual method of presentation. Renal involvement is clinically present in 60% of cases, and is the most common cause of death. *(Ref. 2, pp. 1671–1672)*

682. **(F)** A high percentage of patients with Wegener's develop antineutrophil cytoplasmic antibodies (ANCAs). Particular cytoplasmic or c-ANCAs are 88% sensitive and 95% specific for Wegener's. *(Ref. 2, p. 1675)*

683. **(C)** Henoch–Schönlein purpura, characterized by palpable purpura, arthralgias, GI symptoms, and glomerulonephritis, can be seen in any age group, but is most common in children. It can resolve and recur several times over a period of weeks or months, and can resolve spontaneously. *(Ref. 2, p. 1674)*

684. **(I)** Behçet syndrome is a leukocytoclastic venulitis characterized by episodes of oral ulcers, genital ulcers, iritis, and cutaneous lesions. *(Ref. 2, pp. 1669–1670, 1678)*

CHAPTER 10

Infection
Questions

DIRECTIONS (Questions 685 through 721): Each of the questions or incomplete statements below is followed by five suggested answers or completions. Select the ONE that is best in each case.

685. Complications of infection with *Entamoeba histolytica* include all of the following EXCEPT

    (A) liver abscess
    (B) renal abscess
    (C) meningoencephalitis
    (D) intestinal partial obstruction
    (E) pleural pulmonary amebiasis

686. Which of the following statements is true regarding tetanus?

    (A) tetanus usually develops within two weeks following exposure
    (B) tetanus always develops within four hours following exposure in patients who have not been previously immunized
    (C) tetanus may develop many months or years following exposure in susceptible individuals
    (D) the usual incubation period for tetanus is 48 hours
    (E) tetanus may be prevented with penicillin

687. A 14-year-old with severe hemophilia develops pneumocystis carinii pneumonia. Additional testing is most likely to show

    (A) Hodgkin's disease
    (B) heterophil antibody
    (C) HIV
    (D) lymphocytosis
    (E) pulmonary hemorrhage

688. Primary genital infection with vesicular lesions on an erythematous base associated with bilateral tender lymphadenopathy is most likely due to

    (A) cytomegalovirus
    (B) gonococcus
    (C) herpes simplex virus-2
    (D) herpes simplex virus-1
    (E) varicella zoster

689. Primary atypical pneumonia is caused by a

    (A) bacterium
    (B) mycoplasma
    (C) fungus
    (D) rickettsia
    (E) spirochete

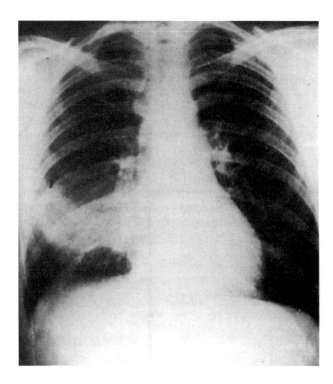

Figure 10.1

690. A 25-year-old man is admitted with fever and rust-colored sputum. The chest x-ray is shown in Figure 10.1. The most likely diagnosis is

(A) right middle lobe pneumonia

(B) loculated pleural effusion

(C) aspergilloma

(D) aspiration pneumonia

(E) right lower lobe pneumonia

691. Pustular lesions at the site of the scratch of a cat, followed by malaise, fever, and lymphadenopathy, are likely to be caused by

(A) gram-negative bacillus

(B) coccobacilli

(C) acid-fast bacilli

(D) rickettsia

(E) fungus

692. Deaths due to measles are almost always due to

(A) pneumonia

(B) mastoiditis

(C) meningitis

(D) dehydration

(E) encephalitis

693. A patient with an indwelling plastic intravenous line who develops subacute bacterial endocarditis is most likely to be infected with

(A) *Staphylococcus aureus*

(B) meningococcus

(C) *Staphylococcus saprophytricus*

(D) pneumococcus

(E) *Staphylococcus epidermidis*

694. Pneumococcal meningitis is usually a complication of

(A) subacute bacterial endocarditis

(B) otitis media

(C) pharyngitis

(D) chorea

(E) cellulitis

695. Which of the following is least likely to cause bacterial meningitis in adults?

(A) pneumococcus

(B) *Clostridium perfringens*

(C) meningococcus

(D) *Staphylococcus*

(E) *Haemophilus influenzae*

696. In pulmonary complications of influenza, the most common bacterial invader is

(A) pneumococcus

(B) *Haemophilus influenzae*

(C) *Streptococcus*

(D) *Staphylococcus*

(E) *Neisseria catarrhalis*

697. Clinical manifestations of enterovirus infections may include all of the following EXCEPT

(A) fever

(B) aseptic meningitis

(C) myalgia

(D) exanthems

(E) Horner syndrome

698. Travelers' diarrhea may be markedly reduced by the prophylactic use of

(A) penicillin

(B) doxycycline

(C) chloramphenicol

(D) erythromycin

(E) chloroquine phosphate

699. Progressive disseminated histoplasmosis may be associated with all of the following EXCEPT

(A) spontaneous regression

(B) nasopharyngeal ulcers

(C) hepatomegaly

(D) meningitis

(E) Addison's disease

700. *Histoplasma capsulatum* may be best characterized as

(A) causing a localized infection

(B) an intracellular organism found in the reticuloendothelial (RE) system

(C) an encapsulated bacterium

(D) sensitive to large doses of penicillin

(E) uniformly fatal with miliary spread

701. Food poisoning that results in motor paralysis within 24 hours is most likely due to

(A) *Clostridium botulinum* toxin

(B) staphylococcal toxin

(C) salmonellosis

(D) brucellosis

(E) shigellosis

702. Cytomegalovirus infection is best characterized as

(A) always fatal

(B) unresponsive to antibiotics

(C) highly infectious

(D) only acquired

(E) only congenital

703. Pulmonary cavitation resulting from fungal infection is most likely to be caused by

(A) ringworm

(B) *Cryptococcus neoformans*

(C) *Candida albicans*

(D) mycobacteria

(E) *Coccidioidomycosis*

704. The most frequent complication of measles is

(A) pneumonia

(B) encephalitis

(C) otitis media

(D) bronchitis

(E) mastoiditis

705. Subacute sclerosing panencephalitis

(A) responds to tetracycline

(B) is usually self-limiting

(C) causes largely sensory symptoms

(D) is a late complication of measles

(E) is a late complication of scarlet fever

706. Live rubella vaccine should be given to

(A) children between one year and puberty

(B) infants less than one year

(C) all adults

(D) pregnant women

(E) all exposed patients

707. Death from influenza is usually due to

(A) encephalitis

(B) tracheobronchitis

(C) pneumonia

(D) myocarditis

(E) adrenal collapse

708. Granuloma inguinale is associated with all of the following clinical findings EXCEPT

(A) ulcerative skin lesions

(B) extensive scarring

(C) limitation to the inguinal area

(D) vegetative lesions

(E) response to amphotericin B

709. A renal transplant patient develops severe cough and dyspnea. Bronchial brushings show clusters of cysts that stain with methenamine silver. The best treatment is

(A) amphotericin B

(B) cephalosporins

(C) co-trimoxazole

(D) aminoglycosides

(E) penicillins

710. A food poisoning epidemic resulting from ingestion of cream-filled pastry is most likely due to

(A) staphylococcal enterotoxin

(B) *Clostridium botulinum*

(C) *Clostridium perfringens*

(D) *Salmonella* species

(E) ptomaine poisoning

711. A young woman complains of hair loss, loss of hair luster, and intense scalp irritation. A Wood's light examination is positive. The most likely cause is

(A) seborrhoeic dermatitis

(B) *Aspergillus*

(C) trichophyton

(D) neurosis

(E) excess androgen levels

712. Coxsackie A viruses may cause any of the following EXCEPT

(A) herpangina

(B) exanthem

(C) aseptic meningitis

(D) basophilia

(E) common cold

713. Which of the following statements is most likely to be true about rabies?

(A) may be transmitted from human to human through exchange of body fluids

(B) transmission from animals is from infected blood

(C) following the first signs of rabies in humans, vaccines may reverse up to 20% of cases

(D) symptoms of rabies uniformly include hyperexcitability

(E) confirmation of the diagnosis is based on finding Negri bodies in nerve cells

714. Although etiology has not necessarily been established, antibodies to Epstein–Barr virus have frequently been found in association with all of the following EXCEPT

(A) infectious mononucleosis

(B) multifocal leukoencephalopathy

(C) nasopharyngeal carcinoma

(D) Burkitt's lymphoma

(E) chronic fatigue syndrome

715. A 40-year-old man develops erythema nodosum, conjunctivitis, and a pleural effusion. Over several weeks, pulmonary lesions lead to cavitation and a large thin-walled cavity. The most likely cause is

(A) *Streptococcus*

(B) *Coccidioidomycosis*

(C) candidiasis

(D) *Staphylococcus*

(E) *Pneumocystis carinii*

716. A patient undergoing emergency surgery for trauma receives 20 blood transfusions during the operation. Four weeks later, she develops a syndrome resembling infectious mononucleosis. The most likely cause is

(A) Epstein–Barr virus

(B) hepatitis C virus

(C) delayed hemolysis

(D) cytomegalovirus

(E) serum sickness

717. Toxic shock syndrome is characteristically associated with

(A) males

(B) *Streptococcus* infection

(C) vomiting and diarrhea

(D) bacteremia

(E) gradual onset

718. Initial management for the neutropenic patient with high fever should include

(A) an aminoglycoside and a cephalosporin

(B) tetracycline

(C) acetaminophen alone until culture results are available

(D) an anthracycline and a folate inhibitor

(E) testing for antibodies to HIV

719. Aspiration pneumonia in the recumbent position is most likely to be associated with

(A) aerobic and anaerobic organisms

(B) an afebrile course

(C) lower lobe infection

(D) *Haemophilus influenzae* infection

(E) sterile pneumonitis

720. Which of the following are characteristic of infection with *Legionella pneumophilia*?

(A) usually very mild disease

(B) heavy sputum production

(C) transmitted by blood transfusion

(D) high fever is common

(E) indigenous to northeastern United States

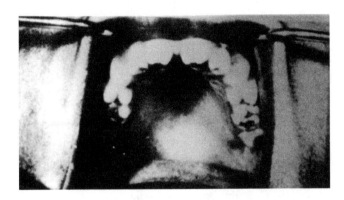

Figure 10.2

721. The dental condition illustrated in Figure 10.2 is usually associated with

(A) osteoporosis

(B) high forehead

(C) Paget's disease of bone

(D) absent radius

(E) anterior bowing of tibiae

722. The following statements about endocarditis in intravenous drug abusers are true EXCEPT

(A) *Streptococcus* organisms are the most common cause

(B) murmurs can be absent

(C) the tricuspid valve is the most common affected

(D) pneumonia can be a presenting problem

(E) the course is usually acute

723. Which of the following statements concerning infective endocarditis is CORRECT?

(A) Janeway lesions are most common in endocarditis with a subacute course

(B) emboli to large arteries (e.g., femoral arteries), usually indicate *Pseudomonas* endocarditis

(C) Roth spots are a sensitive but not specific indicator of infective endocarditis

(D) aortic prosthetic valves are more commonly infected than mitral prosthetic valves

(E) mycotic aneurysms frequently cause severe symptoms in infective endocarditis

724. Which of the following statements concerning spontaneous bacterial peritonitis (SBP) is CORRECT?

(A) pre-existing ascites is present in only 50% of the cases

(B) most cases present with fever

(C) the microbiology reveals a polymicrobial infection

(D) a WBC of less than 1000 PMNs per microliter virtually excludes the diagnosis

(E) over 70% of cirrhotic patients will develop SBP over the course of their illness

725. Which of the following statements concerning Lyme disease is correct?

(A) the incubation period is three months

(B) after an initial brisk immune response, immunity wanes with continuous infection

(C) the disease is caused by a spirochete

(D) the disease is caused by a tick

(E) the characteristic skin lesion of erythema migrans is found in over 95% of cases

DIRECTIONS (Questions 726 through 735): Each group of questions below consists of a list of lettered headings followed by a list of numbered words, phrases, or statements. For each numbered word, phrase, or statement select the one lettered heading that is most closely associated with it. Each lettered heading may be selected once, more than once, or not at all.

Questions 726 through 730

(A) brucellosis

(B) *Coccidioidomycosis*

(C) histoplasmosis

(D) leprosy

(E) leptospirosis

(F) infectious mononucleosis

(G) tuberculosis

(H) tularemia

726. Oropharyngeal ulcerations

727. Thin wall pulmonary cavitation

728. Positive Mantoux test

729. Iowa hog farmers

730. Infected rabbits

Questions 731 through 735

    (A) toxoplasmosis

    (B) tetanus

    (C) syphilis

    (D) *Streptococcus*

    (E) *Staphylococcus*

    (F) smallpox

    (G) salmonellosis

731. Dark field examination

732. Congenital brain calcifications

733. Abdominal pain and diarrhea

734. Preventive measures not used any longer

735. Treated with muscle relaxants

DIRECTIONS (Questions 736 through 745): This section consists of clinical situations, each followed by a series of questions. Study each situation, and select the ONE best answer to each question following it.

Questions 736 through 740: An 18-year-old woman visits her physician because of three weeks of malaise, two weeks of fever, and a sore throat. Physical examination shows pharyngeal infection with enlarged tonsils and a patchy white exudate; enlarged palpable anterior and posterior cervical, axillary, and inguinal lymph nodes; tenderness in the right upper quadrant; and minimal splenomegaly. Laboratory data show: hemoglobin 14% gm; hematocrit 42%; platelets 380,000; white blood count 8500 with 35% segmented neutrophils, 1% eosinophils, and 64% lymphocytes of which 36 were atypical.

736. The most likely diagnosis is

    (A) infectious hepatitis

    (B) lymphocytic leukemia

    (C) infectious mononucleosis

    (D) Hodgkin's disease

    (E) cat-scratch fever

737. The diagnosis is most likely to be proved by

    (A) lymph node biopsy

    (B) bone marrow

    (C) erythrocyte sedimentation rate

    (D) heterophil antibody (sheep cell agglutination) test of Paul–Bunnell

    (E) hepatic biopsy

738. The treatment of choice for this disease is

    (A) gamma globulin

    (B) adequate rest

    (C) leukeran

    (D) chloramphenicol

    (E) radiation therapy

739. Which one of the following rare complications is not usually associated with this disease?

    (A) meningoencephalitis

    (B) Guillain–Barré syndrome

    (C) splenic rupture

    (D) jaundice

    (E) hemorrhage

740. Other manifestations of this disease that the patient may develop include all of the following EXCEPT

    (A) carditis

    (B) maculopapular rash

    (C) herpes zoster

    (D) jaundice

    (E) pinpoint palatal petechiae

Questions 741 through 745: A 20-year-old woman visits your office because of headache, anorexia, chilly sensations, pain and drawing sensations in both sides of her jaw, and pain in both lower abdominal quadrants. Physical examination reveals bilateral enlarged parotid glands that are doughy, elastic, and slightly tender; reddened orifice of Stensen's duct; bilateral lower quadrant abdominal tenderness; a temperature of 102°F; and a pulse rate of 92/minute. Laboratory data show hemoglobin 13% gm; hematocrit 40%; 9000 white blood cells, with 35% segmented neutrophils, 7% monocytes, and 58% lymphocytes.

741. The most likely diagnosis is

    (A) cervical lymphadenitis

    (B) Mikulicz syndrome

    (C) parotid gland tumor

    (D) uveoparotid fever

    (E) mumps

742. The patient's abdominal pain and tenderness is most likely due to

    (A) mesenteric lymphadenitis

    (B) oophoritis

    (C) gonorrhea

    (D) peritoneal metastases

    (E) intestinal hyperperistalsis

743. All of the following are laboratory tests to confirm the diagnosis of epidemic parotitis EXCEPT

    (A) complement fixation test during acute and convalescent stage

    (B) cutaneous test with suspension of heated inactivated virus

    (C) blood culture

    (D) hemagglutination inhibition test

    (E) serum amylase

744. The best treatment for this disease is

    (A) symptomatic

    (B) convalescent serum

    (C) broad spectrum antibiotics

    (D) sulfonamides

    (E) steroids

745. All of the following statements concerning this disease are true EXCEPT

    (A) the disease is caused by a filterable virus, is endemic in most large communities, and occurs in epidemics about every seven years

    (B) complement-fixing antibody in the circulating blood in adequate titer during convalescence denotes recent infection

    (C) the most common complication of this disease in postpubertal boys and men is orchitis

    (D) mastitis, pancreatitis, and meningoencephalitis may occur as complications of this disease

    (E) an increased serum amylase is proof of the existence of pancreatitis as a complication

DIRECTIONS (Questions 746 through 782): For each numbered phrase select the ONE lettered heading that is most closely associated with it. Each lettered heading may be selected once, more than once, or not at all.

Questions 746 through 750

    (A) *Staphylococcus aureus*

    (B) Candida

    (C) *Pneumocystis carinii*

    (D) Giardia lamblia

    (E) gram-negative enteric bacilli

    (F) *Haemophilus influenzae*

    (G) *Neisseria species*

    (H) *Nocardia* species

    (I) *Salmonella*

    (J) rubella virus

746. Cytotoxic chemotherapy

747. Selective IgA deficiency

748. Defect in alternate pathology of complement

749. T lymphocyte deficiency/dysfunction

750. Microbial defect

Questions 751 through 755

    (A) *Staphylococcus aureus*

    (B) *Clostridium perfringens*

    (C) *Vibrio cholerae*

    (D) enterotoxigenic *E. Coli*

    (E) *Salmonella*

    (F) *Shigella*

    (G) *Vibrio parahaemolyticus*

    (H) bacillus cereus

751. Occurs 3 hours after a meal of a ham sandwich and potato salad

752. Most common cause of travelers' diarrhea

753. Causes bloody diarrhea 24 hours after a salad

754. Causes watery diarrhea 24 hours after raw oyster ingestion

755. Can cause both early onset vomiting and later onset diarrhea

Questions 756 through 760

    (A) associated with gonococcal arthritis but *not* nongonococcal septic arthritis

    (B) associated with nongonococcal septic arthritis but *not* gonococcal arthritis

    (C) associated with *both* gonococcal and nongonococcal septic arthritis

    (D) associated with *neither* gonococcal nor nongonococcal septic arthritis

756. Usually presents as a monoarticular arthritis

757. Associated with skin lesions

758. Interphalangeal joints frequently involved

759. Synovial culture usually diagnostic

760. Mucocutaneous lesions usually present

Questions 761 through 765

    (A) associated with *Neisseria gonorrhoeae* but *not Chlamydia trachomatis*

    (B) associated with *Chlamydia trachomatis* but *not Neisseria gonorrhoeae*

    (C) associated with *both Neisseria gonorrhoeae and Chlamydia trachomatis*

    (D) associated with *neither Neisseria gonorrhoeae nor Chlamydia trachomatis*

761. Commonly causes epididymitis in older men and following urinary tract instrumentation

762. Causes vulvovaginitis in the absence of cervicitis

763. Causes ulcerative lesions of the genitalia

764. Can cause mucopurulent cervicitis in women

765. Can be definitively diagnosed by Gram stain of urethral discharge

Questions 766 through 770

    (A) B-lactams (penicillins and cephalosporins)

    (B) vancomycin

    (C) erythromycin

    (D) sulfonamides and trimethoprim

    (E) ciprofloxacin

766. Major cellular target is interference with cell metabolism

767. Work by inhibiting DNA synthesis

768. Resistance can be caused by drug inactivation

769. Work by inhibiting protein synthesis

770. Decreased intracellular accumulation can result in resistance

Questions 771 through 775

    (A) erythromycin

    (B) ciprofloxacin

    (C) tetracycline

    (D) sulfonamides

    (E) metronidazole

    (F) rifampin

771. Can cause unwanted pregnancy

772. Can contribute to hypoglycemia in noninsulin-dependent diabetes mellitus

773. Can cause severe reaction to alcohol

774. Drug interaction can result in rejection for transplant recipients

775. Can result in phenytoin toxicity .

Questions 776 through 782

    (A) associated with *Streptococcus pneumoniae* but *not Mycoplasma pneumoniae*

    (B) associated with *Mycoplasma pneumoniae* but *not Streptococcus pneumoniae*

    (C) associated with *both Streptococcus pneumoniae and Mycoplasma pneumoniae*

    (D) associated with *neither Streptococcus pneumoniae nor Mycoplasma pneumoniae*

776. Tracheobronchitis is the most common manifestation

777. An elevated white blood count with neutrophilia is characteristic

778. Frequently causes dermatological lesions

779. Severe pleuritic pain is characteristic

780. Patients can often pinpoint the start of the illness

781. Productive cough can be present

782. Fever is frequently absent

Infection

Answers and Explanations

685. **(B)** Abscesses develop in the liver, abdominal cavity, spleen, and brain. The most common type of amoebic infection, however, is that of asymptomatic cyst passage. When pathogenic strains are ingested, symptomatic colitis develops 2 to 6 weeks later and is characterized by lower abdominal pain and mild diarrhea. This can progress to malaise, weight loss, and more diffuse pain. Only a minority are febrile, but almost all patients have heme-positive stools. *(Ref. 2, p. 884)*

686. **(A)** In tetanus, an acute onset is usual. The median onset is 7 days, and 90% present within 14 days of injury. The organism is an anaerobic, motile gram-positive rod. It has the ability to survive for years in the form of spores, which are resistant to disinfectants and heat. Tetanus can occur in nonimmunized individuals, or those who have neglected their booster shots. Penicillin is used in treatment, but its efficacy is not clear. *(Ref. 2, p. 633)*

687. **(C)** People with hemophilia are probably exposed to AIDS through the large number of transfusions of pooled plasma products. Pneumocystis carinii pneumonia is a frequent presenting symptom of AIDS. *(Ref. 2, p. 1570)*

688. **(C)** Herpes simplex virus-2 genital infections may be associated with fever, malaise, and anorexia. Vesicular lesions usually ulcerate rapidly and become covered with exudate. *(Ref. 2, p. 78)*

689. **(B)** Mycoplasmas have no cell walls and have filtration characteristics of viruses, but morphologically are closer to bacteria. The typical *Mycoplasma pneumoniae* infection produces an influenza-like respiratory illness characterized by headache, malaise, fever, and cough. If pneumonia occurs, physical exam can be relatively benign despite a grossly abnormal chest x-ray. *(Ref. 2, p. 757)*

690. **(A)** The x-ray shows a silhouette sign indicating right middle lobe pneumonia. The organism is most likely to be pneumococcus, but care must be taken to consider blockage of the right middle lobe bronchus. *(Ref. 2, p. 1185)*

691. **(A)** The cause of cat-scratch fever is thought to be a small gram-negative bacillus. The organism has been assigned the name Afifpia felix. Cats acquire the organism from the soil and inoculate humans via scratches or bites. The disease is generally benign and self-limited, and is treated with analgesics and antipyretics. A variety of antibiotics have been used when immunocompromised patients are affected, but an optimal regime has not been identified. *(Ref. 2, p. 570)*

692. **(A)** Pneumonia is an infrequent complication but accounts for over 90% of measles deaths. Giant cell pneumonia is also seen. This giant cell pneumonia is most commonly seen in children suffering with a severe disease such as leukemia or immunodeficiency. Aerosolized ribavirin has been used to treat severe pneumonia secondary to measles, but its efficacy is still unclear. *(Ref. 2, p. 826)*

693. **(E)** The patient presents with low-grade fever and almost always has a pre-existing organic valvular lesion. *Staphylococcus epidermidis* accounts for about 5% of all cases of subacute endocarditis. *(Ref. 2, p. 615)*

694. **(B)** Otitis media may result from group A infections of the upper respiratory tract, particularly the mastoid after middle ear disease. Of course, many cases of pneumococcal meningitis can develop as a "primary" disease, without obvious evidence of infection elsewhere. Pneumococcal meningitis is treated with 18 to 24 million units of penicillin G daily. All isolates should be tested for sensitivity as reports of pneumococcal resistance are becoming more frequent. *(Ref. 2, p. 609)*

695. (B) *Clostridium* is a rare cause of meningitis, usually secondary to a penetrating injury. Patients with neoplastic disease most commonly have gram-negative infections. *(Ref. 2, p. 639)*

696. (D) *Staphylococcus* is the most common bacterial invader in pulmonary complications of influenza. Pneumonia is the leading cause of death and may also be due to pneumococcus and *H. influenzae*. *(Ref. 2, p. 817)*

697. (E) Horner syndrome. There are about 70 enteroviruses that affect humans. These include polio viruses, coxsackie viruses, echoviruses and others. The spectrum of disease includes paralytic disease, encephalitis, aseptic meningitis, pleurodynia, exanthems, pericarditis, myocarditis, and nonspecific febrile illnesses. They can on occasion cause fulminant disease in the newborn. The most important enteroviruses are the three poliovirus serotypes. *(Ref. 2, pp. 821–822)*

698. (B) Doxycycline, 200 mg on the day of travel, followed by 100 mg daily for three weeks markedly reduced the incidence of diarrhea in Peace Corps volunteers in double-blind studies. Generally prophylactic antibiotics are not recommended. *(Ref. 2, pp. 532–534)*

699. (A) All cases of untreated progressive disseminated histoplasmosis reported to date have been uniformly progressive and fatal. After antifungal treatment, suppressive therapy should be continued indefinitely. Addison's disease can occur in disseminated histoplasmosis, and can cause death. *(Ref. 2, pp. 856–857)*

700. (B) *Histoplasma capsulatum* occurs in yeast cell forms and is ingested by the RE system, where it produces granulomatous reactions. The vast majority of infections are either asymptomatic or mild. Cough, fever, and malaise are the most common symptoms. Hilar adenopathy and pneumonitis can occur on chest x-ray. *(Ref. 2, p. 856)*

701. (A) The incubation period of *C. botulinum* toxin is 18 to 36 hours, but ranges from a few hours to days. There are no sensory symptoms. Food-borne botulinum is associated primarily with home-canned food. Severe food-borne botulinum can produce diplopia, dysarthria, and dysphagia; weakness then can progress rapidly to involve neck, arms, thorax, and legs. There is usually no fever. Nausea, vomiting, and abdominal pain can precede the paralysis or come afterwards. *(Ref. 2, p. 635)*

702. (B) CMV infection is best characterized as unresponsive to antibiotics. In adults, it may be asymptomatic and is not a highly communicable disease. However, in four particular groups, fetuses, organ transplant recipients, bone marrow transplant recipients, and persons with AIDS, the disease can be progressive and cause severe morbidity (e.g., CMV retinitis) or death. There is no treatment for the fetal CMV syndrome, but ganciclovir and/or foscarnet are useful in the other three syndromes. *(Ref. 2, pp. 794–796)*

703. (E) *Coccidioidomycosis* is the usual cause of pulmonary cavitation resulting from fungal infection. A rarefaction may be demonstrable in a pneumonic lesion within 10 days of onset. In the United States, most cases are acquired in California, Arizona, western Texas, and New Mexico. *(Ref. 2, p. 857)*

704. (C) In addition to otitis media, the most common complication of measles, other complications include mastoiditis, pneumonia, bronchitis, encephalitis, and lymphadenitis. The otitis media is usually a bacterial superinfection, and should be treated with antibiotics. *(Ref. 2, p. 826)*

705. (D) Subacute sclerosing panencephalitis causes involuntary spasmodic movements and progressive mental deterioration, frequently ending in death within a year. It usually occurs in children whose measles occurred at an early age (≤ 2 years). It occurs 6 to 8 years after the primary infection. It presents with nonspecific symptoms such as poor school performance or mood and personality changes. It then progresses to intellectual decline, seizures, myoclonus, ataxia, and visual disturbances. Continued deterioration results in inevitable death. *(Ref. 2, p. 2317)*

706. (A) Patients with immune deficiencies or generalized illnesses, pregnant women, infants less than one year old, adults, and all exposed patients should not receive the live rubella vaccine. Patients with immune deficiency secondary to HIV infection may be vaccinated. *(Ref. 2, p. 829)*

707. (C) One-fourth of deaths from influenza are due to pneumonia, with *Staphylococcus*, pneumococcus, and *H. influenzae* the chief organisms. Prophylactic immunization is recommended for those with chronic cardiac or pulmonary (including asthma) disorders, diabetes mellitus, renal disease, hemoglobinopathies or immunosuppression. Individuals over 65 and health care providers are also recommended to receive prophylaxis. *(Ref. 2, p. 817)*

708. (E) Granuloma inguinale is not responsive to amphotericin B. Oral tetracycline, 2 gm daily divided into four doses, is the treatment of choice. The disease is most common in tropical areas and is felt to be sexually transmitted. The early painless ulcer can be mistaken for syphilis. The causative organism is *Calymmatobacterium granulomatis. (Ref. 2, p. 695)*

709. **(C)** The patient is infected with pneumocystis organisms invading an immunocompromised host. The treatment of choice is trimethoprim and sulfamethoxazole, which is equally effective as pentamidine. Co-trimoxazole combines these two drugs. *(Ref. 2, pp. 909–910)*

710. **(A)** Staphylococcal enterotoxin food poisoning is characterized by violent gastrointestinal upset with severe nausea, cramps, vomiting, and diarrhea. *(Ref. 2, p. 533)*

711. **(C)** The patient has tinea capitis, that may be caused by trichophyton or microsporin species. It may be successfully treated with griseofulvin. *(Ref. 2, p. 277)*

712. **(D)** Coxsackie A viruses may cause a number of syndromes, including herpangina, exanthem, aseptic meningitis, common cold, paralysis, pneumonitis, and summer febrile illness. Basophilia in the blood is not seen. *(Ref. 2, p. 824)*

713. **(E)** Rabies is transmitted through the saliva of infected animals. Once clinical signs develop the disease is almost 100% fatal. Symptoms of rabies may include apathy as well as hyperexcitability. *(Ref. 2, p. 833)*

714. **(B)** Epstein–Barr virus may be the causative agent in infectious mononucleosis, but it is unlikely to be the sole agent causing chronic fatigue syndrome. The association with nasopharyngeal carcinoma and Burkitt's lymphoma is strong, but has not been proven to be causative. *(Ref. 2, pp. 790–793)*

715. **(B)** *Coccidioidomycosis* may present with a syndrome of erythema nodosum, fever, and conjunctivitis. Serious complications include cavitating lung lesions or meningitis. *(Ref. 2, p. 857)*

716. **(D)** Cytomegalovirus is probably transmitted in the leukocyte component of transfusions. The syndromes include fever and lymphocytosis. Screening donors for this virus reduces the incidence of transmission. *(Ref. 2, p. 1793)*

717. **(C)** Toxic shock syndrome is most often seen in females using vaginal tampons and is secondary to staphylococcal enterotoxins. Abrupt onset is characteristic. The clinical criteria for diagnosis include high fever, a diffuse rash that desquamates on the palms and soles over the subsequent one to two weeks, hypotension, and in-

volvement in three or more organ systems. This involvement can include GI dysfunction (vomiting and diarrhea), renal insufficiency, hepatic insufficiency, thrombocytopenia, myalgias with elevated CK levels, and delirium. *(Ref. 2, p. 614)*

718. **(A)** Several antibiotic combinations could be used and may vary with the indigenous organisms. An aminoglycoside and a cephalosporin are commonly used in combination. *(Ref. 2, p. 572)*

719. **(A)** The most frequent anaerobic isolates are *Bacteroides* and *Peptostreptococcus*. The most frequent aerobic isolates are *Streptococcus* and *Staphylococcus. (Ref. 2, pp. 702, 1184)*

720. **(D)** Legionnaire's disease is transmitted via infectious aerosols and may cause severe disease characterized by dry cough and fevers. Mild infections and asymptomatic seroconversion also occur. Natural reservoirs for the organisms include streams, hot springs, and stagnant lakes. Amplifiers are man-made water supplies that favor growth of *Legionellae*. Common amplifiers are hot water systems and heat exchange units. *(Ref. 2, pp. 655–656)*

721. **(E)** Figure 10.2 illustrates Hutchinson's teeth, which is a manifestation of late congenital syphilis. This may be associated with cardiovascular and neurologic manifestations as well as "saddle nose" and "saber shins." *(Ref. 2, pp. 731–732)*

722. **(A)** Infective endocarditis in IV drug abusers is usually acute, and caused by *Staphylococcus aureus* infection. The common involvement of the tricuspid valve (> 50% of cases) means that murmurs can be absent and that septic emboli to the lungs causing pulmonary emboli or pneumonia are frequent. *(Ref. 2, pp. 521–522)*

723. **(D)** Aortic valve prostheses are more commonly infected. Janeway lesions, small hemorrhages with a slightly nodular character on the palms and soles, are most commonly seen in acute endocarditis. Large artery emboli are most frequently seen in fungal endocarditis with their large friable vegetations. Roth spots are seen in less than 5% of cases and are also seen in severe anemia and connective tissue disease. These oval, retinal hemorrhages with a clear pale center are therefore neither sensitive nor specific. Mycotic aneurysms occur in only 10% of cases and are generally asymptomatic. Rupture can occur during therapy or even years later. *(Ref. 2. pp. 521–523)*

724. **(B)** As many as 80% of patients with SBP will present with fever. Pre-existing ascites is almost always present, but only 10% of cirrhotics at most will develop SBP. The microbiology is characteristically that of a single organism (*E. coli* most common). Polymicrobial infection should suggest the possibility of secondary peritonitis secondary to a perforation. More than 300 PMNs per microliter of ascitic fluid is said to be diagnostic. (*Ref. 2, pp. 526–527*)

725.   **(C)**   Lyme disease is caused by a spirochete *Borrelia burgdorferi*, a fastidious microaerophilic bacterium. It is a *tick-transmitted* disease, and is not caused by the tick. The incubation period is 3 to 32 days and is associated, initially, with minimal immune response. Perhaps as many as 25% of patients lack the characteristic skin lesion. (*Ref. 2, pp. 745–746*)

726.   **(C)**   In histoplasmosis, oropharyngeal ulcerations begin as solitary indurated plaques with no pain present at first, although eventually pain becomes deep-seated. These oropharyngeal manifestations are usually part of disseminated infection. (*Ref. 2, p. 856*)

727.   **(B)**   In *Coccidioidomycosis*, hemoptysis may call attention to cavitations or patients may complain of pain at the cavity site. Only half of the patients with a thin wall pulmonary cavity secondary to *Coccidioidomycosis* will have symptoms, however. (*Ref. 2, p. 857*)

728.   **(G)**   The intracutaneous tuberculin test with PPD is read for evidence of delayed hypersensitivity at 48 hours. Although induration greater than 10 mm is felt to be positive, interpretation is really dependent on the population being studied. In an HIV-infected patient, any reaction should be considered significant. When testing households contacts, greater than 5 mm is probably enough to warrant prophylactic treatment. (*Ref. 2, pp. 714–715*)

729.   **(A)**   Brucellosis is prevalent in midwestern hog-raising states, in Texas, and in California. Transmission is by contact of *Brucella* organisms with abraded skin, through the conjunctiva or by inhalation. Person-to-person transmission is rare or nonexistent. The disease can be acute, localized, or chronic. It requires prolonged antibiotic treatment with doxycycline or tetracycline. Streptomycin is usually added for the first two weeks. (*Ref. 2, p. 685*)

730.   **(H)**   Tularemia can be acquired through direct contact with an infected rabbit, which may occur in preparation or cooking inadequately. The incubation period is 2 to 5 days and the syndrome includes fevers, chills, headaches, myalgias, and tender hepatosplenomegaly. In addition, specific

syndromes such as ulceroglandular, or oculoglandular, tularemia can accompany the nonspecific syndrome. (*Ref. 2, p. 687*)

731.   **(C)**   On dark field examination, *Treponema pallidum* (the spirochete that causes syphilis) is a thin, delicate organism with tapering ends and 6 to 14 spirals. (*Ref. 2, p. 732*)

732.   **(A)**   Congenital toxoplasmosis is initiated in utero usually as a complication of a primary infection. Infants are usually asymptomatic at birth but later can present with a multitude of signs and symptoms, including chorioretinitis, strabismus, epilepsy and psychomotor retardation. (*Ref. 2, p. 904*)

733.   **(G)**   Salmonellosis is an acute infection resulting from ingestion of food containing bacteria and is characterized by abdominal pain and diarrhea. *Salmonella* gastroenteritis is not usually treated with antibiotics because the length of the illness is not shortened but the length of time the organism is carried is increased. Antibiotics are used for more serious systemic *Salmonella* infections. (*Ref. 2, p. 675*)

734.   **(F)**   Preventive measures are not used as smallpox is thought to be eradicated worldwide, and vaccination may be associated with serious side effects. As humans are the only reservoir for smallpox, there is no longer any risk of infection. (*Ref. 2, p. 798*)

735.   **(B)**   Patients with tetanus develop hypertonus, seizures, respiratory distress, and asphyxia unless they are treated with muscle relaxants. The treatment of tetanus requires muscle relaxants, antitoxin, respiratory care, and managing autonomic dysfunction. Antibiotics are given, but are probably of little help. (*Ref. 2, p. 633*)

736.   **(C)**   Infectious mononucleosis is an acute, self-limited infection of the lymphatic system, probably by the Epstein–Barr (EB) virus. Typical infectious mononucleosis has an incubation period of four to eight weeks. The prodrome includes malaise, anorexia, and chills, and then the classic symptoms of pharyngitis, fever, and lymphadenopathy develop. Headache is also common. (*Ref. 2, p. 791*)

737.   **(D)**   The presence of IgG antibodies by the indirect immunofluorescence test indicates recent or prior EB virus infection. IgM antibodies indicate recent infection only. Heterophil antibodies are present in 50% of children and 90 to 95% of adolescents and adults with infectious mononucleosis. Mono spot tests are the best diagnostic tools but may not turn positive until the second or third week of the illness. Specific EB virus anti-bodies and cultures are rarely used. *(Ref. 2, p. 792)*

738. **(B)** Adequate rest is the treatment of choice, but forced bed rest is not necessary. Glucocorticoids hasten defervescence and resolution of pharyngitis, but are not routinely used. Acyclovir halts oropharyngeal shedding of EB virus but has minimal effect on the clinical disease. Similarly α-interferon and ganciclovir have antiviral efficacy, but have no role to play in uncomplicated infectious mononucleosis. Antibiotics are not helpful, and ampicillin is likely to cause a pruritic maculopapular rash in most patients. *(Ref. 2, p. 791)*

739. **(E)** Hemorrhage is not a usual complication of infectious mononucleosis. Over 90% of cases are benign and uncomplicated, but liver involvement is clinical in 5 to 10%. Splenic rupture occurs during the second or third week of the illness and can be insidious or abrupt in presentation. Surgery is required. Over 85% of EB virus-associated neurologic problems resolve spontaneously. Although hemorrhage does not occur, autoimmune hemolytic anemia can occur. It is usually mediated by IgM antibodies with anti-i specificity. *(Ref. 2, p. 792)*

740. **(C)** Herpes zoster is not a manifestation of infectious mononucleosis. Neurologic manifestations include meningitis and encephalitis in 1 to 2% of cases. *(Ref. 2, p. 792)*

741. **(E)** Mumps is an acute communicable infection with localized swelling of one or more salivary glands. At times, gonads, meninges, pancreas, and other organs can be involved. Up to 25% of infections are inapparent clinically. The virus is transmitted in saliva, but is also found in urine, and this might be another source of transmission. *(Ref. 2, p. 830)*

742. **(B)** Pain referring to either or both lower quadrants is common when oophoritis is present. Fever usually accompanies oophoritis. Sterility is not a consequence of mumps oophoritis. *(Ref. 2, p. 831)*

743. **(C)** Complement fixation tests are run on specimens drawn as soon after onset as possible and then at the end of the third week. Of course, a typical presentation during an epidemic probably does not require any confirmatory tests. Sporadic cases require more active confirmation. Other causes of parotitis requiring specific treatment include calculi, bacterial infections, and drugs. Tumors, sarcoid, tuberculosis, leukemia, Hodgkin's disease, Sjögren's syndrome and lupus

erythematosus can also cause parotid enlargement. *(Ref. 2, p. 831)*

744. **(A)** Antibiotics, sulfas, steroids, and mumps convalescent sera are of no value. Mouth care, analgesics, and a bland diet are usually recommended. Glucocorticoids are usually prescribed for orchitis, although definite evidence of their effectiveness is lacking. Prevention via vaccination is the preferred strategy for mumps. *(Ref. 2, p. 832)*

745. **(E)** Serum amylase is elevated in 96% of cases because of parotitis, not pancreatitis. Other complications include thyroiditis, myocarditis, and polyarthritis. *(Ref. 2, p. 831)*

746. **(E)** Cytotoxic chemotherapy frequently results in neutropenia and subsequently gram-negative bacillary infection. *Pseudomonas*, staphylococcal, *Candida*, and *Aspergillus* infections are also common. *(Ref. 2, pp. 496–497)*

747. **(D)** Selective IgA deficiency predisposes to *Giardia lamblia* infection, hepatitis virus, and *Streptococcus pneumoniae*. *Hemophilus influenzae* infection occurs, but this is not as characteristic as *Giardia*. *(Ref. 2, pp. 496–497)*

748. **(I)** Defects in the alternate pathway of complement (e.g., sickle cell disease) predispose to *Salmonella* infections. *(Ref. 2, pp. 496–497)*

749. **(B)** All forms of T lymphocyte deficiency/dysfunction are characterized by candidal infections. Pneumocystis infections are of course particularly common in AIDS. *(Ref. 2, pp. 496–497)*

750. **(A)** Microbicidal defects (chronic granulomatous disease, Chédiak–Higashi disease) predispose to staphylococcal infections. *(Ref. 2, pp. 496–497)*

751. **(A)** The preformed toxin of *Staphylococcus* causes nausea within 1 to 6 hours of ingestion. Ham, poultry, potato and egg salad, mayonnaise, and cream pastries are common food sources. *(Ref. 2, p. 533)*

752. **(D)** Enterotoxigenic *E. coli* causes 15 to 50% of travelers' diarrhea, depending on geographical location. The incubation period is > 16 hours, and water and many foods can be the source. *(Ref. 2, p. 532)*

753. **(F)** *Shigella* causes an invasive diarrhea with blood with an incubation period greater than 16 hours. Potato and egg salad, lettuce, and raw vegetables are common food sources. *(Ref. 2, p. 533)*

754. **(C)** *Vibro cholerae* cause profuse watery diarrhea with an incubation period > 16 hours. Shellfish are a common source. *(Ref. 2, pp. 532–533)*

755. **(H)** Bacillus cereus causes an early onset of food poisoning when found in fried rice. This occurs within 1 to 6 hours and like staphylococcal food poisoning is characterized by vomiting. The enteric form of bacillus cereus food poisoning is characterized by watery diarrhea and occurs 8 to 16 hours after ingestion of contaminated food such as meat, vegetable, dried beans, or cereals. *(Ref. 2, p. 533)*

756. **(B)** Septic arthritis usually presents as a monoarticular arthritis with a predilection for large weight-bearing joints. After the initial diffuse tenosynovitis and arthralgia stage disseminated gonococcal infection (DGI) can localize to one or more joints. *(Ref. 2, pp. 555–556)*

757. **(A)** Gonococcal arthritis is characterized by vesiculopustular skin lesion. *(Ref. 2, p. 556)*

758. **(A)** Gonococcal arthritis frequently involves interphalangeal joints, whereas other septic arthritides rarely do, except for mycobacterial infections. *(Ref. 2, pp. 555–556)*

759. **(B)** The majority of synovial cultures in gonococcal arthritis are negative, whereas they are frequently positive in nongonococcal disease. *(Ref. 2, pp. 555–556)*

760. **(D)** The presence of mucocutaneous lesions suggests Reiter syndrome. *(Ref. 2, p. 556)*

761. **(D)** Although *C. trachomatis* and *N. gonorrhoeae* are the most common causes of acute epididymitis in young men, gram-negative bacilli or other urinary pathogens are the most common causes in older men, or following instrumentation. *(Ref. 2, p. 536)*

762. **(D)** The bacteria causing vulvovaginitis are not well characterized but probably include *G. vaginalis, Mycoplasma hominis* and several anaerobic bacteria. As well, yeasts (e.g., *Candida albicans*) and *Trichomonas vaginalis* can cause the syndrome. *(Ref. 2, p. 538)*

763. **(B)** The lymphogranuloma venereum (LGV) strains of *C. trachomatis* are rare in North America. *(Ref. 2, pp. 536, 541)*

764. **(C)** Mucopurulent cervicitis is a common syndrome in both *N. gonorrhoeae* and *C. trachomatis* infection. *(Ref. 2, p. 540)*

765. **(A)** Presence of typical gram-negative diplococci within neutrophils confirms the diagnosis of gonococcal infection. There are no characteristic Gram-stain findings for *C. trachomatis,* and it makes up less than half the cases of nongonococcal urethritis. *(Ref. 2, p. 536)*

766. **(D)** Sulfonamides and trimethoprim competitively inhibit enzymes involved in folic acid biosynthesis. *(Ref. 2, p. 594)*

767. **(E)** Ciprofloxacin, rifampin, and metronidazole inhibit DNA synthesis, albeit by different mechanisms. *(Ref. 2, p. 594)*

768. **(A)** Beta lactams can be inactivated by beta lactamase. *(Ref. 2, p. 594)*

769. **(C)** Macrolides (erythromycin), lincosamides (clindamycin), and chloramphenicol inhibit protein synthesis by binding to the 50S ribosomal subunit. Tetracyclines and aminoglycosides inhibit protein synthesis by binding to the 30S ribosomal subunit. *(Ref. 2, p. 594)*

770. **(E)** Some gram-negative bacteria acquire mutations in their outer-membrane pori so they are no longer permeable to ciprofloxacin. Some gram-positive bacteria develop a mutation that allows them to actively pump the drug out. The most common form of resistance however, is a mutation in the DNA gyrase, which is the target of ciprofloxacin action. *(Ref. 2, p. 596)*

771. **(F)** Rifampin is an excellent inducer of many cytochrome P450 enzymes and increases the hepatic clearance of a number of drugs including oral contraceptives. *(Ref. 2, p. 605)*

772. **(D)** Sulfonamides potentiate the effects of oral hypoglycemics through reduction in metabolism or displacement from serum protein. *(Ref. 2, p. 605)*

773. **(E)** Metronidazole can cause a disulfiram-like syndrome when alcohol is ingested. Instructions to avoid alcohol should be given when this drug is prescribed. *(Ref. 2, p. 605)*

774. **(F)** Rifampin's enzyme induction properties can result in increased metabolism of cyclosporin with resultant organ rejection. In contrast, erythromycin inhibits the enzyme involved in cyclosporin metabolism and can result in enhanced toxicity. *(Ref. 2, pp. 604–605)*

775. **(D)** Sulfonamides may potentiate the effects of phenytoin through reduction in metabolism or displacement from serum protein. *(Ref. 2, p. 605)*

776. (B) Tracheobronchitis is the most common manifestation of *Mycoplasma pneumoniae* infection, whereas pneumonia is the most common form of pneumococcal infection. *(Ref. 2, pp. 608, 758)*

777. (A) Neutrophilia is characteristic in pneumococcal infection, but the white blood count and differential are usually normal in *M. pneumoniae* infections. *(Ref. 2, pp. 609, 758)*

778. (B) *M. pneumoniae* frequently causes a maculopapular rash in children and has been associated with erythema multiforme and the Stevens–Johnson syndrome. *(Ref. 2, p. 758)*

779. (A) About 75% of patients with pneumococcal pneumonia will develop pleuritic chest pain. *(Ref. 2, p. 608)*

780. (A) The onset of a single sudden shaking chill in more than 80% of cases and a rapid rise in temperature allow many patients to state the exact hour that illness began with *Streptococcus pneumoniae*. *(Ref. 2, p. 608)*

781. (C) A pinkish or "rusty" mucoid sputum is an early symptom of pneumococcal pneumonia. The cough of *M. pneumoniae* is initially nonproductive, but a cough productive of mucoid or mucopurulent sputum may gradually develop. *(Ref. 2, pp. 608, 758)*

782. (D) High fever (39.2 to 40.5°C) is a characteristic of pneumococcal pneumonia. Low-grade fever (rarely exceeding 38.9°C) is the most common physical finding in *M. pneumoniae* infection. *(Ref. 2, pp. 608, 758)*

Immunology and Allergy
Questions

783. Laboratory findings in serum sickness may include all of the following EXCEPT

    (A) circulating immune complexes
    (B) albuminuria
    (C) casts in the urine
    (D) rapid sedimentation rate
    (E) eosinophilia

784. Delayed hypersensitivity reactions are characterized by

    (A) possible transference to another individual by means of serum injections
    (B) absence of serum antibody
    (C) effect primarily on smooth muscle
    (D) presence of high titers of circulating antibody
    (E) severe life-threatening reactions

785. Large granular lymphoid cells that are mediators of antibody-dependent cellular cytotoxicity are known as

    (A) macrophages
    (B) natural killer cells
    (C) T lymphocytes, suppressor subset
    (D) B lymphocytes
    (E) granulocytes

786. Patients with hay fever

    (A) may develop asthma
    (B) are not improved by moving to different locations
    (C) are not more prone to develop upper respiratory infections
    (D) are severely disturbed emotionally
    (E) can be improved symptomatically only with steroids

787. In deaths from the hereditary form of angioneurotic edema, death is usually

    (A) not related to the allergy
    (B) an anaphylactic shock reaction
    (C) from edema of the glottis
    (D) caused by over-treatment
    (E) related to stress

788. The peripheral blood cell counts in acquired immune deficiency syndrome are best characterized by

    (A) granulocytosis
    (B) lymphopenia
    (C) increased helper T cells
    (D) monocytosis
    (E) decreased natural killer cells

789. A 30-year-old woman with myasthenia gravis is found to have an autoimmune hemolytic anemia. Chest x-ray reveals an anterior mediastinal mass. The most likely diagnosis is

    (A) thymoma
    (B) nodular sclerosing Hodgkin's disease
    (C) small cleaved cell nonHodgkin's lymphoma
    (D) teratoma
    (E) bronchogenic carcinoma, small cell undifferentiated type

790. Autoantibodies to basement membranes have been well demonstrated to play a role in the pathogenesis of

    (A) thyroiditis
    (B) myasthenia gravis
    (C) Goodpasture syndrome
    (D) thrombocytopenia
    (E) hemolytic anemia

791. Antigen–antibody complex disease may play a part in the pathogenesis of renal disease in all of the following EXCEPT

    (A) acute tubular necrosis
    (B) systemic lupus erythematosus
    (C) bacterial endocarditis
    (D) chronic glomerulonephritis
    (E) mixed cryoglobulin syndromes

792. Proper therapy for a systemic reaction following the subcutaneous injection of an allergen should include

    (A) discontinuation of subsequent injections for three weeks
    (B) application of a tourniquet distal to the injection site
    (C) administration of steroids prior to the next injection
    (D) administration of aminophylline subcutaneously
    (E) administration of epinephrine (1:1000) subcutaneously

793. Significant factors in the pathophysiology of asthma include all of the following EXCEPT

    (A) acute peribronchiolar inflammation
    (B) swelling of bronchiolar mucosa
    (C) narrowing of the lumen by thick sputum
    (D) subacute bronchiolar inflammation
    (E) microthrombi in the pulmonary capillary bed

794. All of the following represent allergens that may be responsible for extrinsic asthma EXCEPT

    (A) inhaled organic dusts
    (B) house dusts
    (C) chocolate
    (D) high-molecular-weight drugs
    (E) shellfish

795. Which of the following is characteristic of serum sickness?

    (A) usually requires corticosteroids
    (B) symptoms last several months
    (C) may recur after apparent recovery
    (D) may be transferred by leukocyte infusions
    (E) most patients are children

796. In a patient with suspected immunodeficiency secondary to impaired T-cell function the most cost-effective screening test is

    (A) quantification of serum IgA
    (B) lymphocyte enumeration on a cell sorter
    (C) lymphocyte responses to mitogens
    (D) nitroblue tetrazolium assay
    (E) intradermal skin test with *Candida albicans* extract

797. All the following statements about urticaria are true EXCEPT

    (A) is most common on the palms and soles
    (B) is associated with increased blood flow
    (C) is generally itchy
    (D) is caused by an ongoing immediate hypersensitivity
    (E) the lesions blanch on pressure

798. A 27-year-old man develops small (several millimeters) pruritic wheals when he goes jogging and when he takes very hot showers. Management will include

    (A) discontinuation of all vigorous exercises
    (B) counseling regarding recognition and treatment of anaphylactic reactions
    (C) treatment with anticholinergic medications
    (D) treatment with hydroxyzine
    (E) cool baths rather than hot showers

799. Angioedema is characterized by

    (A) invariably severe itching
    (B) prolonged nature of the edema
    (C) fluid extravasation from subcutaneous and intradermal postcapillary venules
    (D) involvement of lips, tongue, eyelids, genitalia, and dorsum of hands or feet
    (E) fluid accumulation in the most dependent areas of the body

800. The following have all been implicated in anaphylactic reactions EXCEPT

    (A) hymenoptera venom
    (B) nuts
    (C) radiographic contrast media
    (D) penicillin
    (E) horse serum

801. All the following statements concerning drug allergy are true EXCEPT

    (A) multiple courses of treatment increases the likelihood of allergy
    (B) parenteral administration is the most likely cause of sensitization
    (C) parenteral administration causes the most severe drug allergies
    (D) genetic factors in drug metabolism influence the likelihood of allergy
    (E) men are less frequently affected than women

802. Penicillin allergy can be characterized by all the following EXCEPT

(A) interstitial nephritis

(B) IgG reactions

(C) availability of reliable tests for predicting immediate penicillin allergy

(D) asthma

(E) invariable reactions to cephalosporins when true penicillin allergy is present

803. Which of the following statements concerning the life cycle of the human immunodeficiency virus, (HIV-1) is correct?

(A) the virus preferentially attacks killer T cells

(B) after infection is established, there is a latent period of little or no viral replication, during which the patient remains asymptomatic

(C) surface expression of CD8 molecule is required before the virus can infect a lymphocyte

(D) cytomegalovirus (CMV) infection may increase virus production by infected cells

(E) after a cell is infected, viral DNA can be directly integrated into the host cell's DNA

804. All of the following statements concerning HIV-induced immunosuppression are correct EXCEPT

(A) qualitative defects in T-lymphocytes precede quantitative problems

(B) the low CD4 count in advanced disease is secondary to the direct cytotoxic effects of virus infection

(C) B-lymphocyte abnormalities can occur early in the disease

(D) macrophages are important in viral dissemination

(E) circulating immune complexes are invariably present

DIRECTIONS (Questions 805 through 811): Match the following diseases with the appropriate HLA antigen

(A) HLA B27

(B) HLA DR4

(C) HLA DR3

(D) HLA B17

(E) HLA B8

805. Ankylosing spondylitis

806. Lupus erythematosus (S.L.E.)

807. Juvenile rheumatoid arthritis

808. Insulin-dependent diabetes mellitus

809. Reiter's syndrome

810. Rheumatoid arthritis

811. Reactive arthritis (yersinia)

DIRECTIONS (Questions 812 through 817): Each question below lists a defect in inflammatory or immunologic response. For each question select the ONE lettered heading that is most closely associated with it. Each lettered heading may be selected once, more than once, or not at all.

(A) B cell deficiency/dysfunction

(B) mixed T and B cell deficiency/dysfunction

(C) T-lymphocyte deficiency/dysfunction

(D) neutropenia

(E) chemotaxis

(F) C_3 deficiency (complement 3)

812. Multiple myeloma

813. Hodgkin's disease

814. Chronic lymphocytic leukemia

815. Systemic lupus erythematous

816. Hematologic malignancies

817. Ataxia–telangiectasia

Immunology and Allergy
Answers and Explanations

783. **(E)** Leukocytosis and circulating plasma cells may be seen, but eosinophilia is uncommon. Drug hypersensitivity is the most common cause of serum sickness. It is felt that the drug acts as a hapten binding to a plasma protein. The resultant drug–protein complex induces an immune response. Common signs and symptoms include fever, skin rash (urticarial or morbilliform), arthralgias, lymphadenopathy and albuminuria. Arthritis, nephritis, neuropathy, and vasculitis are less common. Primary sensitization requires 1 to 3 weeks, but symptoms can occur rapidly on re-exposure. *(Ref. 2, p. 1641)*

784. **(B)** Delayed hypersensitivity is a reaction of T cells, which have been stimulated by antigen to react against infectious agents, grafts, and tumors. They occur 48 to 72 hours after antigen exposure. A classic example is the response to the tuberculin skin test in a person previously exposed to *M. tuberculosis* organisms. *(Ref. 2, pp. 1557–1558)*

785. **(B)** Natural killer cells may be of T cell lineage or monocyte–macrophage lineage. They appear to play an important role in surveillance mechanisms. *(Ref. 2, pp. 1545–1546)*

786. **(A)** Allergic asthma is often associated with a personal and/or family history of allergic diseases. It is dependent on an IgE response controlled by T- and B-lymphocytes and activated when antigens interact with mast cell-bound IgE molecules. Most provoking allergens are airborne. Allergic asthma can be seasonal. *(Ref. 2, p. 1167)*

787. **(C)** In hereditary and angioneurotic edema, the lesions are tense, rounded, nonpitting, and several centimeters in diameter. Edema of the glottis is the usual cause of death. *(Ref. 2, pp. 1634–1636)*

788. **(B)** The acquired immune deficiency syndrome is characterized by lymphopenia, with a selective diminution of helper T cells. Likely infectious complications and their appropriate prophylaxis can be predicted by the CD4+ T-lymphocyte count. Lymphocyte dysfunction can occur even when severe lymphopenia is not yet present. *(Ref. 2, p. 1577)*

789. **(A)** Thymic tumors may be associated with myasthenia gravis, red cell aplasia, polymyositis, hemolytic anemia, pemphigus, and agranulocytosis. There is also an association with immunodeficiency and thymoma. These patients have B-lymphocyte deficiency and have bacterial infections and diarrhea. Erythroid aplasia may develop as well. *(Ref. 2, pp. 286, 1565, 1879)*

790. **(C)** Autoantibodies can be demonstrated by immunofluorescence or electron microscopy on the basement membranes of glomeruli and alveoli in Goodpasture syndrome. The disease is most common in young men, but can strike at any age. The hemoptysis can be minimal or massive. The course of the hemoptysis is variable, but renal involvement is often progressive. Current therapy includes intensive plasma exchange, cytotoxic agents, and glucocorticoids. Other causes of lung–renal syndromes such as various vasculitides, Wegener's granulomatosis, mixed essential cryoglobulinemia, Henoch–Schönlein purpura, and SLE are not characterized by antibodies to basement membranes. *(Ref. 2, p. 1309)*

791. **(A)** Acute tubular necrosis is usually the result of an ischemic insult such as hypovolemia, low cardiac output, renal vasoconstriction, or systemic vasodilation. The other common cause is toxins. Exogenous toxins includes x-ray contrast material, cyclosporin, antibiotics (e.g., aminoglycosides), chemotherapeutic agents (e.g., cisplatin), ethylene glycol, and acetaminophen. Intrinsic toxins include myoglobin (in rhabdomyolysis), hemoglobin (hemolysis), uric acid, oxalate, and abnormal proteins (e.g., multiple myeloma). *(Ref. 2, p. 1266)*

792. (E) These systemic reactions are uncommon and easily managed in the office if detected, but if the patient leaves too soon, it could be dangerous. The exact mechanism of benefit for hyposensitization therapy is unclear. One hypothesis is that the stimulation of IgG antibody production results in reduction or neutralization of the amount of allergen available for interaction with tissue mast cells. This type of therapy is reserved for clearly seasonal diseases that cannot be adequately managed with drugs. *(Ref. 2, p. 1638)*

793. (E) There is a constant state of hyperreactivity of the bronchi, during which exposure to an irritant precipitates an asthmatic attack. A following subacute phase has been described that can lead to late complications. The presence of inflammation in the airways has resulted in increased usage of inhaled corticosteroids for maintenance therapy. *(Ref. 2, p. 1167)*

794. (D) Low-molecular-weight drugs rather than high-molecular-weight drugs may lead to asthma by acting as haptens in antigen–antibody reactions. Examples include aspirin, tartrazine, and sulphating agents. Tartrazine is a coloring agent that is widely present in the environment. Sulphating agents are also frequently encountered as they are used as sanitizing and preserving agents (e.g., in salad bars). Aspirin-sensitive individuals may react to many other nonsteroidal anti-inflammatory drugs. *(Ref. 2, p. 1168)*

795. (C) The symptoms of serum sickness are usually self-limited and may recur after apparent recovery. The natural course is 1 to 3 weeks. Recurrence can occur rapidly (12 to 36 hours) if repeat exposure to the offending antigen occurs. *(Ref. 2, p. 1641)*

796. (E) A positive skin test with *Candida albicans* extract (erythema and induration of 10 mm or more at 48 hr) excludes virtually all primary T-cell defects. Lymphocyte enumeration and responses to mitogens are much costlier tests. Serum IgA levels are a good screening test for agammaglobulinemia and the nitroblue tetrazolium assay is useful to detect killing defects of phagocyte cells. *(Ref. 1, p. 1449)*

797. (A) Although urticaria can involve any epidermal or mucosal surface, the palms and soles are usually spared. The associated itching indicates stimulation of nociceptive nerves. The increased blood flow results in erythema that blanches on pressure. An ongoing, immediate, hypersensitivity reaction in association with degranulation of mast cells is the most common cause. *(Ref. 1, p. 1453)*

798. (D) This represents a case of generalized heat urticaria or cholinergic urticaria rather than exercise-induced urticaria. The latter is characterized by larger lesions, possible anaphylactic reactions and is not triggered by hot showers. Although thought to be cholinergically mediated, atropine does not block symptoms in generalized heat urticaria. Because anaphylaxis does not occur, and hydroxyzine is so effective, hot showers are not a great danger. *(Ref. 1, p. 1455)*

799. (D) Angioedema is often not itchy, and like urticaria is transient; manifestation peaks in minutes to hours and disappears over hours to days. The fluid extravasates from deeper areas such as dermal and subdermal sites. Unlike other causes of edema, angioedema is not dependent and can involve all epidermal and submucosal surfaces, although the above-mentioned areas are the most common. *(Ref. 1, pp. 1453–1456)*

800. (C) Anaphylaxis is characterized by an initial exposure followed by the formation of specific IgE antibody. Repeat exposure results in antigen combining with IgE bound to basophils and mast cells and subsequent degranulation. Anaphylactoid reactions such as those to radiographic contrast media are generally not immune-mediated and do not require prior exposure. *(Ref. 1, pp. 1462–1463)*

801. (B) Although parenteral administration results in the most severe reactions, topical administration is the most likely to sensitize. Multiple courses of treatment increase the chances of reactions. As reactions often occur to metabolites rather than the parent drug, genetic factors can influence the likelihood of reactions (for example procainamide-induced systemic lupus erythematosus). Children and men have fewer reactions than women. *(Ref. 1, p. 1479)*

802. (E) Penicillin can cause numerous reactions including anaphylaxis, interstitial nephritis, rashes, urticaria, fever, pneumonitis, dermatitis, and even asthma in workers exposed to airborne penicillin. Hemolytic anemia is often IgG-mediated. Skin tests are reliable in predicting low risk (similar to general population) for those claiming previous penicillin reactions. The frequency of reactions to cephalosporins in penicillin-allergic patients is not definitely known. *(Ref. 1, p. 1482)*

803. (D) Infection with CMV, Epstein–Barr virus, human herpes virus VI, and others increases in vitro viral production. HIV-I is a retrovirus and requires the action of reverse transcriptase to transcribe viral RNA into DNA before it can be incorporated into the host cell DNA. HIV-I preferentially attacks helper–inducer lymphocytes which express the CD4 molecule on their surface. There seems to be no latent period once a cell is infected. *(Ref. 1, pp. 1908–1909)*

804. **(B)** Even in advanced disease only a minority of CD4 lymphocytes are actually infected. Numerous other factors, including "innocent bystander destruction" and autoimmune phenomena, might be implicated. Impaired soluble antigen recognition by T-lymphocytes can occur when absolute counts are still normal. Polyclonal activation of B cells, which occurs early in the disease, is unlikely to be triggered by direct HIV infection of B cells. Macrophages are felt to be particularly important in carrying the virus across the blood–brain barrier. Circulating immune complexes might help explain arthralgias, myalgias, renal disease, and vasculitis that occurs in infected individuals. *(Ref. 1, pp. 1909–1910)*

805. **(A)** **806.** **(C)** **807.** **(B)** **808.** **(C)** **809.** **(A)** **810.** **(B).** **811.** **(A)** The relationship between HLA antigens and diseases is not absolute, but rather one of increased relative risk. The pres-

ence of HLA B27 increased the relative risk of ankylosing spondylitis by a factor of 82, of Reiter syndrome by a factor of 40, and reactive arthritis by a factor of approximately 18. The presence of HLA DR4 increased the likelihood of juvenile rheumatoid arthritis by a factor of 7 and rheumatoid arthritis by a factor of 6. The presence of HLA DR3 increased the likelihood of both SLE and insulin-dependent diabetes mellitus by a factor of approximately 3. *(Ref. 1, p. 1478)*

812. **(A)** **813.** **(C)** **814.** **(A)** **815.** **(F)** **816.** **(D)** **817.** **(B)** Multiple myeloma and chronic lymphocytic leukemia are two of the more common causes of B cell deficiency/dysfunction. Hodgkin's disease, acquired immunodeficiency syndrome, sarcoidosis, and thymic aplasia or hypoplasia result in T-lymphocyte depletion/dysfunction. SLE has been associated with C3 deficiency but most severe complement deficiencies result from inherited disorders. Ataxia–telangiectasia, common variable hypogammaglobulinemia, severe combined immunodeficiency, and Wiskott–Aldrich syndrome have mixed T and B cell deficiency

CHAPTER 12

Diseases of the Respiratory System
Questions

DIRECTIONS (Questions 818 through 849): Each of the questions or incomplete statements below is followed by five suggested answers or completions. Select the ONE that is best in each case.

818. In primary pulmonary hypertension the disease process involves

    (A) pathology that varies with patient age
    (B) large pulmonary arteries
    (C) pulmonary capillaries predominantly
    (D) fibrosis of the alveolar wall
    (E) organic cardiac disease

819. Management of aspiration pneumonia includes all of the following EXCEPT

    (A) antibiotics
    (B) steroids
    (C) oxygen
    (D) sedation
    (E) bronchoscopy

820. Most lung abscesses are likely to contain

    (A) oropharyngeal flora
    (B) *Nocardia*
    (C) *Staphylococcus aureus*
    (D) *Pseudomonas aeruginosa*
    (E) *Candida albicans*

821. Which one of the following is characteristic of farmer's lung?

    (A) symptoms appear a few days after exposure
    (B) it is caused by exposure to oxides of nitrogen
    (C) it is usually followed by complete recovery
    (D) it usually progresses to diffuse fibrosis
    (E) it usually progresses to diffuse obstructive emphysema

822. Etiologic studies indicate that obstructive pulmonary emphysema is usually

    (A) caused by bronchial asthma
    (B) preceded by bronchitis
    (C) due to childhood mucoviscidosis

    (D) due to elastic tissue degeneration
    (E) a forerunner of pulmonary carcinoma

823. Treatment for severe or prolonged attacks of asthma requiring hospitalization should avoid

    (A) theophylline
    (B) sedatives
    (C) corticosteroids
    (D) sympathomimetic amines
    (E) intravenous fluids

824. The syndrome of carbon dioxide narcosis

    (A) occurs only with CO_2 inhalation
    (B) does not occur in obstructive lung disease
    (C) does not occur in restrictive lung disease
    (D) may worsen with oxygen administration
    (E) occurs with chronic hypocapnia

825. Pulmonary embolism may be ruled out in the presence of a normal

    (A) chest x-ray
    (B) electrocardiogram
    (C) perfusion lung scan
    (D) CT scan
    (E) magnetic resonance image

826. Pulmonary infiltrates with eosinophilia are seen in all of the following EXCEPT

    (A) ascaris infestation
    (B) malaria
    (C) allergic granulomatosis of Churg and Strauss
    (D) bronchial asthma
    (E) penicillin sensitivity

827. Hypercapnia at rest in most individuals is most indicative of

    (A) ventilation–perfusion ratio inequality
    (B) right-to-left shunt
    (C) impaired diffusion
    (D) hypoventilation
    (E) carbon monoxide poisoning

828. The emphysematous type of chronic obstructive pulmonary disease (COPD) usually demonstrates

(A) copious, purulent sputum
(B) early cor pulmonale
(C) decreased total lung capacity
(D) normal or low arterial P_{CO_2}
(E) normal diffusing capacity

829. The most common primary posterior mediastinal tumor is

(A) lipoma
(B) neurogenic tumor
(C) esophageal cyst
(D) fibroma
(E) bronchogenic cyst

830. Familial emphysema may be associated with

(A) α_{-1}-antitrypsin deficiency
(B) β-glycosidase deficiency
(C) glucose-6-phosphatase deficiency
(D) glucocerebrosides deficiency
(E) growth hormone deficiency

831. Pulmonary features of ankylosing spondylitis can include

(A) fibrocavitary disease
(B) air flow obstruction
(C) bilateral lower lobe involvement
(D) pleural effusions
(E) hilar adenopathy

832. A patient with hypoxemia, hypercapnia, and polycythemia is able to restore his blood gases to normal by voluntary hyperventilation. The primary pathology is likely to be located in the

(A) cerebral cortex
(B) bone marrow
(C) ventricular septum
(D) medullary respiratory center
(E) cerebellum

833. Intrinsic asthma is usually characterized by all of the following EXCEPT

(A) begins with antigenic stimulus
(B) onset usually in adults
(C) other allergies are uncommon
(D) immediate skin test negative
(E) IgE levels normal or low

834. All of the following systemic syndromes are associated with lung cancer EXCEPT

(A) inappropriate ADH secretion
(B) acanthosis nigricans
(C) Cushing syndrome
(D) leukemoid reaction
(E) Stevens–Johnson syndrome

835. Carbon dioxide retention is commonly seen in

(A) impaired diffusion syndromes
(B) right-to-left shunt
(C) hyperventilation
(D) ventilation–perfusion ratio inequality
(E) mechanical ventilation at fixed volume

836. Interstitial lung disease is associated with treatment involving all of the following EXCEPT

(A) bleomycin
(B) diazepam
(C) hydralazine
(D) busulfan
(E) cyclophosphamide

837. Symptoms of acute pulmonary thromboembolism include all of the following EXCEPT

(A) dyspnea
(B) seizures
(C) syncope
(D) substernal pressure
(E) palpitations

838. Prolonged hyperventilation syndrome may be associated with all of the following EXCEPT

(A) hyperkalemia
(B) parasthesias
(C) low bicarbonate
(D) tetany
(E) palpitations

839. Adult respiratory distress syndrome may be characterized by

(A) increased compliance
(B) responsiveness to antibiotics
(C) intrapulmonary shunting
(D) consolidation pattern on x-ray
(E) decreased ventilatory dead space

840. The treatment of chronic airway obstruction includes

(A) long-term steroids
(B) calorie reduction

(C) intravenous aminophylline

(D) antibiotics for infection

(E) α-adrenergic blockage

841. Mediastinal emphysema is most likely to be caused by

(A) apical tuberculosis

(B) pericarditis

(C) tension pneumothorax

(D) Hodgkin's disease

(E) aspergillosis

842. Cystic fibrosis in the adult patient is most likely to be associated with

(A) spontaneous remission

(B) good pancreatic exocrine function

(C) hemoptysis

(D) rectal polyps

(E) normal sweat chloride

843. Hypoxemia while receiving 100% oxygen indicates

(A) ventilation–perfusion ratio inequality

(B) right-to-left shunt

(C) hypoventilation

(D) impaired diffusion

(E) interstitial lung disease

844. A 50-year-old man with severe kyphoscoliosis is most likely to have

(A) enlarged overall lung volume

(B) alveolar hyperventilation

(C) left rather than right ventricular failure

(D) increased compliance

(E) recurrent pulmonary infections

845. Reduction of the ratio of forced expiratory volume to vital capacity (FEV/VC) is seen in

(A) emphysema

(B) ankylosing spondylitis

(C) pickwickian syndrome

(D) scleroderma of the chest wall

(E) lobar pneumonia

846. Which of the following statements concerning asbestosis is CORRECT?

(A) the type of asbestos fiber is crucial in determining whether asbestos-related lung disease occurs

(B) moderate rather than severe obstruction to air flow is characteristic of asbestosis

(C) mesothelioma is the common malignancy associated with asbestosis

(D) pleural effusions are invariably associated with malignancy in asbestosis

(E) short-term (i.e., 1 to 2 years) exposure can result in serious sequelae decades later

847. Which of the following statements concerning pulmonary embolism is CORRECT?

(A) continuous intravenous heparin therapy is more effective than intermittent intravenous or intermittent subcutaneous therapy.

(B) the most common ECG change is that of acute pulmonary hypertension (rightward shift of the QRS axis, tall peaked P wave)

(C) if symptoms occur, pleuritic chest pain is the most common symptom

(D) long delays in diagnosis and treatment of symptomatic pulmonary emboli are the major cause of death in this syndrome

(E) can be associated with petechiae

848. A 50-year-old man presents with excessive daytime sleepiness and a history of snoring. He is obese and has moderate hypertension. All of the following statements concerning this syndrome are correct EXCEPT

(A) altering medications can improve symptoms

(B) surgery can be effective treatment

(C) nocturnal oxygen will reverse sequelae of this syndrome

(D) effective treatment will improve the quality of sleep

(E) the syndrome can cause sudden death

849. Which of the following statements concerning hypoxemia in obstructive airways disease is CORRECT?

(A) erythrocytosis is an appropriate compensation for hypoxemia, and phlebotomy will worsen symptoms

(B) nocturnal oxygen therapy is effective in producing symptomatic and hemodynamic improvement in severe hypoxia

(C) a pO_2 of 58 mm Hg is an indication for continuous oxygen therapy

(D) a pO_2 of 65 mm Hg or below is an indication for supplemental oxygen during air travel

(E) continuous supplemental oxygen improves functional ability, but does not alter the natural history of obstructive airways disease with severe hypoxemia.

DIRECTIONS (Questions 850 through 865): This section consists of clinical situations, each followed by a question or a series of questions. Study each situation, and select the ONE best answer to each question following it.

Questions 850 through 854: A black woman presents with mild dyspnea on exertion, arthralgia, fever, and erythema nodosum. Physical examination reveals hepatosplenomegaly, generalized lymphadenopathy, and corneal opacities. X-ray of the chest shows bilaterally symmetrical hilar adenopathy.

850. The most likely diagnosis is

    (A) Hodgkin's disease
    (B) tuberculosis
    (C) rheumatic fever
    (D) sarcoidosis
    (E) rheumatoid arthritis

851. All of the following laboratory results are likely to be present EXCEPT

    (A) hyperglobulinemia
    (B) hypocalcemia
    (C) elevated sedimentation rate
    (D) normal serum phosphorus
    (E) mild anemia

852. Which of the following laboratory tests would be most likely to be positive?

    (A) tuberculin test
    (B) alcohol tolerance test
    (C) latex fixation
    (D) antistreptolysin-O (ASLO) titer
    (E) Kveim test

853. The eye lesion is probably due to

    (A) uveitis
    (B) diabetic complications
    (C) steroids
    (D) congenital origin
    (E) infectious infiltration

854. This disease is best treated with

    (A) aspirin
    (B) isoniazid and streptomycin
    (C) steroids
    (D) nitrogen mustard
    (E) no therapy

Questions 855 through 859: A 30-year-old man presents with a history of recurrent pneumonias and a chronic cough productive of foul-smelling, purulent sputum, occasionally blood-tinged, which is worse in the morning and on lying down. On physical examination, the patient appears chronically ill with clubbing of the fingers. Wet inspiratory rales are heard at the lung bases posteriorly.

855. The most likely diagnosis is

    (A) bronchiectasis
    (B) chronic bronchitis
    (C) disseminated pulmonary tuberculosis
    (D) pulmonary neoplasm
    (E) chronic obstructive emphysema

856. The most commonly involved area is likely to be the

    (A) apical segment of the upper lobe
    (B) posterior basal segments of the lower lobes
    (C) lingula
    (D) right middle lobe
    (E) superior segments of the lower lobes

857. The most likely precursor of the above condition was

    (A) bronchial asthma
    (B) endobronchial tuberculosis
    (C) pertussis
    (D) bronchopneumonia
    (E) influenza

858. The most important procedure necessary to define the extent of the disease would be

    (A) computed tomography
    (B) bronchoscopy
    (C) bronchography
    (D) open thoracotomy
    (E) gastric washings

859. Therapy for this disease might include

    (A) antibiotics and postural drainage
    (B) steroids
    (C) radiotherapy
    (D) aerosols
    (E) isoniazid

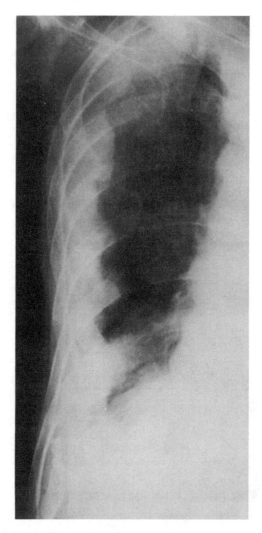

Figure 12.1

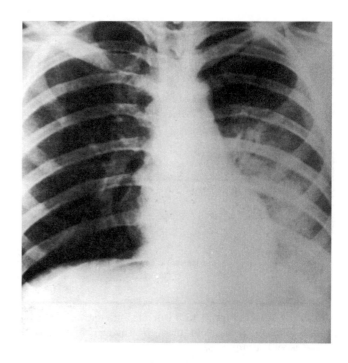

Figure 12.2

Question 861: (Figure 12.2): Cough with blood-tinged sputum, chills, and fever of two days' duration brought a 24-year-old man to the hospital. Physical findings revealed dullness and moist rales in the left lower chest. What is your diagnosis?

    (A) pneumonia, left lower lobe

    (B) atelectasis, left lower lobe

    (C) pulmonary embolism

    (D) tuberculosis

    (E) sarcoidosis

Question 860: (Figure 12.1): A 58-year-old steampipe worker had vague ache in the right chest and mild dyspnea of several months' duration. There was flatness on percussion of the right chest associated with diminished breath sounds. What is your diagnosis?

    (A) pleural metastases

    (B) Paget's disease

    (C) mesothelioma and asbestosis

    (D) pleural effusion

    (E) multiple myeloma

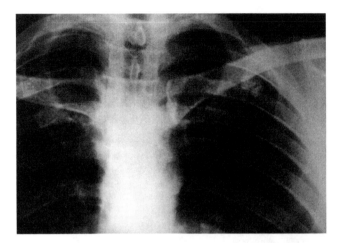

Figure 12.3

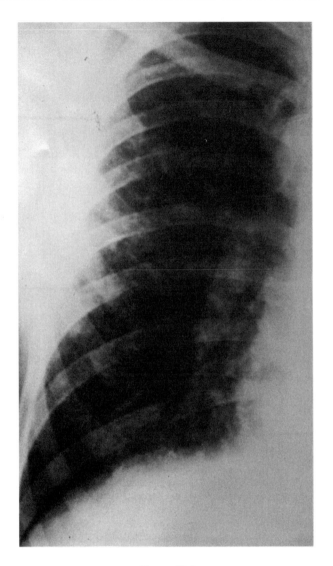

Figure 12.4

Question 862: Figure 12.3 is a close-up view of a chest x-ray from a 40-year-old man for insurance checkup. What is your diagnosis?

    (A) hamartoma of the lung

    (B) tuberculous granuloma of the left apex

    (C) osteochondroma of the left fourth rib

    (D) bronchogenic carcinoma

    (E) pulmonary metastases

Question 863: (Figure 12.4): A 17-year-old boy had slight tightness of the chest on heavy breathing, of two days' duration. He had pain in the left arm, which showed a lytic lesion on x-ray. What is your diagnosis?

    (A) eosinophilic granuloma

    (B) cystic fibrosis

    (C) pulmonary metastases

    (D) bronchiectasis

    (E) tuberculosis

TABLE 12.1 PULMONARY FUNCTION STUDIES

Chronic $Paco_2$ mm Hg	35
Chronic Pao_2 mm Hg	70
Hematocrit %	35
Pulmonary hypertension	
Rest	None
Exercise	Moderate
Elastic recoil	Severely decreased
Resistance	Normal
Diffusing capacity	Decreased

Question 864: The pulmonary function studies shown in Table 12.1 are of a 65-year-old man with severe dyspnea and cough. The most likely diagnosis is

(A) emphysema

(B) lobar pneumonia

(C) chronic bronchitis

(D) acute bronchitis

(E) congestive heart failure

Question 865: A 33-year-old woman, otherwise perfectly well, presents with recurrent episodes of hemoptysis. Investigation is likely to reveal

(A) a peripheral lesion with "popcorn" calcification

(B) a benign lesion, centrally located on CXR

(C) ring shadows, tram lines, and cyst formation on the CXR

(D) significant airflow reduction on pulmonary function tests

(E) a large left atrium on CXR

DIRECTIONS (Questions 866 through 875): Each group of questions below consists of a list of lettered headings, followed by a list of numbered words, phrases, or statements. For each numbered word, phrase, or statement, select the ONE lettered heading that is most closely associated with it. Each lettered heading may be selected once, more than once, or not at all.

Questions 866 through 870

(A) decreased fremitus, low diaphragms, prolonged expiration

(B) absent fremitus, hyperresonant, absent breath sounds

(C) decreased fremitus, tracheal shift away from affected side, flat percussion, absent breath sounds

(D) decreased fremitus, tracheal shift towards affected side, dull or flat percussion, absent breath sounds

(E) increased fremitus, dull to percussion, bronchophony

866. atelectasis

867. complete pneumothorax

868. acute asthmatic attack

869. large pleural effusion

870. lobar pneumonia

Questions 871 through 875

(A) epidermoid carcinoma

(B) adenocarcinoma

(C) large cell carcinoma

(D) small cell carcinoma

(E) bronchiolo-alveolar carcinoma

871. The most common type of lung cancer associated with hypercalcemia

872. Most responsive to cytotoxic chemotherapy

873. Overall best survival by natural history or after surgery

874. Most commonly associated with ectopic endocrine syndromes

875. This variety of lung cancer is frequently diffuse at presentation and may be associated with profuse sputum production

Diseases of the Respiratory System

Answers and Explanations

818. **(A)** In young women (plexogenic arteriopathy) is different than in older women and men (thrombotic arteriopathy). Small vessels are involved, but capillary involvement is rare. The plexogenic arteriopathy is characterized by medial hypertrophy associated with laminar intimal fibrosis and plexiform lesions. The thrombotic arteriopathy is characterized by eccentric intimal fibrosis with medial hypertrophy, fibroelastic intimal pads in the arteries and arterioles, and evidence of old recanalized thrombi. There is a female predominance and the third or fourth decade is the most common age at presentation. By the time of diagnosis the pulmonary hypertension is usually severe. *(Ref. 2, p. 1211)*

819. **(D)** An acute inflammation of the lungs is produced by hydrochloric acid, and obstructive atelectasis results from inhaled solid material. Sedation is best avoided in pulmonary disease as respiratory drive may be affected. Of course, sedation is frequently required in ventilated patients. *(Ref. 2, p. 1190)*

820. **(A)** Most lung abscesses and all anaerobic abscesses involve the normal flora of the oropharynx. Septic embolic usually contain *S. aureus*. Factors that predispose to gram-negative colonization of the oropharynx include hospitalization, debility, severe underlying diseases, alcoholism, diabetes, and advanced age. Impaired consciousness, neurologic disease, swallowing disorders, nasogastric or endotracheal tubes, all increase the likelihood of aspiration. *(Ref. 2, p. 1184)*

821. **(C)** When exposure to mouldy hay is stopped, symptoms and signs of farmer's lung all tend to abate and complete recovery usually follows. In acute syndromes the presentation is 4 to 8 hours after exposure. Symptoms include fever, chills, malaise, cough, and dyspnea without wheezing. The rate of disease depends on rainfall (which promotes fungal growth) and agricultural practices related to turning and stacking hay. *(Ref. 2, p. 1181)*

822. **(B)** Emphysema and chronic bronchitis are closely related and the term chronic obstructive lung disease (COLD) is often used to encompass both. Chronic bronchitis is a clinical syndrome defined as excessive tracheobronchial mucus production severe enough to cause productive cough for at least three months of the year for at least two consecutive years. Emphysema is defined as distention of the air spaces distal to the terminale bronchiole with destruction of alveolar septa. It is primarily a histologic diagnosis. *(Ref. 2, p. 1197)*

823. **(B)** Tranquilizers and sedatives should be avoided in prolonged asthma attacks. Bronchodilators, fluids, aminophylline, and steroids may be used. In acute situations intravenous glucocorticoids are frequently used. Results of therapy should be monitored in an objective manner with peak expiratory flow rates or FEV_1. In acute asthmatic attacks hypocarbia is usual on blood gas analysis. Normal or elevated $Paco_2$ is a bad sign and requires intensive monitoring and aggressive treatment. *(Ref. 2, pp. 1170–1172)*

824. **(D)** Administration of oxygen may worsen the syndrome of carbon dioxide narcosis because the chief stimulus to ventilation is often hypoxia, and when this is suddenly relieved the ventilation may drop quickly. Causes of the chronic hypoventilation syndrome include impaired respiratory drive (e.g., prolonged hypoxia, CNS disease), neuromuscular disorders (e.g., motor neuron disease, myasthenia gravis), or impaired ventilatory apparatus (e.g., kyphoscoliosis, chronic obstructive lung disease). *(Ref. 2, p. 1235)*

825. (C) The perfusion lung scan is most valuable in ruling out a pulmonary embolism. If properly performed early in the course of symptoms, a normal scan rules out the diagnosis. High probability scans are usually considered enough evidence of pulmonary embolism to warrant definitive treatment. Intermediate or low probability scans may require further investigation with pulmonary angiography, depending on the prior probability of disease. *(Ref. 2, p. 1217)*

826. (B) Etiology remains obscure in most cases of pulmonary eosinophilia, but infestation is often suspect. Malaria is not seen in these cases. Allergic bronchopulmonary aspergillosis (in asthmatics), parasitic reactions, and drugs are known causes of pulmonary eosinophilia. Idiopathic causes include Loeffler syndrome (benign, acute eosinophilic pneumonia), chronic eosinophilic pneumonia, hypereosinophilic syndrome, and the allergic granulomatosis of Churg and Strauss. *(Ref. 2, p. 1175)*

827. (D) Hypoventilation always causes both hypoxemia and hypercapnia. If the hypoventilation syndrome is caused exclusively by impaired respiratory drive (e.g., drug overdose) then the alveolar-arterial PaO_2 gradient remains normal. Often hypoventilation results from more than one disorder in the respiratory system (e.g., chronic obstructive lung disease plus metabolic alkalosis secondary to diuretics and glucocorticoids). *(Ref. 2, p. 1234)*

828. (D) Emphysematous COPD usually demonstrates scanty mucoid sputum, late onset of heart failure, increased total lung capacity, and markedly reduced diffusing capacity. Hypercarbia and hypoxemia are not as marked as in the chronic bronchitic type. The cough is not very productive and follows the onset of dyspnea. The body build is thin, usually with evidence of weight loss. *(Ref. 2, p. 1201)*

829. (B) Neurogenic tumors are the most common posterior mediastinal masses. Other posterior mediastinal masses include meningoceles, meningomyeloceles, gastroenteric cysts, and esophageal diverticula. Common anterior mediastinal masses include thymomas, lymphomas, teratomas, and thyroid masses. Middle mediastinal masses include vascular lesions, lymph nodes, and pleuropericardial and bronchogenic cysts. *(Ref. 2, p. 1233)*

830. (A) Most people have two MM genes and a resultant α-$_1$-antitrypsin level in excess of 2.5 g/L. Homozygotes with ZZ or SS genotypes have severe α-$_1$-antitrypsin deficiency and develop severe panacinar emphysema in the third or fourth decade of life. Heterozygotes (MZ or MS) have intermediate levels of α-$_1$-antitrypsin (i.e., genetic expression is that of an autosomal co-dominant allele). This heterozygous state is common (5 to 14% of general population), but it is unclear whether it is associated with lung function abnormalities. *(Ref. 2, p. 1199)*

831. (A) Ankylosing spondylitis is characterized by bilateral upper lobe fibrosis which may be complicated by fibrocavitary disease. The pulmonary involvement is rare and is usually very slowly progressive. The cavities can be colonized by *Aspergillus*. *(Ref. 2, pp. 1209, 1666)*

832. (D) The primary pathology is likely to be located in the medullary respiratory center. Cyanosis, especially when asleep, is caused by a combination of polycythemia and hypoxia. The symptoms of alveolar hypoventilation are caused by both hypercarbia and hypoxemia. *(Ref. 2, p. 1235)*

833. (A) Extrinsic asthma usually begins with an antigenic stimulus, whereas intrinsic asthma usually begins with infection, exercise, or cold. The major categories of stimuli that incite acute episodes of asthma are as follows: allergenic, pharmacologic, environmental, occupational, infectious, exercise-related, and emotional. *(Ref. 2, pp. 1167–1169)*

834. (E) Syndromes are classified as metabolic, neuromuscular, connective tissue, dermatologic, and vascular. Stevens–Johnson syndrome usually follows drug allergy. Acanthosis nigricans and other cutaneous manifestations (e.g., dermatomyositis) are rare (< 1%). Clubbing is common and occurs in up to 30% of nonsmall cell lung cancer. The various endocrine syndromes occur in 12% of cases. At times, paraneoplastic syndromes may be the presenting finding in lung cancer or be the first sign of recurrence. *(Ref. 2, p. 1223)*

835. (D) Carbon dioxide retention is seen in right-to-left shunt only with exercise and is uncommon in impaired diffusion syndromes. Disorders of the chest wall, lower airways, and lungs can cause an increased $PaCO_2$ because of severe ventilation–perfusion mismatching despite normal or increased minute volume of ventilation. *(Ref. 2, p. 1234)*

836. (B) Drug-induced interstitial lung disease is seen with various antineoplastic agents, antibiotics, and cardiovascular drugs. The presence of tumors, infections, granulocytopenia, or left ventricular dysfunction, make accurate diagnosis very difficult in these cases. *(Ref. 2, p. 1206)*

837. **(B)** In acute pulmonary thromboembolism, pleuritic chest pain and hemoptysis are present only when infarction has occurred. Palpitations may accompany arrhythmias. The sudden onset of unexplained dyspnea is the most common and often the only symptom of pulmonary embolism. *(Ref. 2, p. 1216)*

838. **(A)** Prolonged hyperventilation may be associated with hypokalemia, but not hyperkalemia. The patient is often nervous and anxious with other functional disturbances. Alkalemia, as well as causing hypokalemia, causes arrhythmias, parasthesias, and tetany (decreased free calcium), and neurologic symptoms secondary to cerebral vasoconstriction (dizziness, syncope, seizure). *(Ref. 2, p. 1239)*

839. **(C)** Grossly, the lung is edematous and hemorrhagic. Microscopically, there is intra-alveolar collection of proteinaceous fluid. Some common causes of ARDS include infection, aspiration, toxins, narcotics, drugs, immunologic responses, trauma with hypotension, and postcardiopulmonary bypass. *(Ref. 2, p. 1240)*

840. **(D)** Treatment includes antibiotics such as tetracycline. Some patients respond to steroids, but these are used only in strictly controlled circumstances. Steroid use is usually confined to acute exacerbations. Dietary support to prevent malnutrition and improve muscle strength can be helpful. Exercise programs seem to provide subjective improvement as well. *(Ref. 2, p. 1198)*

841. **(C)** Mediastinal emphysema may also result from thoracocentesis, trauma to the trachea or esophagus, rupture of the alveoli, or dissection of the retroperitoneum. Clinical presentation may include substernal chest pain, subcutaneous emphysema and Hamman's signs, a crunching or clicking noise synchronous with the heart beat. *(Ref. 2, p. 1233)*

842. **(C)** Approximately 60% of patients have hemoptysis. Pancreatic exocrine function is poor. Nasal polyps are common, but not rectal polyps. About 3% of cases of cystic fibrosis are diagnosed as adults. Because of improved therapy, cystic fibrosis is no longer just a pediatric disease. About 25% of patients reach adulthood, and over 9% live past thirty years of age. *(Ref. 2, p. 1196)*

843. **(B)** Hypoxemia while receiving 100% oxygen indicates right-to-left shunt. Shunts permit circulation of blood that never passes through the ventilated lung. Shunting can occur within the lung (atelectasis, vascular abnormalities) or outside the lung (congenital cardiac malformations). The hypoxemia of ventilation–perfusion mis-

match is more easily correctable by 100% oxygen. *(Ref. 2, p. 179)*

844. **(E)** Bony deformities of the chest can lead to respiratory failure with raised Pco_2, as well as recurrent pulmonary infection. The pattern on pulmonary function testing is usually that of a restrictive pattern. *(Ref. 2, pp. 1154, 1234)*

845. **(A)** The vital capacity is reduced in emphysema, but the FEV_1 is grossly reduced because of high airway resistance. In predominant emphysema diffusing capacity is more profoundly decreased than in predominant bronchitis. *(Ref. 2, pp. 1199–1201)*

846. **(E)** All forms of asbestos fiber have been associated with lung disease. Restrictive, not obstructive, disease is characteristic. Lung cancer, either squamous cell or adenocarcinoma, is the most common malignancy and the risk is greatly increased by smoking. Benign pleural effusions can occur in both symptomatic and asymptomatic individuals. Reports of mesothelioma 30 to 35 years after brief exposure to asbestos emphasize the importance of a complete occupational/environmental history. *(Ref. 2, pp. 1177–1178)*

847. **(E)** Pulmonary embolism secondary to fat emboli is characterized by petechiae on the upper thorax and arms. Although continuous heparin therapy with an infusion pump is the most popular method of acute treatment, other methods can also be effective. The common ECG change is tachycardia. Sudden onset of dyspnea is the most common symptom of pulmonary embolism. Pleuritic pain (and hemoptysis) only occur when infarction, an uncommon event, occurs. Some 90% of deaths related to pulmonary embolism occur in the first hour or two, too quickly to allow effective diagnosis and therapy. The thrust of management is therefore prevention. *(Ref. 2, pp. 1214–1220)*

848. **(C)** The description of a middle-aged man with daytime sleepiness, obesity, hypertension, and snoring suggests obstructive sleep apnea. Although nasal continuous positive airway pressure is effective treatment, simple O_2 therapy is not. Stopping sedative medications and avoiding alcohol improves symptoms. Restless sleep and sudden death have been described as part of the syndrome and surgery (uvulopalatopharyngoplasty or tracheostomy) has been used in severe cases. *(Ref. 2, pp. 1236–1238)*

849. **(B)** Nocturnal oxygen supplementation improves symptoms, but is not as effective as continuous supplementation in prolonging life and decreasing hospitalization. Some symptoms of

erythrocytosis, headaches, and fullness, can be relieved by phlebotomy. In prolonged air travel, even those with a pO_2 in the mid 70s should be considered for oxygen therapy. A pO_2 below 55 mm Hg is an indication for oxygen therapy but between 55 to 60 mm Hg associated evidence of right heart dysfunction should also be present before therapy is commenced. *(Ref. 2, p. 1203)*

850. (D) Sarcoidosis is the most likely diagnosis. Granulomatous inflammatory changes of sarcoidosis may occur in almost any organ. About 90% of patients with sarcoid will have an abnormal chest x-ray at some point. *(Ref. 2, pp. 1681–1683)*

851. (B) Hypocalcemia is not a laboratory result. Hypercalcemia occurs infrequently, but may result from increased intestinal absorption of calcium. *(Ref. 2, p. 1683)*

852. (E) The Kveim test requires six weeks' incubation and must be biopsied to be interpreted. The material for the test is not widely available and with easy availability of transbronchial biopsy the test is rarely used. It is only positive in 70 to 80% of people with sarcoid, and has a 5% false-positive rate. *(Ref. 2, p. 1683)*

853. (A) Acute granulomatous uveitis may be the initial manifestation of sarcoidosis. It can cause blindness. About 25% of patients with sarcoid have eye involvement; three quarters have anterior uveitis and one quarter have posterior uveitis. Involvement of lacrimal glands can lead to dry, sore eyes. *(Ref. 2, p. 1682)*

854. (C) Relatively asymptomatic patients often require no treatment. Steroids are used with ocular, central nervous system, or other serious complications. Although 50% of patients are left with permanent organ impairment, these are usually not symptomatic or significant. Only in 15 to 20% of cases does the disease remain active or recur. Glucocorticoids are the treatment of choice, but numerous other agents have been used. *(Ref. 2, p. 1684)*

855. (A) Bronchiectasis is defined as a permanent abnormal dilatation of large bronchi due to destruction of the wall. It is a consequence of inflammation, usually an infection. Other causes include toxins or immune response. Persistent cough and purulent sputum production are the hallmark symptoms. *(Ref. 2, p. 1193)*

856. (B) The posterior basal segments of the lower lobes are likely to be the most commonly involved area. True bronchiectasis is not re-

versible, but reversible conditions such as tracheobronchitis may simulate it. *(Ref. 2, p. 1193)*

857. (E) In the pre-antibiotic era, bacterial bronchopneumonia was the most common cause of bronchiectasis. Now, it is felt that influenza and adenoviruses are the most common causes. Of the bacterial causes, *Staphylococcus aureus, Klebsiella,* and anaerobes are the most common. *(Ref. 2, p. 1192)*

858. (A) Bronchography has been superseded by CT scan in defining the extent of bronchiectasis. Occasionally, advanced cases of saccular bronchiectasis can be diagnosed by routine chest x-ray. The use of high resolution CT scanning in which the images are 1.5-mm thick has resulted in excellent diagnostic accuracy. *(Ref. 2, p. 1193)*

859. (A) Antibiotics and postural drainage might be included in therapy. The choice of antimicrobial agents is guided by the sputum culture, but ampicillin and tetracycline are used if normal flora are found. The general principles of therapy include eliminating underlying problems, improved clearance of secretions, control of infections, and reversal of airflow obstruction. *(Ref. 2, p. 1193)*

860. (C) There is moderate pleural thickening, with scalloped margins from apex to base. There is a similar finding in the mediastinal and diaphragmatic pleura. Furthermore, there is a plaque of pleural calcification in the base. The association of asbestosis with mesothelioma has long been known. As the neoplasm progresses, it may envelope the thorax. *(Ref. 2, p. 1231)*

861. (A) The diagnosis is pneumonia. There is consolidation of the left lower lobe. The increased density, presence of air bronchogram, and the silhouetting of the left diaphragm point to a parenchymal lesion. Pneumococcal infection, as in this patient, is still the most common etiology, although other bacterial infections such as *Klebsiella* streptococcus, or *Staphylococcus* are often encountered. Viral and arthropod-bone diseases are also seen. *(Ref. 2, p. 1185)*

862. (B) There is a calcified nodule in the left apex. Obviously, a calcified tuberculous granuloma is the most common lesion. This may be from reinfection tuberculosis, where its preference for the apicoposterior segment is well known. It is also possible that it may be a calcified Ghon's lesion. *(Ref. 2, p. 710)*

863. (A) Eosinophilic granuloma is the diagnosis. There is a course, reticular pattern in the whole lung—somewhat more prominent in the upper lobes—suggesting a honeycomb appearance. It is the density here that is abnormal and not the lucency. *(Ref. 2, pp. 1210–1211)*

864. **(A)** Because of the maintained increase in minute volume and the maintenance of arterial PaO_2, patients with emphysema are referred to as "pink puffers." The relatively high PaO_2 and relatively low hemoglobin as compared to chronic bronchitis, make cyanosis unusual in emphysema. *(Ref. 2, p. 1201)*

865. **(B)** This history suggests a benign bronchial adenoma. These are usually centrally located on CXR. A peripheral lesion with "popcorn" calcification suggests a hamartoma, not an adenoma, and does not usually present with hemoptysis. Bronchiectasis (tram line, cysts) chronic obstructive pulmonary disease (airflow reduction), and mitral stenosis (enlarged left atrium) although potential causes of hemoptysis, rarely present without other symptoms as well. *(Ref. 2, pp. 173, 1229)*

866. **(D)** **867. (B)** **868. (A)** **869. (C)** **870. (E)** Careful physical examination can be very useful in diagnosing many common pulmonary disorders. Atelectasis and large pleural effusions both can present with decreased fremitus, dullness or flatness to percussion, and absent breath sounds. In atelectasis tracheal shift, if present, is *towards* the affected side, the opposite for a large pleural effusion. Asthma's most typical manifestations are prolonged expiration and diffuse wheezing. However, impaired expansion, decreased fremitus, hyperresonance, and low di-aphragms can also be found. A complete pneumothorax results in absent fremitus, hyperresonance or tympany, and absent breath sounds. Lobar pneumonia is characterized by consolidation with increased fremitus, dullness, and auscultatory findings of bronchial breathing, bronchophony, pectoriloquy, and crackles. *(Ref. 2, pp. 1146–1147)*

871. **(A)** Hypercalcemia may be due to metastatic destruction of bone, ectopic formation of parathyroid hormone, or formation of other osteolytic substances. *(Ref. 2, pp. 1222–1223)*

872. **(D)** Combination chemotherapy has produced promising results in lung cancer, particularly of the small cell anaplastic type. Alkylating agents and anthracyclines are active among other agents. *(Ref. 2, pp. 1227–1228)*

873. **(A)** The two-year survival of patients with epidermoid carcinoma is 46% for stage I and 40% for stage II. Adenocarcinoma is also associated with a relatively good stage I survival, but a much worse stage II survival. *(Ref. 2, p. 1226)*

874. **(D)** The most commonly encountered syndromes are inappropriate antidiuretic hormone secretion, Cushing syndrome, and gynecomastia. *(Ref. 2, p. 1223)*

875. **(E)** Bronchiolo-alveolar carcinoma is a variety of adenocarcinoma but spreads in a diffuse pattern throughout the lungs. It is associated with a particularly poor prognosis. *(Ref. 2, p. 1227)*

CHAPTER 13

Clinical Pharmacology
Questions

DIRECTIONS (Questions 876 through 908): Each of the questions or incomplete statements below is followed by five suggested answers or completions. Select the ONE that is best in each case.

876. The administration of hydrochlorothiazide may cause

    (A) increased serum potassium
    (B) metabolic acidosis
    (C) potassium loss and alkalosis
    (D) respiratory alkalosis
    (E) sodium retention

877. Ranitidine may be characterized as follows

    (A) blocks H_1 receptors
    (B) contains an imidazole ring
    (C) crosses the blood–brain barrier
    (D) peak effect at two hours
    (E) effective with once or twice daily administration

878. Antidiuretic hormone (ADH) acts by

    (A) increasing the permeability of the proximal renal tubule to water
    (B) increasing the permeability of the distal renal tubule to water
    (C) decreasing the glomerular filtration rate
    (D) increasing sodium excretion
    (E) causing active reabsorption of water from the loop of Henle

879. Methemazole (Tapazole) interferes with thyroid function mainly by

    (A) inhibition of iodine uptake
    (B) inhibition of thyroidal organic-binding and coupling reactions
    (C) immunologic means
    (D) destruction of thyroid cells
    (E) the same mechanism as perchlorate

880. Nifedipine produces its vasodilating effect by

    (A) β-adrenergic stimulation
    (B) interfering with calcium flux

    (C) inhibition of angiotensin 1
    (D) α-adrenergic blockade
    (E) direct smooth muscle relaxation

881. Ampicillin (α-aminobenzyl penicillin) is

    (A) not effective orally
    (B) not inactivated by penicillinase
    (C) acid-stable
    (D) not effective against coliform organisms
    (E) not allergenic

882. Untoward side effects of phenothiazines include all of the following EXCEPT

    (A) sensory loss
    (B) parkinsonism-like symptoms
    (C) dystonic movements
    (D) hypotensive episodes
    (E) convulsive seizures

883. Quinidine produces a decrease in all of the following electrophysiologic properties of the myocardium EXCEPT

    (A) the effective refractory period
    (B) automaticity
    (C) membrane responsiveness
    (D) the conduction velocity
    (E) excitability

884. Which of the following drugs requires a major adjustment in dosage in the presence of renal disease?

    (A) tetracycline
    (B) methicillin
    (C) erythromycin
    (D) chloramphenicol
    (E) ampicillin

885. Bronchodilators include all of the following EXCEPT

(A) ephedrine

(B) aminophylline

(C) isoproterenol hydrochloride

(D) potassium iodide

(E) epinephrine

886. All of the following stimulate gastric secretion EXCEPT

(A) ethyl alcohol

(B) acetylcholine

(C) reserpine

(D) caffeine

(E) fats

887. Xerostomia or dryness of the mouth may result from all of the following EXCEPT

(A) infection of salivary glands

(B) atropine

(C) gingivitis

(D) antihistamines

(E) Sjögren syndrome

888. Thiocyanate and perchlorate are examples of agents that

(A) inhibit thyroglobulin release

(B) increase BMR

(C) inhibit iodide transport

(D) inhibit thyroid organic binding

(E) increase thyroxin synthesis

889. Estimation of barbiturates in the blood

(A) may be diagnostic in a patient in a coma of unknown etiology

(B) revealing a level of 2 mg/dL in a comatose patient is usually due to poisoning with long-acting barbiturates

(C) revealing a level of 12 mg/dL in a comatose patient is usually due to poisoning with long-acting barbiturates

(D) is quite reliable with the methods available

(E) correlates with salicylate levels

890. Propranolol may be used in the presence of

(A) asthma

(B) hypertrophic subaortic stenosis

(C) sinus bradycardia

(D) heart block

(E) cardiogenic shock

891. Folic acid is best absorbed

(A) as a monoglutamate

(B) in the distal ileum

(C) with alcohol

(D) in pernicious anemia

(E) in the presence of abnormal gut bacteria

892. Vitamin B_{12} absorption is characteristically

(A) totally dependent on the intrinsic factor

(B) best in the duodenum

(C) improved in folic acid deficiency

(D) best in the distal ileum

(E) prevented by anti-parietal cell antibodies

893. All of the following are properties of insulin EXCEPT

(A) increase in the permeability of some cells to glucose

(B) stimulation of RNA formation

(C) movement of potassium into cells

(D) promotion of fat synthesis

(E) effectiveness in the absence of intact cells

894. An overdose of lysergic acid diethylamide (LSD) is most likely to be associated with

(A) pupillary dilatation

(B) pupillary constriction

(C) bradycardia

(D) blindness

(E) deafness

895. The major side effects in patients receiving tetracycline have been

(A) neutropenia

(B) allergic reactions

(C) hepatitis

(D) gastrointestinal symptoms

(E) polyuria

896. In quinidine-induced thrombocytopenic purpura

(A) there is a relation of dose to thrombocytopenia

(B) there is a more common incidence in males

(C) thrombocytopenia lasts three weeks following cessation of the drug

(D) antibodies may be demonstrated for as long as six months

(E) there is cross-reactivity with penicillin

897. Plasma lithium concentrations greater than 2 mEq/L can lead to all of the following EXCEPT

(A) mania
(B) disorientation
(C) tremor
(D) diarrhea
(E) leukocytosis

898. Nitroglycerin has the effect of

(A) dilating coronary arteries
(B) increasing cardiac venous return
(C) increasing cardiac output
(D) constricting peripheral veins and capillaries
(E) raising blood pressure

899. Allopurinol effectively

(A) increases uric acid production
(B) blocks excretion of uric acid by renal tubular mechanism
(C) inhibits xanthine oxidase
(D) diminishes inflammation of acute gouty arthritis
(E) stabilizes lysozymes

900. Heparin therapy

(A) is active by mouth
(B) affects hepatic synthesis of factors
(C) is monitored by prothrombin time
(D) is contraindicated in pregnancy
(E) may be neutralized by protamine

901. Acute physiologic effects of cannabis one hour after inhalation includes

(A) decrease in heart rate
(B) increase in intraocular pressure
(C) fine tremor of fingers
(D) peripheral vasoconstriction
(E) increase in intelligence quotient

902. Excessive use of furosemide may lead to

(A) acidosis
(B) edema
(C) alkalosis
(D) hyperkalemia
(E) hypernatremia

903. Antibiotics that distribute well to cerebrospinal fluid include

(A) streptomycin
(B) sulfonamides
(C) tetracycline
(D) tobramycin
(E) doxycycline

904. Cimetidine is beneficial in the treatment of peptic ulcer because it

(A) almost totally abolishes secretion
(B) blocks histamine-H_1 receptors
(C) is well absorbed in the stomach
(D) must be taken four times per day
(E) has no neurologic side effects

905. Which of the following correctly describes furosemide?

(A) no effect in the presence of hypoalbuminemia
(B) affects only the proximal tubules
(C) may cause acidosis
(D) chemically related to sulfonamides
(E) not indicated in the presence of oliguria

906. Which of the following is true in reference to anthracyclines?

(A) major site of metabolism is in tumor tissue
(B) DNA but not RNA is affected, after administration in vivo
(C) acute cardiac arrhythmias may occur
(D) extravasation is not harmful
(E) best used as a single agent

907. Biotransformation of medications is influenced by all of the following EXCEPT

(A) liver disease
(B) other medications
(C) renal function
(D) genetically determined polymorphisms
(E) environmental influences

908. Amiodarone is known to have

(A) excellent oral absorption
(B) short half-life
(C) active metabolite
(D) few drug interactions
(E) small volume of distribution

DIRECTIONS (Questions 909 through 940): For each numbered phrase select the ONE lettered heading that is most closely associated with it. Each lettered heading may be selected once, more than once, or not at all.

(A) associated with H_2 blockers (cimetidine) but *not* proton pump inhibitors (omeprazole)

(B) associated with proton pump inhibitors but *not* H_2 blockers

(C) associated with *both* H_2 blockers and proton pump inhibitors

(D) associated with *neither* H_2 blockers nor proton pump inhibitors

909. Can be used in some patients with urticaria

910. Useful in short bowel syndrome

911. Drug of choice in esophageal ulceration

912. May cause impotence

913. May cause CNS disturbance

Questions 914 through 918

(A) true of epinephrine but *not* norepinephrine

(B) true of norepinephrine but *not* epinephrine

(C) true of *both* epinephrine and norepinephrine

(D) true of *neither* epinephrine nor norepinephrine

914. Increased cardiac output

915. Increased renal blood flow

916. Increased diastolic blood pressure

917. Increased blood glucose

918. Increased systolic blood pressure

Questions 919 through 922

(A) true of dopamine but *not* dobutamine

(B) true of dobutamine but *not* dopamine

(C) true of *both* dopamine and dobutamine

(D) true of *neither* dopamine nor dobutamine

919. Stimulates dopaminergic receptors

920. Less tachycardia than isoproterenol

921. Can have marked effect on peripheral vascular resistance

922. In low doses selectively improves renal perfusion

Questions 923 through 927

(A) combines with cytochromes and catalase to block hydrogen and electron transport, thus producing tissue asphyxia

(B) methemoglobinemia

(C) vertigo, hyperventilation, tinnitus, and deafness

(D) bone marrow depression

(E) acute hepatic insufficiency

923. Chlorinated hydrocarbons

924. Salicylates

925. Cyanide

926. Benzene

927. Aniline dyes

Questions 928 through 932

(A) associated with alcohol but *not* heroin

(B) associated with heroin but *not* alcohol

(C) associated with *both* alcohol and heroin

(D) associated with *neither* alcohol nor heroin

928. High incidence of addiction

929. Pancreatitis

930. Nutritional value

931. Amblyopia

932. Methadone treatment

Questions 933 through 936

(A) true of verapamil but *not* bretylium

(B) true of bretylium but *not* verapamil

(C) true of *both* verapamil and bretylium

(D) true of *neither* verapamil nor bretylium

933. Interferes with the movement of calcium

934. Following administration there is a transient increase in heart rate and blood pressure

935. Permits conversion of refractory ventricular fibrillation when DC cardioversion has failed

936. May be the treatment of choice in acute paroxysmal AV junctional tachycardia

Questions 937 through 940

(A) true of cyclophosphamide but *not* nitrogen mustard

(B) true of nitrogen mustard but *not* cyclophosphamide

(C) true of *both* cyclophosphamide and nitrogen mustard

(D) true of *neither* cyclophosphamide nor nitrogen mustard

937. Requires hepatic activation

938. Causes severe local tissue injury

939. Belongs structurally to the nitrosoureas

940. Forms covalent bonds with nucleic acids

Clinical Pharmacology
Answers and Explanations

876. **(C)** Administration of hydrochlorothiazide may cause potassium loss and alkalosis. The mechanism is most probably increased delivery of sodium to sites where secretion of hydrogen and potassium occur. Other side effects include hyperglycemia, worsening of pre-existing diabetes mellitus, and increases in plasma lipids. Rare instances of purpura, dermatitis, pancreatitis, and necrotizing vasculitis have been reported. *(Ref. 8, p. 721)*

877. **(E)** Ranitidine possesses a furan ring, blocks H_2 receptors, and does not cross the blood–brain barrier well; hence does not cause the confusion seen with cimetidine. If given as a single daily dose, the best timing is before bedtime. Most H_2 blockers are very well tolerated, and often price is the determining factor in the choice of a specific agent. *(Ref. 8, p. 899)*

878. **(B)** No direct effect of ADH on sodium excretion has been observed in humans, but water retention may secondarily induce sodium excretion. ADH can also act as a neurotransmitter. Autonomic effects of ADH in the central nervous system include bradycardia, increase in respiratory rate, suppression of fever, and alteration of sleep patterns. *(Ref. 8, p. 739)*

879. **(B)** Methemazole interferes with thyroid function mainly by inhibition of thyroidal organic-binding and coupling reactions. In contrast to other agents such as perchlorate, the action of thioamides is not prevented by large doses of iodide. *(Ref. 8, p. 1374)*

880. **(B)** Nifedipine is a synthetic agent that is a potent, long-acting systemic vasodilator for treatment of coronary vasospasm. At doses used clinically, nifedipine does not block transmission through the AV node. The vasodilatation can result in a reflex increase in heart rate. *(Ref. 8, p. 774)*

881. **(C)** Polar side chains added to penicillin molecules made these compounds acid stable and, therefore, improved absorption. Intake of food prior to ingestion of ampicillin will decrease absorption. In cases of severe renal impairment, the dose should be adjusted downwards. *(Ref. 8, p. 1078)*

882. **(A)** Sensory loss is not a side effect of phenothiazines. Parkinsonism-like symptoms disappear when phenothiazine is withdrawn. Dystonic movements involve the mouth, tongue, and shoulder girdle. As well as having useful antipsychotic effects, phenothiazines are useful as antiemetics and antinausea agents. They can also potentiate the effects of sedatives, analgesics, and general anesthetics. *(Ref. 8, p. 386)*

883. **(A)** The refractory period increase accounts for the effect on tachycardia. Similar effects are seen with procainamide. The slowed repolarization can result in a prolonged QT interval. Life-threatening polymorphic ventricular tachycardias (Torsade de pointes) can be provoked by quinidine. *(Ref. 8, p. 848)*

884. **(A)** Tetracycline requires a major adjustment in dosage in the presence of renal disease. An injection may accentuate azotemia by its catabolic effect in increasing nitrogen turnover. Doxycycline, however, is different from other tetracyclines in that blood levels are not affected by renal failure. Thus it is the safest member of the tetracycline family for use in patients with renal failure. *(Ref. 8, p. 1117)*

885. **(D)** Potassium iodide is not a bronchodilator. It assists in the liquefaction of sputum, as does glyceryl guaiacolate. Potassium iodide is also used to treat the lymphocutaneous form of sporotrichosis. It has been used for treatment of erythema nodosum and nodular vasculitis as well. *(Ref. 8, pp. 625, 1585)*

886. **(E)** Fats release cholecystokinin, which inhibits gastric secretion. The increased gastric acid production may result in an increased prevalence of peptic ulcer disease. Ulcers are also common with drugs that impair mucosal protection (i.e., NSAIDs). *(Ref. 8, p. 125)*

887. **(C)** Xerostomia does not result from gingivitis. Radiation of salivary glands may cause permanent dryness secondary to gland atrophy. Atropine is a muscarinic cholinergic blocking agent. Besides depression of salivary and bronchial secretions, atropine causes dilation of the pupil, tachycardia, and numerous other signs and symptoms of parasympathetic blockade. *(Ref. 8, p. 150)*

888. **(C)** Because of their toxicity, neither drug is widely used in treatment, but both are effective in inhibiting iodide transport. They work by preventing the thyroid gland from concentrating iodide. Thiocyanate is produced following enzymatic hydrolysis of certain plant glycosides (e.g., cabbage) and may be a contributing factor to endemic goiter in certain parts of the world where iodide intake is low. *(Ref. 8, p. 1377)*

889. **(A)** Estimation of barbiturates in the blood may be diagnostic in a patient in a coma of unknown etiology. The production of barbiturates by drug companies greatly exceeds the amount needed for therapeutic purposes, so that addiction and overdose are common problems. *(Ref. 8, p. 357)*

890. **(B)** Propranolol may be used in the presence of hypertrophic subaortic stenosis. Beta-adrenergic blockade will exacerbate asthma, bradycardias, and myocardial dysfunction. They are probably also not first-line drugs for patients with insulin-dependent diabetes mellitus. They are effective and well tolerated during pregnancy, and there appears to be no increase in adverse outcomes for newborns. *(Ref. 8, p. 796)*

891. **(A)** Folic acid is present in food as polyglutamates and is deconjugated to a monoglutamate by intestinal enzymes. Common causes of folate deficiency include malnutrition, hemolytic anemia, and drugs (e.g., methotrexate, anticonvulsants). The folate deficiency in alcoholism is primarily caused by poor intake, but is exacerbated by an impaired enterohepatic cycle for the vitamin. *(Ref. 8, p. 1303)*

892. **(D)** Vitamin B_{12} absorption is best in the distal ileum. Receptors for the intrinsic factor are present in the distal ileum, but mass action absorption also occurs with large doses. The Schilling test, with and without intrinsic factor, can help

diagnose the exact cause of B_{12} deficiency. *(Ref. 8, p. 1298)*

893. **(E)** Insulin is not effective in the absence of intact cells. Insulin is synthesized as proinsulin with 86 amino acids and is then split into two chains connected by sulfur bridges. Insulin acts by binding to cell surface receptors that are present in virtually all mammalian cells. While some cells, such as erythrocytes, have few receptors, the prime target cells for insulin, such as hepatocytes and adipose cells, can have up to 300,000 receptors per cell. *(Ref. 8, p. 1463)*

894. **(A)** Sympathomimetic effects such as pupillary dilatation, piloerection, hyperthermia, and tachycardia are common in an overdosage of LSD. Other symptoms include dizziness, weakness, drowsiness, nausea, and parasthesias. The hallucinogenic effects can last for hours, and are mainly visual. *(Ref. 8, p. 554)*

895. **(D)** Gastrointestinal symptoms are the major side effects of tetracycline. Stomatitis, glossitis, and diarrhea are seen and may be related to superinfections. Hepatic toxicity has been reported, but is rare except in massive doses or during pregnancy. Tetracyclines can cause discoloration of teeth in children and in fetuses of mothers given the drug during pregnancy. *(Ref. 8, p. 1117)*

896. **(D)** Thrombocytopenia usually occurs after weeks or months of therapy. It is due to formation of drug–platelet complexes that evoke a circulating antibody. Thrombocytopenia and bleeding can be severe. The antibody is long lasting, and reintroduction of quinidine, even in a small dose, can rapidly cause thrombocytopenia. Other hypersensitivity reactions to quinidine include fever, anaphylactic reactions, and asthma. The most common side effects of quinidine, however, are gastrointestinal and include nausea, vomiting, and diarrhea. *(Ref. 8, p. 856)*

897. **(A)** Lithium is used primarily for bipolar affective disorder, either to treat mania or prevent recurrences of the bipolar disorder. It has also been used in severe unipolar depression. Acute intoxication can result in vomiting, diarrhea, tremor, ataxia, coma, and convulsions. Both acute and chronic intoxication can be lethal. The toxic and therapeutic levels of lithium are very close, and patients on lithium require close medical observation, including measurement of serum lithium levels. *(Ref. 8, p. 418)*

898. **(A)** The benefit of nitroglycerin is probably due to diminution in cardiac output and work of the heart and to dilation of coronary arteries. Nitroglycerin generally dilates most veins and arteries, and this results in both a decreased preload and a decreased afterload for the heart. This results in decreased myocardial oxygen requirements. *(Ref. 8, p. 764)*

899. **(C)** Allopurinol effectively blocks uric acid production and inhibits xanthine oxidase. Allopurinol is indicated in patients with a history of uric acid calculi of the urinary tract. As well, it is often used in patients with malignancy (e.g., leukemia, lymphoma) particularly when chemotherapy or radiation therapy is being used. *(Ref. 8, p. 676)*

900. **(E)** Heparin must be given parenterally (usually intravenously or subcutaneously) to be active, and its activity is monitored by the partial thromboplastin time (PTT), not the prothrombin time. It is safer than oral anticoagulants in pregnancy, and does not deplete clotting factors as its mode of action. Rather it potentiates the effect of antithrombin III on the clotting cascade. It can be neutralized by administration of protamine. As protamine can cause a bleeding tendency by its own actions, it is used only when bleeding is severe, and in the lowest possible dose. *(Ref. 3, p. 1316)*

901. **(C)** Peak effects at one hour after inhalation include increase in heart rate, decrease in intraocular pressure, and peripheral vasodilatation. The most common therapeutic use of cannabis is as an antiemetic during cancer chemotherapy. It might have some analgesic and anticonvulsant properties. Its ability to lower intraocular pressure has not been therapeutically useful in glaucoma. *(Ref. 8, p. 549)*

902. **(C)** In addition to dehydration, hypokalemia, hypochloremia, and alkalosis also result from excessive use of furosemide. Loop diuretics such as furosemide act primarily to inhibit electrolyte reabsorption in the thick ascending limb of the loop of Henle. The degree of diuresis is greater than in other classes of diuretics. *(Ref. 8, p. 721)*

903. **(B)** Some drugs such as penicillin, tetracycline, or streptomycin distribute in the CSF only during meningeal infection. Unfortunately, the therapeutic value of sulfonamides in meningitis is limited because many strains of *Neisseria meningitidis* are resistant. For prophylaxis in an outbreak where sulfonamide sensitivity has been demonstrated sulfisoxazole can be used. Generally, however, rifampin is the preferred agent for chemoprophylaxis. *(Ref. 8, p. 1050)*

904. **(A)** Cimetidine blocks histamine-H_2 to receptors and is well absorbed in the small intestine.

Initially it was thought to require adminstration four times per day, but has now been shown to be effective if given twice a day, or even once at night. It decreases all gastric secretion, not just acid, and is helpful in short bowel syndromes whereas omeprazole is not. *(Ref. 8, p. 899)*

905. **(D)** Furosemide is effective despite gross electrolyte disturbances or hypoalbuminemia. Excretion of large volumes of bicarbonate-poor urine leads to alkalosis. Furosemide increases the excretion of titratable acid and ammonia. This is felt to be caused by effects on the distal nephron and is one of the factors causing diuretic-induced metabolic alkalosis. *(Ref. 8, p. 721)*

906. **(C)** Anthracyclines include daunorubicin and doxorubicin. The major site of metabolism is the liver, and the mechanism of action includes inhibition of DNA-dependent RNA metabolism. The cardiomyopathy is characteristic of these drugs and is characterized by arrhythmias and cumulative dose-related congestive heart failure. *(Ref. 8, p. 1241)*

907. **(C)** Renal function influences excretion of drugs, not biotransformation. The common factors in altering biotransformation in man are genetic variability (e.g., P_{450} enzymes), liver disease (especially with malnutrition), other drugs, and environmental influences. *(Ref. 8, p. 170)*

908. **(C)** With prolonged treatment the active desethyl derivative of amiodarone accumulates in plasma, and its concentration may exceed that of the parent compound. Amiodarone is poorly (approximately 45%) absorbed and there is marked inter-individual variability. The half-life is long, 25 to 60 days, presumably because it is extensively bound to tissues, resulting in a large volume of distribution and a reservoir of drug. *(Ref. 8, p. 867)*

909. **(A)** Most patients with urticaria respond to H_1 blockers. Some patients with urticaria resistant to H_1 blockers alone will respond to a combination of H_1 and H_2 blockers. *(Ref. 8, p. 902)*

910. **(A)** H_2 blockers decrease the volume of gastric secretions and are useful in short bowel syndromes. Proton pump inhibitors such as omeprazole have only small and inconsistent effects on the volume of gastric secretions. *(Ref. 8, pp. 901–903)*

911. **(B)** Omeprazole is only marginally more effective than H_2 blockers in healing peptic ulcers. However, it is significantly more effective in the treatment of reflux esophagitis. *(Ref. 8, p. 904)*

912. **(A)** Cimetidine can cause loss of libido, impotence and gynecomastia when used long term in high doses. These adverse effects may be to enhanced prolactin secretion and to binding to androgen receptors. *(Ref. 8, p. 900)*

913. **(C)** With cimetidine CNS symptoms such as headache and dizziness are more common in the elderly and those with renal impairment. Omeprazole can infrequently cause headache, dizziness, and somnolence. *(Ref. 8, pp. 900, 904)*

914. **(A)** Epinephrine results in an increase in heart rate, a shorter and more powerful cardiac systole, and thus an increase in cardiac output (with a resultant increase in the work of the heart and its O_2 consumption). Norepinephrine causes no change or a decrease in cardiac output. *(Ref. 8, pp. 194–195, 199)*

915. **(D)** Both epinephrine and norepinephrine result in a decrease in renal blood flow. However epinephrine causes a marked increase in splanchnic blood flow, whereas norepinephrine has little or no effect. *(Ref. 8, p. 194)*

916. **(B)** Epinephrine results in little or no change in diastolic blood pressure; the total peripheral vascular resistance is decreased. Norepinephrine increases peripheral vascular resistance and diastolic blood pressure. *(Ref. 8, pp. 193–194, 199)*

917. **(A)** Epinephrine causes glycogenolysis in skeletal muscle and liver, causes gluconeogenesis in the liver, and decreases insulin secretion to elevate blood sugar. Norepinephrine has little or no effect on blood sugar. *(Ref. 8, pp. 108, 194)*

918. **(C)** Both epinephrine and norepinephrine increase systolic blood pressure. *(Ref. 8, p. 194)*

919. **(A)** Dopamine stimulates D_1-dopaminergic receptors at low dose. As infusion rates increase, activation of β_1-adrenergic receptors and then α_1-adrenergic receptors occurs. *(Ref. 8, p. 200)*

920. **(C)** Both dopamine and dobutamine cause less tachycardia than isoproterenol. The mechanism for this is unknown. *(Ref. 8, pp. 200, 202)*

921. **(A)** Dobutamine has relatively little effect on peripheral vascular resistance. At high doses dopamine activates α_1-adrenergic receptors, leading to vasoconstriction that can be clinically deleterious. *(Ref. 8, pp. 200, 202)*

922. **(A)** At low doses dopamine selectively stimulates D_1-dopaminergic receptors resulting in an increase in glomerular filtration rate and renal blood flow. This is useful in the management of low cardiac output associated with impaired renal function. Dobutamine has no such effect. *(Ref. 8, p. 200)*

923. **(E)** In chronically poisoned patients, cerebellar symptoms and evidence of liver damage may develop, especially with hexachlorobenzene. Many industrial solvents are chlorinated hydrocarbons and have been implicated in several deaths. Carbon tetrachloride was once used widely for medical purposes and as a cleaning agent. It has been replaced by safer alternatives. Hepatotoxicity of these compounds is exacerbated by concurrent ethanol ingestion. *(Ref. 8, p. 1622)*

924. **(C)** Salicylates are associated with vertigo, hyperventilation, tinnitus, and deafness. Excretion of salicylates is renal, and in the presence of normal renal function about 50% will be excreted in 24 hours. Severe toxicity can cause severe acid-base abnormalities. It can be difficult to diagnose when the toxicity is secondary to a therapeutic regimen. *(Ref. 8, p. 651)*

925. **(A)** Inhalation of hydrogen cyanide may cause death within a minute; oral doses act more slowly, requiring several minutes to hours. Cyanide combines with cytochromes and catalase to produce tissue asphyxia. The treatment for cyanide poisoning includes the administration of intravenous sodium thiosulfate, which hastens the transformation of the cyanide to thiocyanate which is excreted in the urine. *(Ref. 8, p. 1630)*

926. **(D)** Benzene is associated with bone marrow depression. Benzene is present to some extent in most gasolines, and poisoning may result from ingestion or from vapors. Acute benzene poisoning can cause severe CNS symptoms such as blurred vision, tremors, shallow and rapid respiration, ventricular irregularities, paralysis, and loss of consciousness. *(Ref. 8, p. 1625)*

927. **(B)** Headaches, dizziness, hypotension, convulsions, and coma may occur in methemoglobinemia, and jaundice and anemia may be late sequelae. Aniline derivatives are used as herbicides as well. Methemoglobinemia can also be caused by acetaminophen, a related compound. *(Ref. 8, pp. 657, 1634)*

928. **(C)** Both alcohol and opiates have a high incidence of addiction. Children may exhibit an increased susceptibility to opiates, so that relatively small doses may prove toxic. As well, alcohol is the most frequent cause of teratogenically induced mental deficiency in Western society. Even moderate alcohol ingestion is contraindicated in pregnancy. *(Ref. 8, pp. 370, 500)*

929. **(A)** Alcohol is associated with pancreatitis. The mildest forms may go unnoticed unless revealed by a transient elevation of the serum amylase level. The acute pancreatitis is felt to be caused by increased secretion accompanied by pancreatic duct obstruction. Chronic pancreatic insufficiency can also occur. *(Ref. 8, pp. 370, 500)*

930. **(D)** Opiates have no nutritional value and contrary to prevailing opinion, beers and liquors have too low a vitamin B content to be of nutritional value. In chronic alcoholics, nutritional deficiencies can be very common. *(Ref. 8, pp. 370, 500)*

931. **(C)** Amblyopia is associated with both. In heroin addicts, it is probably due to the toxic effects of quinine in the mixtures. Other neurologic sequelae of ethanol include memory loss, psychoses, polyneuritis, Wernicke's encephalopathy, and Korsakoff's psychosis. The classic overdose signs of heroin include coma, pinpoint pupils, and depressed respirations. *(Ref. 8, pp. 370, 500)*

932. **(B)** Methadone is used to control the addiction to heroin, but it requires daily administration and the patient is dependent on the methadone. Methadone is useful in treating addicts because it is an effective analgesic, long acting, and effective orally. *(Ref. 8, pp. 370, 500)*

933. **(A)** Verapamil appears to exert its effect by interfering with movement of calcium through the so-called slow channel. Verapamil also depresses the rate of the sinus node pacemaker, and slows AV conduction. This latter effect is the basis for its use in the treatment of supraventricular tachyarrhythmias. *(Ref. 8, pp. 774, 866)*

934. **(B)** Bretylium initially causes a release of catecholamines followed by sympathetic blockade. It is considered a class III antiarrhythmic. It has the capacity, in Purkinje and ventricular muscle fibers, to prolong the duration of action potentials and refractoriness. *(Ref. 8, pp. 774, 866)*

935. **(B)** Bretylium prolongs the refractoriness of tissues in the His–Purkinje system as well as the ventricles. Bretylium is recommended only for treatment of life-threatening ventricular arrhythmias that fail to respond to a first-line drug. It should be used only in an intensive care unit. *(Ref. 8, pp. 774, 866)*

936. **(A)** The slow channel calcium blockade has considerable importance in the region of the sinus node and the AV node. Verapamil is also useful in slowing the ventricular response to atrial fibrillation in the absence of Wolff–Parkinson–White syndrome. Verapamil does not have a major role in the treatment of ventricular arrhythmias. *(Ref. 8, pp. 774, 866)*

937. **(A)** Hepatic activation of cyclophosphamide produces the active compound phosphoamide mustard and a side product, acrolein. It is activated by the cytochrome P_{450} system. It is well absorbed orally, and can also be given by the intravenous route. It has more effect than other "mustard" agents on hair follicles, so alopecia is a common side effect. The hemorrhagic cystitis seen with cyclophosphamide may be caused by the acrolein metabolite. *(Ref. 8, p. 1209)*

938. **(B)** High chemical reactivity causes the local injury on infusion. Positively charged carbonium ions are formed. If extravasation should occur, the involved area should be infiltrated with sodium thiosulfate which will provide an ion that reacts avidly with the nitrogen mustard, and thereby protects tissue constituents. *(Ref. 8, p. 1209)*

939. **(D)** The nitrosoureas are distinct structures that are highly lipid-soluble, chemically reactive compounds. The nitrosoureas include carmustine (BCNU), lomustine (CCNU), semustine (methyl-CCNU) and streptozocin (a naturally occurring nitrosurea). *(Ref. 8, p. 1209)*

940. **(C)** By attaching to DNA, alkylating agents lead to single strand breakage and misreading of the DNA code. The major classes of alkylating agents are nitrogen mustards (cyclophosphamide, melphalan, chlorambucil, and classic nitrogen mustard or mechlorethamine), ethylenimines and methylmelamines, alkyl sulfonates (busulfan), nitrosoureas, and triazenes. *(Ref. 8, p. 1209)*

CHAPTER 14

Legal Medicine
Questions

DIRECTIONS (Questions 941 through 956): Each of the questions or incomplete statements below is followed by five suggested answers or completions. Select the ONE that is best in each case.

941. All of the following will probably constitute a coroner's case EXCEPT

(A) deaths associated with violence
(B) deaths in a chronic hospital
(C) cremation of a body before pronouncement
(D) nonattendance by a physician
(E) moving a body out of state

942. Actions in tort alleging cardiac injury most commonly arise from

(A) motor vehicle accidents
(B) food poisoning
(C) cardiac catheterization
(D) ECG stress tests
(E) office visits

943. To establish time of death during the first 24 hours, assume a rate of cooling in average temperatures of

(A) 2°C per minute
(B) 10°C per hour
(C) 10°C per minute
(D) 2°C per hour
(E) 10°C per day

944. In seeking evidence to document rape, after more than six hours have elapsed, the most likely specimen for detecting intact spermatozoa is

(A) vaginal aspirates
(B) seminal fluid dried on clothing or skin
(C) vulvar aspirates
(D) rectal aspirates
(E) oral aspirates

945. The physician who testifies as an expert witness

(A) must be the defendant's physician
(B) must be the plaintiff's physician
(C) will have seen the claimant after the incident
(D) might never have seen the claimant
(E) may not review a hospital record

946. The treating physician is generally prohibited from signing a death certificate in cases that involve

(A) infectious disease
(B) suicide
(C) platelet emboli
(D) epilepsy
(E) venereal disease

947. In arranging artificial insemination, all of the following points should be covered in the agreement with the parties EXCEPT

(A) the wife should consent in writing
(B) written consent of the donor's wife should be obtained
(C) the physician should have permission to select the donor
(D) the donor should consent in writing
(E) the success rate should be written into the agreement

948. Consent for surgery may be invalid in all of these cases EXCEPT when

(A) the act consented to is unlawful
(B) it is not an informed consent
(C) it was obtained by misinterpretation
(D) the consenter is incompetent
(E) a parent signs for a child

949. In order to comply with federal regulations concerning narcotics prescriptions, every practicing physician should

(A) register with the Federal Bureau of Narcotics every five years
(B) utilize a state narcotics form to secure an office supply
(C) order narcotics by telephone only if he or she knows the pharmacist
(D) list his or her registry number on every prescription
(E) only prescribe narcotics once to a given patient

950. Which criterion is necessary for the diagnosis of "brain death"?

(A) no response to external stimuli
(B) only occasional breathing
(C) no reflexes for a four-hour period
(D) a flat isoelectric electroencephalogram
(E) response only to deep pain

951. If a patient's fractured arm is set poorly but the patient refuses to allow the physician to reset the arm, liability for negligence rests with

(A) the physician
(B) the patient
(C) the hospital
(D) the patient's next of kin
(E) the assisting nurse

952. Under actions in tort in common law, recovery of damages requires that the injured party show

(A) the plaintiff owed the defendant a duty
(B) the plaintiff suffered injuries
(C) the plaintiff's conduct breached a duty
(D) the victim's negligence contributed to the injury
(E) the plaintiff neglected the defendant

953. The legal judgment of sanity or insanity is relevant to cases of

(A) impaired driving
(B) capability to make a will
(C) ownership of property
(D) ability to receive treatment
(E) qualification as a plaintiff

954. Revocation of the license to practice medicine commonly occurs with any of the following problems EXCEPT

(A) practicing chiropractic
(B) conviction of a felony
(C) drug addiction
(D) professional liability
(E) conviction of malpractice

955. Statutes of limitation, providing periods of time during which legal action must be instituted, may be delayed in onset by the

(A) death of a patient
(B) death of a physician
(C) request of the patient's lawyer
(D) fraudulent concealment of the wrongful act
(E) request of the hospital

956. Investigation of body fluid stains may include all of the following EXCEPT

(A) isoenzyme phenotype analysis
(B) ABO substance detection
(C) PH determination
(D) sex chromatin determination
(E) species origin determination

DIRECTIONS (Questions 957 through 961): The group of questions below consists of five lettered headings followed by a list of numbered words, phrases, or statements. For each numbered word, phrase, or statement, select the ONE lettered heading that is most closely associated with it. Each lettered heading may be selected once, more than once, or not at all.

(A) abrasion
(B) contusion
(C) laceration
(D) blunt trauma
(E) penetrating wounds

957. Displacement of the epidermis by friction

958. The severity of the injury cannot be estimated by the size of the cutaneous defect

959. Internal organs may be lacerated without damage to the surface of the body

960. Extravasated blood diffusely distributed through the tissue spaces

961. Most commonly seen in areas where the skin is stretched over bony eminences

Legal Medicine

Answers and Explanations

941. **(B)** Between 15 and 20% of all deaths that occur in the United States are related to violence, or to unexplained or unexpected causes. Deaths in a chronic care hospital will not constitute a coroner's case. *(Ref. 3, p. 6)*

942. **(A)** It is claimed that a myocardial contusion, coronary occlusion, or ischemia has resulted from mechanical or psychological trauma. *(Ref. 3, p. 1564)*

943. **(D)** Assume a rate of cooling in average temperatures of 2°C per hour. Postmortem heat loss is accelerated in cold environments and by passage of air currents over the body or by low humidity. *(Ref. 3, p. 16)*

944. **(B)** The most likely specimen is seminal fluid dried on clothing or skin. Ordinarily, spermatozoa have either migrated out of the vagina or have disintegrated after a lapse of 6 to 12 hours. *(Ref. 3, p. 72)*

945. **(D)** The medical expert need never have seen the claimant and may testify based on a review of the records. *(Ref. 9, p. 2464)*

946. **(B)** A death certificate should not be signed if there is any violent or suspicious death whether homicidal, suicidal, or accidental. *(Ref. 3, pp. 7–8)*

947. **(E)** A physician should also establish to his own satisfaction that, from the medical point of view, the husband is sterile. *(Ref. 3, p. 187)*

948. **(E)** Consent should be explained to the patient in understandable, nontechnical terms. Authority may come from a legally appointed guardian, as well as from a parent signing for a child. *(Ref. 3, p. 213)*

949. **(D)** Telephone orders for narcotics are prohibited whether a prescription is subsequently received or not. The physician should use a federal narcotics order form to secure an office supply, and should list his or her registry number on every prescription. *(Ref. 3, p. 281)*

950. **(C)** In addition, signs must be absent for 24 hours. The patient must not be on sedatives, and the temperature should be over 90°F. *(Ref. 3, p. 293)*

951. **(A)** A patient's negligence is not "contributory" if it merely aggravates an injury caused by the doctor's negligence. Liability for negligence rests with the physician. *(Ref. 3, p. 196)*

952. **(B)** The plaintiff must show that the defendant's conduct breached a duty, and that the victim's negligence did not contribute to the injury. *(Ref. 9, p. 2463)*

953 **(B)** Legal judgment is relevant to cases of capability to make a will, and competence to testify. There is no mental disease called "insanity." Insanity is a legal term for certain people who exhibit particular symptoms of mental disease. *(Ref. 3, p. 167)*

954. **(A)** Other grounds for revocation include gross indecency, false advertising, fraud in application, and alcoholism. *(Ref. 3, p. 223)*

955. **(D)** The statutory period is delayed also in the case of a minor, until the patient attains the age of majority. *(Ref. 3, p. 315)*

956. **(C)** Body fluids can be studied also from the point of view of MN, Lewis, secretor status, immunoglobulin isotypes, and time lapse since formation of the stain. *(Ref. 3, p. 145)*

957. **(A)** An abrasion displaces the epidermis by friction. The location and character of an abrasion may help to establish the circumstances in which more severe injuries were sustained. *(Ref. 3, p. 31)*

958. **(E)** In penetrating wounds, the severity of the injury cannot be estimated by the size of the cutaneous defect. Firearm injuries comprise the majority of penetrating wounds other than stab wounds. *(Ref. 3, p. 33)*

959. **(D)** The internal structures most frequently damaged include bones, ligaments, meningeal vessels, the brain, and the spinal cord. In blunt trauma, internal organs may be lacerated without damage to the surface of the body. *(Ref. 3, p. 32)*

960. **(B)** In contusions, extravasated blood is diffusely distributed through the tissue spaces. Multiple contusions from minor trauma are often encountered in alcoholic females and may lend false importance to the role of physical violence. *(Ref. 3, p. 31)*

961. **(C)** Lacerations are most commonly seen in areas where the skin is stretched over bony eminences. The skin on the side of the wound opposite to the direction of motion is usually undermined for a variable distance. *(Ref. 3, p. 32)*

CHAPTER 15

Comprehensive Review
Questions

DIRECTIONS (Questions 962 through 1052): Each of the questions or incomplete statements below is followed by five suggested answers or completions. Select the ONE that is best in each case.

962. Which of the following characteristics best characterizes a feature of geriatric patients compared to younger patients?

(A) medical problems are less complex
(B) they spend less money on housing
(C) homeostasis is impaired
(D) hepatic enzyme deterioration is a result of aging
(E) senile dementia is a result of aging

963. Uncomplicated urethral gonococcal infection is best treated with

(A) intramuscular ceftriaxone plus oral doxycycline
(B) oral penicillin G
(C) intramuscular penicillin V
(D) ampicillin intramuscularly and oral penicillin V
(E) intravenous tobramycin

964. In patients suspected of having Alzheimer's disease, a search for reversible causes of dementia might include all of the following EXCEPT

(A) blood sugar
(B) serum calcium
(C) thyroid function tests
(D) serum B_{12}
(E) urinary and plasma amino acids

965. In patients with cardiac insufficiency, clues to the presence of thyrotoxicosis include all of these features EXCEPT

(A) atrial fibrillation
(B) relatively rapid circulation time
(C) increased cardiac output
(D) response to low doses of digitalis
(E) high-output failure

966. Which of the following has NOT been identified as a mediator of tumor-associated hypercalcemia?

(A) osteoclast activation factor
(B) colony-stimulating factor
(C) tumor necrosis factor
(D) interleukin-1
(E) prostaglandin E

967. A 30-year-old woman develops acute onset of erythema nodosum, fever, malaise, and anorexia. Chest x-ray reveals bilateral hilar lymphadenopathy and a left paratracheal lymph node. The most likely diagnosis is

(A) AIDS
(B) rheumatic fever
(C) sarcoidosis
(D) tuberculosis
(E) bronchogenic carcinoma

968. The imaging technique that is best able to measure regional myocardial substrate uptake and metabolic kinetics is

(A) magnetic resonance imaging
(B) computed axial tomography
(C) positron emission tomography
(D) serial thallium scintigrams
(E) Doppler ultrasound

969. A sudden overwhelming sepsis, associated with high fever and a high mortality rate (toxic shock-like syndrome) is most likely due to infection with

(A) *C. diphtheriae*
(B) *Streptococcus* group C
(C) *N. gonorrhoeae*
(D) *Streptococcus* group A
(E) *Salmonella enteritidis*

970. In malignant hypertension, the agent that best reduces blood pressure immediately is

(A) hydralazine
(B) labetalol
(C) methyldopa
(D) diazoxide
(E) nifedipine

971. Vacuolization of proximal tubular epithelium and loss of urinary concentrating ability is most likely to be associated with

(A) severe potassium depletion
(B) hypercalcemia
(C) gouty nephropathy
(D) diabetic nephropathy
(E) rheumatoid arthritis

972. Which of the following drugs is NOT usually of value in controlling grand mal seizures?

(A) phenytoin
(B) carbamazepine
(C) phenobarbital
(D) valproic acid
(E) ethosuximide

973. The classification of low-grade lymphomas in the Working Formulation would include

(A) lymphoblastic type
(B) follicular, small cleaved-cell type
(C) diffuse large cell type
(D) Burkitt's lymphoma
(E) small noncleaved-cell type

974. A patient with HIV infection may be considered to have progressed to frank AIDS with the onset of

(A) antibodies to HIV
(B) palpable lymphadenopathy
(C) invasive cervical cancer
(D) fever
(E) urticaria

975. Which of the following is more characteristic of ulcerative colitis when compared to regional enteritis?

(A) segmental involvement
(B) granulomas
(C) lymph node involvement
(D) rectal bleeding
(E) palpable abdominal mass

976. A 28-year-old pregnant woman develops sudden onset of dyspnea and tachycardia with no other physical findings. The most likely explanation is

(A) pulmonary emphysema
(B) pulmonary embolism
(C) myocardial infarction
(D) ventricular tachycardia
(E) lobar pneumonia

977. A 60-year-old man from a poor socioeconomic environment is admitted with an acute illness characterized by mental disturbances, bilateral sixth nerve palsy, and ataxias of gait. He may require emergency treatment with

(A) thiamine
(B) lecithin
(C) vitamin D
(D) phenytoin
(E) diazepam

978. Which of the following is most characteristic of calcitonin?

(A) increases bone resorption
(B) decreases renal calcium clearance
(C) produced by hepatocytes
(D) raises blood phosphate
(E) binds to osteoclasts

979. Which of the following is most characteristic of rheumatic fever?

(A) chronic arthritis
(B) involvement of spinal joints
(C) subcutaneous nodules
(D) erythema nodosum
(E) meningeal irritation

980. A home parenteral nutrition program is most likely to be useful for patients with

(A) an untreatable disease
(B) a four-day requirement for nutrition
(C) severe radiation enteritis
(D) neoplasms with bowel obstruction
(E) anorexia nervosa

981. The most important factor in selecting a patient as a potential heart transplant recipient is

(A) absence of long-standing pulmonary hypertension
(B) survival on mechanical assistance devices
(C) availability of an HLA compatible donor
(D) age under 20 years
(E) ventricular ejection fraction over 80%

982. Chronic lymphocytic leukemia can be best characterized as

(A) usually a T cell disorder

(B) a disease of children

(C) responsive to splenectomy

(D) frequently asymptomatic

(E) most common in orientals

983. All of the following are common precipitants of hepatic encephalopathy EXCEPT

(A) gastrointestinal bleeding

(B) intravenous antibiotics

(C) hypokalemia

(D) constipation

(E) hypoxia

984. An asymptomatic patient with glomerular hematuria is most likely to have

(A) diabetes mellitus

(B) amyloidosis

(C) Berger's disease

(D) focal glomerulosclerosis

(E) thalassemia minor

985. Chronic obstructive lung disease that is primarily due to emphysema is best characterized by

(A) mild dyspnea

(B) copious purulent sputum

(C) hematocrit over 55%

(D) severe pulmonary hypertension at rest

(E) decreasing diffusing capacity

986. All of the following are generally found in rheumatoid arthritis EXCEPT

(A) symmetric joint involvement

(B) restriction to large joints

(C) involvement of small joints

(D) sparing of the lower axial skeleton

(E) morning stiffness

987. α-thalassemia leads to increased formation of

(A) hemoglobin H

(B) hemoglobin A

(C) hemoglobin F

(D) hemoglobin A_2

(E) hemoglobin C

988. Which of the following is most characteristic of diabetic neuropathy?

(A) usually bilateral

(B) pain is not a feature

(C) most commonly affects the brain

(D) spares the autonomic system

(E) responds to meticulous control of blood glucose

989. Which of the following agents is NOT used in the treatment of acute gouty arthritis?

(A) indomethacin

(B) colchicine

(C) phenylbutazone

(D) allopurinol

(E) naproxen

990. Of the following the most common cause of ischemic stroke is

(A) vasovagal faint

(B) cerebral embolism

(C) arteritis

(D) dissecting aneurysm

(E) hemorrhage into atherosclerosis

991. Transfusion-related hepatitis that is not due to hepatitis B is most likely due to

(A) hepatitis A

(B) Epstein–Barr hepatitis

(C) hepatitis C

(D) δ hepatitis

(E) enteric hepatitis

992. A 20-year-old man with abrupt onset of hematuria and proteinuria, accompanied by azotemia and salt and water retention most likely has

(A) nephrotic syndrome

(B) multiple myeloma

(C) diabetic nephropathy

(D) nephrolithiasis

(E) acute glomerulonephritis

993. The most common symptom of duodenal ulcer is

(A) epigastric pain

(B) nausea

(C) melena

(D) anorexia

(E) mid-back pain

994. An elderly patient receiving a blood transfusion for myelodysplastic syndrome, develops tachypnea, lumbar pain, tachycardia, and nausea. The most likely explanation is

(A) anxiety
(B) fluid overload
(C) hemolysis
(D) pulmonary embolism
(E) acute leukemia

995. Treatment of hyperthyroidism during pregnancy could use any of the following EXCEPT

(A) thyroid surgery
(B) propylthiouracil
(C) drugs that cross the placenta
(D) propranolol
(E) glucocorticoids

996. All of the following have been common side effects of tricyclic antidepressants EXCEPT

(A) dry mouth
(B) nausea and vomiting
(C) postural hypotension
(D) drowsiness
(E) slow, coarse tremor

997. Mitral valve prolapse is most likely to be characterized by

(A) a pansystolic murmur
(B) a life-long benign course
(C) sudden death
(D) infective endocarditis
(E) highest incidence in men over age 50

998. An 18-year-old man develops nephrotic syndrome. A renal biopsy shows foot process fusion and no deposits on the membranes under electron microscopy. The most likely lesion is

(A) mesangial proliferative glomerulonephritis
(B) minimal change disease
(C) focal glomerulosclerosis
(D) membranous glomerulonephritis
(E) Goodpasture syndrome

999. A 65-year-old man with positive sputum cytology for malignant cells, but a normal chest x-ray is best managed with

(A) annual chest x-ray
(B) unilateral pneumonectomy
(C) blind percutaneous needle biopsies
(D) bronchoscopic brushings and biopsies
(E) mediastinoscopy and biopsy

1000. A dyspneic patient manifests a 20 mm Hg decrease in systolic arterial pressure during slow inspiration. The most likely cause is

(A) cardiac tamponade
(B) pulmonary hypertension
(C) ventricular septal defect
(D) coarctation of the aorta
(E) malignant hypertension

1001. Suppression of immune rejection of the transplanted kidney is best accomplished with

(A) splenectomy and irradiation
(B) plasmapheresis and steroids
(C) cyclosporin and steroids
(D) azathioprine and plasmapheresis
(E) steroids and thymectomy

1002. A 42-year-old woman has a history of loss of vision and eye pain that spontaneously reversed. She now has diplopia and weakness and spasticity in her right leg. The most likely diagnosis is

(A) cerebral emboli
(B) subclavian steal syndrome
(C) Guillain–Barré syndrome
(D) recurrent transient ischemic attacks
(E) multiple sclerosis

1003. A 16-year-old female presents with abdominal pain and purpuric spots on the skin. Laboratory investigation reveals a normal platelet count, with hematuria and proteinuria. The most likely diagnosis is

(A) hemolytic–uremic syndrome
(B) thrombotic thrombocytopenic purpura
(C) heavy metal poisoning
(D) subacute bacterial endocarditis
(E) Henoch–Schönlein purpura

1004. Which of the following drugs causes an increase in the effective refractory period of the AV node?

(A) bretylium
(B) amiodarone
(C) procainamide
(D) quinidine
(E) disopyramide

1005. Postmenopausal women with hyperparathyroidism, who are unable to undergo surgery, may benefit from

(A) estrogen therapy
(B) androgen therapy
(C) calcium therapy

(D) radioiodine

(E) intravenous phosphate

1006. All of the following drugs may cause hemolysis in patients deficient in glucose-6-phosphate dehydrogenase (G6PD) EXCEPT

(A) chloroquine

(B) sulfisoxazole

(C) vitamin K

(D) tobramycin

(E) nitrofurantoin

1007. Community-acquired pneumonia in a previously healthy 20-year-old woman is best initially treated with

(A) carbenicillin

(B) tobramycin

(C) erythromycin

(D) methicillin

(E) tetracycline

1008. A 60-year-old man with polyuria, nocturia, and renal transport defects is most likely to have

(A) acute nephritis

(B) acute renal failure

(C) renal tubular defects

(D) nephrolithiasis

(E) systolic hypertension

1009. Ranitidine is useful in treatment of peptic ulcer disease because it

(A) binds to the ulcer bed

(B) antagonizes H_2 receptors

(C) inhibits acetylcholine

(D) stimulates mucin secretion

(E) inhibits parietal cell proton pump

1010. A 70-year-old woman, previously in good health, is found to have an asymptomatic monoclonal immunoglobulin peak on serum electrophoresis. The most likely diagnosis is

(A) monoclonal gammopathy of uncertain significance (MGUS)

(B) multiple myeloma

(C) Waldenström's macroglobulinemia

(D) amyloidosis

(E) non-Hodgkin's lymphoma

1011. A 30-year-old woman with dryness of the mouth and cutaneous palpable purpura, probably has

(A) ankylosing spondylitis

(B) mixed connective tissue disease

(C) systemic sclerosis

(D) thrombotic thrombocytopenic purpura

(E) Sjögren syndrome

1012. In an extreme emergency, patients may be transfused with unmatched blood from a donor who is

(A) type AB

(B) polycythemic

(C) a sibling of the recipient

(D) type O

(E) Lewis A positive

1013. In mild mitral stenosis, the earliest change on chest x-ray is

(A) general enlargement of the heart

(B) Kerley B lines

(C) attenuation of pulmonary arteries

(D) straightening of the left heart border

(E) diffuse modulation of the lower lung fields

1014. A 25-year-old woman with diplopia, ptosis, weakness, and fatigability of muscles on repeated use is most likely to have

(A) myasthenia gravis

(B) multiple sclerosis

(C) transient ischemic attacks

(D) muscular dystrophy

(E) cerebral palsy

1015. The group of women with the highest risk of developing breast cancer are

(A) cousins of breast cancer patients

(B) those receiving chest x-rays as children

(C) those with late onset menarche

(D) multiparous

(E) those who have already had one breast cancer

1016. Patients with cystic fibrosis are more likely to be diagnosed for the first time as adults if

(A) the reproductive system is not involved

(B) heat stroke occurs

(C) pulmonary hypertension is avoided

(D) gastrointestinal disease is minimal

(E) hypersplenism is prominent

1017. A 25-year-old nonsmoking man has a 2-cm solitary pulmonary nodule in the left lower lobe, with a "popcorn ball" calcification. The best management would be

(A) left lower lobe resection

(B) serial chest x-rays

(C) needle aspiration biopsy

(D) left pneumonectomy

(E) mediastinoscopy

1018. A 60-year-old man with unstable angina pectoris fails to respond to heparin, nitroglycerin, β-adrenergic blockers, and calcium channel antagonists. The best management includes

(A) intravenous streptokinase

(B) coronary artery bypass grafting

(C) exercise testing

(D) oral aspirin

(E) antihypertensive therapy

1019. The major effect of glucocorticoids in asthma is

(A) anti-inflammatory

(B) bronchodilatory

(C) sedative

(D) mucus dissolving

(E) antibacterial

1020. Immunofluorescence studies of focal glomerulosclerosis demonstrate

(A) nodular deposits of IgM and C_3

(B) linear deposits of IgG

(C) no basement membrane changes

(D) granular deposits of IgG and C_4

(E) extensive fibrin strands

1021. Burning retrosternal chest pain, radiating to the sides of the chest and aggravated by bending forward, is most likely to arise from the

(A) heart

(B) lumbar spine

(C) intercostal nerves

(D) pancreas

(E) esophagus

1022. Raynaud's phenomenon associated with systemic sclerosis is best managed with

(A) amphetamines

(B) ergotamines

(C) β-blocking drugs

(D) warmth

(E) surgical sympathectomy

1023. Transmission of human immunodeficiency virus to patients with factor VIII deficiency (hemophilia A) is reduced by all of the following EXCEPT

(A) heating of factor VIII concentrates

(B) use of antibody purified factor VIII

(C) freezing and thawing factor VIII preparations

(D) use of recombinant factor VIII

(E) use of EACA or DDAVP

1024. Three weeks after surgery to implant a mechanical aortic valve, a 70-year-old man develops chest pain, fever, leukocytosis, and increased jugular venous pressure. The most likely diagnosis is

(A) infection in the aortic valve

(B) postpericardiotomy syndrome

(C) cytomegalovirus infection

(D) pulmonary embolism

(E) acute myocardial infarction

1025. All of the following typically cause a hypochromic microcytic anemia EXCEPT

(A) blind loop syndrome

(B) iron deficiency

(C) thalassemia

(D) chronic inflammation

(E) sideroblastic anemia

1026. An 18-year-old woman develops weakness, weight gain, amenorrhea, abdominal striae, and behavioral abnormalities. Physical examination reveals lateral visual field loss. The most likely diagnosis is

(A) a functional pituitary tumor

(B) adrenal hyperplasia

(C) anorexia nervosa with bulimia

(D) glioblastoma multiforme

(E) multiple sclerosis

1027. Lipoprotein measurements in diabetes mellitus are likely to demonstrate

(A) marked increase in chylomicrons

(B) increase in intermediate-density lipoproteins (IDL)

(C) increase in low-density lipoproteins (LDL)

(D) lipoprotein lipase deficiency

(E) an abnormal ratio of lipoproteins

1028. A 62-year-old woman, previously asymptomatic, presents with sudden onset of severe mid-back pain. X-rays reveal an anterior compression fracture of T10. Other vertebral bodies show decreased density and prominent vertical striations. The most likely diagnosis is

(A) multiple myeloma

(B) metastatic breast cancer

(C) vitamin D deficiency

(D) osteoporosis

(E) Paget's disease of bone

1029. A 70-year-old-man, with no evidence of heart disease, develops transient ischemic attacks, and investigations suggest carotid artery involvement. The best nonsurgical management would include long-term

(A) heparin

(B) aspirin

(C) β-blockers

(D) nonsteroidal anti-inflammatory drugs

(E) calcium channel antagonists

1030. A 60-year-old woman being investigated for menorrhagia is found, on history, to have lethargy, constipation, cold intolerance, and muscle stiffness. The most likely diagnosis is

(A) uterine carcinoma

(B) systemic lupus

(C) hypothyroidism

(D) severe iron deficiency

(E) hypercalcemia

1031. A 20-year-old patient with asymptomatic lymphadenopathy in the right supraclavicular area is found to have nodular sclerosing Hodgkin's disease on biopsy. There is no other evidence of disease. The best management is

(A) combination chemotherapy with MOPP

(B) wide surgical excision following radiotherapy

(C) combination chemotherapy with ABVD

(D) radiotherapy alone

(E) observation until symptoms occur

1032. A 45-year-old man presents with weakness, fever, weight loss, and abdominal pain, and is found to be hypertensive and in renal failure. While being investigated, he has a focal seizure. Laboratory studies show a high ESR, anemia, and a positive test for hepatitis B surface antigen. The most likely diagnosis is

(A) polyarteritis nodosa

(B) acute hepatitis B

(C) subacute bacterial endocarditis

(D) multiple staphylococcal abscesses

(E) chronic active hepatitis

1033. Patients with AIDS can have chorioretinitis with blindness, enteritis with intractable diarrhea, interstitial pneumonitis, and adrenalitis, all caused by infection with

(A) cryptosporidium

(B) herpes zoster

(C) toxoplasma

(D) pneumocystis carinii pneumonia

(E) cytomegalovirus

1034. A patient with extrahepatic biliary obstruction is most likely to have

(A) negative urine bilirubin

(B) marked increase in conjugated bilirubin

(C) normal unconjugated bilirubin

(D) painless jaundice

(E) decrease in glucuronyl transferase

1035. On inspection of a skin lesion, a diagnosis of malignant melanoma is favored by all of the following characteristics EXCEPT

(A) irregular border

(B) hair arising from the lesion

(C) nodularity

(D) reniform outline

(E) variegation of color

1036. In distinguishing prerenal azotemia from acute renal failure, the urine findings in prerenal azotemia should show

(A) urine osmolality less than 400

(B) brown granular casts

(C) urine creatinine less than 20

(D) a high fractional excretion of filtered sodium

(E) urine sodium of less than 20

1037. Which of the following results of blood gas analysis is most likely in a patient with hyperventilation caused by anxiety?

(A) increased P_{CO_2}

(B) decreased P_{O_2}

(C) decreased pH

(D) decreased P_{CO_2}

(E) increased P_{O_2}

1038. Following an acute myocardial infarct, the early injury pattern on ECG is likely to show

(A) tall P waves
(B) prominent U waves
(C) small QRS complex
(D) elevated ST segments
(E) widened QRS complex

1039. An emergency room patient with extreme lethargy admits to taking a large number of long-acting barbiturates. Management might include all of the following EXCEPT

(A) acidification of urine to pH 3.0
(B) repetitive administration of activated charcoal
(C) fluid administration
(D) hemoperfusion
(E) hemodialysis

1040. Five years after exposure to radiation from a nuclear reactor accident, the exposed population is in the greatest danger from

(A) aplastic anemia
(B) radiation dermatitis
(C) lung cancer
(D) multiple myeloma
(E) leukemia

1041. All of the following are common, serious side effects of phenothiazine antipsychotic medication EXCEPT

(A) postural hypotension
(B) urinary retention
(C) parkinsonism
(D) tardive dyskinesia
(E) red cell aplasia

1042. Which of the following diuretics will continue to induce significant diuresis after return of blood volume to normal levels?

(A) hydrochlorothiazide
(B) spironolactone
(C) triamterene
(D) furosemide
(E) metolazone

1043. The polyneuropathy that occurs in association with isoniazid (INH) can best be described as

(A) acute
(B) demyelinating
(C) pure sensory
(D) chronic axonal
(E) pure motor

1044. A patient with recurrent arthritis of the knees recalls an acute illness with fever and severe dermatitis one year earlier. The most likely diagnosis is

(A) rheumatoid arthritis
(B) Lyme disease
(C) syphilis
(D) polyarteritis nodosa
(E) systemic lupus

1045. Zidovudine (AZT) is indicated for treatment of

(A) retroviral infection
(B) pneumocystis carinii pneumonia
(C) Kaposi's sarcoma
(D) toxoplasmosis
(E) herpes simplex of the genitals

1046. Which of the following statements about sleep in the elderly is correct?

(A) the elderly sleep more than younger adults
(B) the time required to fall asleep (sleep latency) increases with advancing age
(C) slow wave sleep increases as a proportion of total sleep with advancing age
(D) sleep efficiency (time sleeping as a percentage of time in bed) improves in the elderly
(E) the elderly are more likely to awaken in the night

1047. All the following statements about the aging of the American population are true EXCEPT

(A) age-adjusted mortality rates are decreasing for all age groups including those over 80
(B) the population is getting older, and the elderly are living longer
(C) the increase in those over age 85 has a dramatic effect on the average age of the population
(D) the increase in those over the age of 85 has a dramatic effect on the utilization of medical resources
(E) the major increases in the average American's life expectancy at birth since the mid 1800s are the result of decreased infant mortality

1048. Which of the following statements concerning women's health issues is correct?

(A) breast cancer is the leading cause of death in US women
(B) men benefit more from thrombolytic therapy than women
(C) the mortality from acute myocardial infarction is greater in women than men

(D) estrogen therapy decreases mortality in post-menopausal women primarily by its ability to prevent osteoporosis-related fractures

(E) immune-related disorders are less common in women

1049. Which of the following statements concerning hypertension during pregnancy is correct?

(A) pre-eclampsia becomes manifest during the end of the middle trimester

(B) angiotensin-converting enzymes (ACE) inhibitors are useful antihypertensives in the pregnant woman

(C) pregnancy increases the risk for future renal impairment in the woman with essential hypertension

(D) α-methyldopa is a useful antihypertensive in the pregnant woman

(E) gestational hypertension infrequently recurs in subsequent pregnancies

1050. Which of the following statements concerning pregnancy and infection is correct?

(A) rubella is the most common cause of congenital viral infection

(B) postpartum infections are the most common cause of maternal mortality in the United States

(C) *Neisseria gonorrhoeae* infection is transmitted to the child only during delivery

(D) asymptomatic bacteriuria is common, but unimportant in pregnant women

(E) cytomegalovirus (CMV) infection in newborns is invariably associated with severe deformities

1051. A 35-year-old man presents with left-sided periorbital headaches of severe intensity. He has been awakened from sleep for three nights in a row. He had similar headaches a year ago. These headaches

(A) are likely tension headaches

(B) are typical of common migraine (without an aura)

(C) may be relieved by the vasodilation of alcohol

(D) usually recur in cycles lasting several months to years

(E) can be relieved by administration of oxygen

1052. A 75-year-old woman presents with sudden onset of a communication disorder. She speaks fluently, but in a series of incomprehensible syllables. She cannot read or repeat sounds or words. This syndrome is

(A) unlikely to improve with time

(B) usually associated with hemiparesis of the dominant side

(C) usually associated with hemiparesis of the nondominant side

(D) usually in the distribution of the posterior cerebral artery

(E) frequently associated with parietal lobe sensory defects

DIRECTIONS (Questions 1053 through 1067): The group of questions below consists of lettered headings followed by a list of numbered phrases. For each numbered phrase, select the ONE lettered heading that is most closely associated with it. Each lettered heading may be selected once, more than once, or not at all.

(A) increased sensitivity with aging

(B) decreased sensitivity with aging

(C) altered excretion with aging

(D) altered metabolism with aging

(E) altered distribution with aging

Questions 1053 through 1057: Match the appropriate statement about pharmacology with each of the following medications.

1053. β Blockers

1054. Metaclorpromide

1055. Morphine

1056. Lithium

1057. Aminophylline

Questions 1058 through 1062

(A) antipsychotics

(B) mineral oil

(C) diuretics

(D) isoniazid

(E) phenytoin and phenobarbital

(F) salicylates

(G) corticosteroids

(H) L-dopa

1058. Disinterest in food with protein/calorie malnutrition

1059. Magnesium and zinc deficiency

1060. Vitamin B$_6$ deficiency

1061. Impaired calcium absorption

1062. Altered vitamin D metabolism

Questions 1063 through 1067

    (A) true of delirium but *not* dementia
    (B) true of dementia but *not* delirium
    (C) true of *both* delirium and dementia
    (D) true of *neither* delirium nor dementia

1063. More common in the elderly

1064. Impaired long-term memory

1065. Impaired attention early in course

1066. Impaired level of consciousness

1067. No effect on mood

Comprehensive Review
Answers and Explanations

962. **(C)** The impaired physiological reserve of every organ system is characteristic of aging. The term homeostenosis has been used to describe this phenomenon. Decline in most systems starts in the third decade and is gradual and progressive. Decrements in each organ system seem independent of other systems and are influenced by diet, environment, personal habits (e.g., exercise), and genetic factors as well as just chronological age. At times, it can be difficult to differentiate between age-related physiologic change and age-related diseases. *(Ref. 2, p. 31)*

963. **(A)** Since 1986 increasing penicillin resistance has meant that penicillin/ampicillin are no longer drugs of choice. Alternatives to ceftriaxone include ciprofloxacin, ofloxacin or cefixine given orally, or IM spectinomycin, with seven days of doxycycline. In pregnant women erythromycin replaces doxycycline. Disseminated gonococcal infection should be treated in hospital with intravenous antibiotics. *(Ref. 2, p. 648)*

964. **(E)** Other tests to rule out reversible disease should include chest x-ray, EEG, liver function tests, and serum electrolytes. Diagnosis of Alzheimer's disease remains a diagnosis of exclusion. However, the insidious and subtle onset, with few focal signs (except for higher mental functioning) and a slowly progressive course are characteristic. The intensity of investigation will depend on numerous factors including age, presence of atypical findings, and the timing of presentation. *(Ref. 2, p. 2270)*

965. **(D)** These complications are more common in the elderly patient, and may dominate the clinical presentation. There is often a wide pulse pressure, systolic murmurs, increased intensity of the first heart sound, and cardiomegaly. Sinus tachycardia and atrial fibrillation are the most common arrhythmias. A to-and-fro high-pitched sound in the pulmonic area (Means–Lerman scratch) can mimic a pericardial friction rub. *(Ref. 2, p. 1943)*

966. **(B)** Other mediators of tumor-associated hypercalcemia include lymphotoxin, vitamin D, and parathormone. Hypercalcemia may occur in 10% of lung carcinoma. Local bone destruction with osteoclast activating factor, interleukin-1, tumor necrosis factor, and lymphotoxin occurs in hematologic malignancies such as lymphoma and multiple myeloma. As well, lymphomas can cause hypercalcemia by humoral mediators such as $1,25(OH)_2$ and parathyroid hormone-related protein (PTH-rP). Some breast cancers cause local bone destruction and hypercalcemia via prostaglandins of the E series. Other breast cancers and kidney, urogenital, and squamous cell lung cancers cause hypercalcemia by humoral mediation (with PTH-rP and other mediators). *(Ref. 2, p. 2157)*

967. **(C)** Sarcoidosis is asymptomatic in at least 10 to 20% of cases. At least 40% of patients present with acute symptoms and hilar lymphadenopathy. Approximately 90% will have an abnormal chest x-ray at some point in their illness. Only a small proportion develop progressive disease. *(Ref. 2, p. 1681)*

968. **(C)** PET has been used to measure regional myocardial uptake of exogenous glucose and free fatty acid and to evaluate myocardial chemical receptor sites. Although not widely clinically available, PET scanning can detect ischemic myocardium and demonstrate potentially viable tissue in the presence of both acute and chronic ischemia. *(Ref. 2, p. 978)*

969. **(D)** *Streptococcus* group A can cause a toxic shock-like syndrome, and has been increasing in frequency in North America. Streptococcal toxic shock-like syndrome was so named because of its similarity to staphylococcal toxic shock syndrome. The illness includes fever, hypotension, renal impairment, and the respiratory distress syndrome. It is usually caused by strains that produce exotoxin. It may be associated with localized infection as well; the most common associated infection is a soft tissue infection such as necrotizing fasciitis. The mortality is high (up to 30%), usually secondary to shock and respiratory failure. The rapid progression of the disease and its high mortality demand early recognition and aggressive treatment. Management includes fluid resuscitation, pressor agents, mechanical ventilation, antibodies, and, if necrotizing fasciitis is present, surgical debridement. *(Ref. 2, p. 621)*

970. (D) Diazoxide acts immediately in malignant hypertension and is the easiest to administer for no individual titration of dosage is required. Labetalol is also useful, but has more contraindications. Regardless of which drug is selected, early administration of medications for long-term control is mandatory. *(Ref. 2, p. 1131)*

971. (A) Hypokalemia, if severe and protracted, leads to tubular vacuolization and ultimately glomerular loss. Early changes are reversible with potassium repletion. Nocturia, polyuria, and polydipsia are common symptoms in hypokalemic nephropathy. Urinalysis is not remarkable, and urea and creatinine are not remarkable. After correction of hypokalemia, maximal urinary concentrating ability might not return to normal for several months. *(Ref. 2, p. 1317)*

972. (E) Ethosuximide (Zarontin) is usually reserved for cases of petit mal. All four of the recommended drugs have neurologic side effects at high doses. Decisions to use one of these drugs instead of the others usually relate to potential side effects and possible drug interactions rather than efficacy. *(Ref. 2, pp. 2230–2231)*

973. (B) Other low-grade lymphomas in the Working Formulation include small lymphocytic cell and follicular mixed-cell types. The working formulation divides lymphomas into low-grade, intermediate-grade, and high-grade lymphomas. Low-grade lymphomas include: small lymphocytic, follicular predominantly small-cleaved cell, and follicular mixed small-cleaved and large-cell. Most low-grade lymphomas are of B cell lineage. *(Ref. 2, p. 1774)*

974. (C) Invasive cervical cancer in a patient with HIV infection satisfies the CDC definition for AIDS. Other recent additions (1993) to the case definition in HIV-positive patients include pulmonary tuberculosis, recurrent pneumonia, or CD4+ T-lymphocyte count < 200. *(Ref. 2, p. 1567)*

975. (D) Rectal bleeding is more characteristic of ulcerative colitis, as is malignancy with long-standing disease, but both can occur in regional enteritis. Transmural involvement, lymph node involvement, skip lesions, granulomas, and anorectal complications (abscesses, fistulas, fissures) are characteristic of Crohn's disease. *(Ref. 2, pp. 1405–1407)*

976. (B) Sudden onset of unexplained dyspnea is the most common and often the only symptom of pulmonary embolism. Findings on physical examination may be deceptively normal, but tachycardia is a consistent finding. Pleuritic chest pain and hemoptysis only occur with infarction, an uncommon event. *(Ref. 2, p. 1216)*

977. (A) The patient has Wernicke–Korsakoff syndrome and requires treatment with thiamine. A delay of a few hours may permit progression to psychosis. The eye findings in Wernicke–Korsakoff syndrome include bilateral (but not necessarily symmetrical) abductor weakness or paralysis, horizontal diplopia, strabismus, and nystagmus. The nystagmus is most frequently horizontal or vertical gaze-evoked nystagmus. *(Ref. 2, pp. 2329–2331)*

978. (E) Calcitonin is secreted by cells in the thyroid. Calcitonin reduces bone resorption and increases renal calcium clearance. The inhibition of osteoclast-mediated bone resorption and the stimulation of renal calcium clearance are mediated by receptors on osteoclasts and renal tubular cells. Other receptors to calcitonin are present in brain, gastrointestinal tract, and immune system. *(Ref. 2, pp. 2149–2150)*

979. (C) Major manifestations of rheumatic fever include carditis, polyarthritis, chorea, erythema, marginatum, and subcutaneous nodules. Minor manifestations include arthralgia, fever, elevated acute phase reactants (ESR, C-reactive protein), and prolonged P–R interval. The diagnosis is made with two major or one major and two minor criteria, and evidence of group A streptococcal infection (positive throat culture or rapid streptococcal antigen test, or rising antibody titers). *(Ref. 2, pp. 1048–1049)*

980. (C) Home parenteral nutrition is usually helpful in extreme short-bowel syndrome, chronic obstruction due to adhesions, and severe radiation enteritis. Placement of a central venous catheter, careful calculation of fluid and nutritional requirements, and meticulous monitoring are required in a long-term parenteral nutrition program. *(Ref. 2, p. 467)*

981. (A) In selecting a heart for transplantation, size, ABO match, negative lymphocyte crossmatch, and other disease states, are important factors. The presence of severe pulmonary hypertension can result in intraoperative death. In the

United States it is estimated that only 2,000 potential donor hearts become available each year for 20,000 potential recipients. This means that careful recipient selection is very important. The optimal candidates will have a high likelihood of return to a high level of function, to be mentally vigorous and medically compliant. *(Ref. 2, p. 1009)*

982. **(D)** Chronic lymphocytic leukemia is frequently discovered on routine evaluation of elderly patients and may not require treatment for several years. Splenomegaly, when present, rarely leads to symptoms. It is a disorder of B cells and is very indolent in its course. Most therapeutic regimens are designed for symptom control, not cure. Common reasons for treatment include hemolytic anemia, cytopenias, disfiguring lymphadenopathy, symptomatic organomegaly, or systemic symptoms. Alkylating agents are still the cornerstone of treatment. Maintenance therapy is not helpful. *(Ref. 2, p. 1772)*

983. **(B)** Other common precipitations of hepatic encephalopathy include excess dietary protein, azotemia, alkalosis, and hypovolemia. Management includes general supportive measures, eliminating the predisposing factors, and lowering blood ammonia levels. Lowering blood ammonia levels is achieved by removing any blood from the GI tract, restricting dietary protein intake, and treating and/or preventing constipation. *(Ref. 2, p. 1493)*

984. **(C)** Other causes of asymptomatic hematuria, with or without proteinuria, include sickle cell disease, Alport syndrome, resolving glomerulonephritis, and thin basement disease. Berger's disease is characterized by IgA deposits in the mesangium. It most commonly affects older children and young adults, mostly male. Macroscopic hematuria may occur with intercurrent illness or vigorous exercise. The prognosis is variable, but tends to progress slowly. Spontaneous remissions are more common in children than in adults. About 50% of patients develop end-stage renal disease within 25 years of diagnosis. *(Ref. 2, p. 1305)*

985. **(E)** Chronic obstructive lung disease due to emphysema usually demonstrates severe dyspnea, scanty mucoid sputum, and normal hematocrit. Chronic bronchitis is characterized by milder dyspnea, greater sputum production, more frequent hypercarbia and polycythemia, and more evidence of cor pulmonale and pulmonary hypertension. *(Ref. 2, p. 1201)*

986. **(B)** The typical picture of rheumatoid arthritis includes bilateral symmetrical involvement of large and small joints in both the lower and upper extremities. The onset can be insidious, with fatigue, anorexia and generalized weakness, and vague musculoskeletal symptoms. Initially the pain and swelling may be poorly localized to the joints. *(Ref. 2, p. 1651)*

987. **(A)** α-Thalassemia involves a decrease in α-chain production and leads to the formation of β-globin tetramers known as hemoglobin H. Individuals normally inherit four α-chain genes. The clinical syndrome depends on how many genes are deleted. Deletion of one gene results in a silent carrier state. Deletion of all four is the most severe, and presents as hydrops fetalis. This condition is incompatible with life. *(Ref. 2, p. 1741)*

988. **(A)** Diabetic neuropathy usually presents as peripheral polyneuropathy, usually bilateral, including symptoms of numbness, paresthesia, severe hyperesthesia, and pain. Impairment of proprioceptive fibers can lead to gait abnormalities and Charcot joints. Mononeuropathy is less common and is often spontaneously reversible. Common syndromes include wrist or foot drop and third, fourth, or sixth cranial nerve palsies. Autonomic neuropathy may cause gastroesophageal dysfunction, bladder dysfunction, and orthostatic hypotension. *(Ref. 2, p. 1995)*

989. **(D)** Uricosuric drugs and allopurinol have no role in the treatment of acute gouty arthritis. Salicylates are also not used in the treatment of gout. The treatments of choice are colchicine, nonsteroidal anti-inflammatory drugs, and intra-articular steroid injection. Response is best when initiated early in the disease. Colchicine is fairly specific for gouty arthritis, and is useful in cases where the diagnosis is not definitely established. It can be given intravenously to avoid GI distress. Allopurinol is only started when all inflammation is gone and colchicine prophylaxis has been started. It is not always required. *(Ref. 2, p. 2085)*

990. **(B)** The two broad categories of ischemic stroke are embolic and thrombotic. Emboli can originate from an arterial atheroma (e.g., common carotid bifurcation) or from the heart. In the latter case, anticoagulants are often indicated. On occasion emboli occur without obvious source (e.g., hypercoagulable states, malignancy, eclampsia). *(Ref. 2, p. 2234)*

991. (C) Screening for antibodies to hepatitis C will reduce the incidence of this infection. There is no specific treatment as yet for this infection. The hepatitis C virus is a linear, single-stranded RNA virus. There are at least five distinct genotypes. *(Ref. 2, p. 1463)*

992. (E) Causes of acute glomerulonephritis include infectious diseases, especially *Streptococcus*, vasculitides, and primary glomerular disease. The "acute nephritic syndrome" consists of the abrupt onset of hematuria and proteinuria, often accompanied by azotemia and renal salt and water retention. Oliguria may be present. *(Ref. 2, p. 1295)*

993. (A) The pain may be described as sharp, burning, or gnawing, usually 90 minutes to 3 hours after eating, relieved by food or antacids. The pain frequently awakens the patient at night. Symptoms are usually episodic and recurrent. Periods of remission are usually longer than periods with pain. The ulcer crater can recur or persist in the absence of pain. *(Ref. 2, p. 1367)*

994. (C) Intravascular hemolysis from blood transfusion is usually due to ABO incompatibility, often from human error. Symptoms of intravascular hemolysis include flushing, pain at the infusion site, chest or back pain, restlessness, anxiety, nausea, and diarrhea. Signs include fever and chills, shock, and renal failure. In comatose patients hemoglobulinuria or bleeding from disseminated intravascular coagulation can be the first signs. Management is supportive. *(Ref. 2, p. 1792)*

995. (D) Propranolol should not be used during pregnancy as fetal growth retardation and neonatal respiratory depression have been reported. Radioactive iodine is absolutely contraindicated. Propylthiouracil (PTU) crosses the placenta, but is effective and safe. The major risk is hypothyroidism in the fetus. Thyroxine does not cross the blood–brain barrier, therefore only relatively low doses of PTU can be used in pregnancy. If this strategy is not successful, subtotal thyroidectomy must be considered. *(Ref. 2, p. 1946)*

996. (E) The tremor associated with tricyclic antidepressants is fine and rapid. Other side effects include dizziness, ataxia, and postural hypertension. Selective serotonin uptake inhibitors, while not more effective than tricyclics, are frequently preferred because of fewer side effects. However, even with these agents bothersome tremor, insomnia, and weight loss can occur. *(Ref. 2, p. 2407)*

997. (B) The most common pathogenic mechanism is thought to be excessive or redundant mitral leaflet tissue, with the posterior leaflet more commonly involved. Myxomatous degeneration can also be seen on pathological examination. Reassurance regarding the benign nature of the disease is the mainstay of management. When a murmur is present, antibiotic prophylaxis for endocarditis is warranted. *(Ref. 2, p. 1058)*

998. (B) Little or no changes are seen on light microscopy in this syndrome. The disease is most common in children. Spontaneous remission is common in children and is enhanced by steroid therapy. Over 95% of children achieve remission within 8 weeks of institution of prednisone therapy. Therefore, in children with nephrotic syndrome, empiric therapy is frequently employed, rather than initial renal biopsy. Only 50% of adults will remit, and thus biopsy is more frequently required. Relapse is common in both children and adults. *(Ref. 2, pp. 1300–1301)*

999. (D) Over 90% of lesions can be localized by fiberoptic bronchoscope under general anesthesia and collection of a series of differential brushings and biopsies. When lesions are found, conservative resection is usually performed. Five-year cure rates in such lesions approach 60%, but second primaries are common (5% per patient per year). *(Ref. 2, p. 1226)*

1000. (A) This is an important clue to cardiac tamponade, called paradoxical pulse. When severe, the arterial pulse may weaken on palpation during inspiration. Pulsus paradoxus is uncommon in constrictive pericarditis and rare in restrictive cardiomyopathy. It is commonly found in severe asthma as well. *(Ref. 2, p. 1097)*

1001. (C) Cyclosporin A blocks production of IL-2 by helper–inducer (CD4+) T cells. It works alone, but is more effective in combination with glucocorticoids. The use of cyclosporine has improved 1-year cadaveric survival rates to the 80% range. Side effects include hepatotoxicity, hirsutism, tremor, and gingival hyperplasia, but only the nephrotoxicity presents a serious management problem. *(Ref. 2, p. 1286)*

1002. (E) Typically, multiple sclerosis presents with optic neuritis. There is usually a history of at least two episodes of neurologic deficit at more than one site. Other common presenting symptoms include weakness, sensory loss, and parasthesias. *(Ref. 2, pp. 2288–2289)*

1003. (E) Other symptoms include arthralgia and gastrointestinal function abnormalities. Renal biopsy shows immunoglobulin deposits. There is an underlying vasculitis. The prognosis is generally good, although relapses can occur before the final remission. *(Ref. 2, p. 1674)*

1004. (B) Amiodarone causes a decrease in the sinus rate and an increase in the effective refractory period in the atrium, the AV node, and the ventricle. The pharmacology of amiodarone is complex and incompletely understood. *(Ref. 2, pp. 1026–1027)*

1005. (A) Estrogen therapy may retard demineralization of the skeleton and may also reduce blood and urinary calcium levels. There is no clear consensus on when asymptomatic hyperparathyroidism requires surgery. Many experts will elect to follow elderly patients with mild hyperparathyroidism who are asymptomatic and have normal renal function and bone mass. *(Ref. 2, p. 2154)*

1006. (D) Other drugs that precipitate hemolysis in G6PD deficiency include dapsone, phenacetin, doxorubicin, and nalidixic acid. The disease is sex-linked and thus most common in males. Female heterozygotes have a dual population of red cells, and depending on the proportion, may develop symptoms. During hemolysis older red cells with the lowest enzyme levels are destroyed, and diagnostic tests done at this time may be falsely normal. They should be repeated some time after the hemolysis has resolved. *(Ref. 2, p. 1747)*

1007. (C) Erythromycin would be effective for most strains of *S. pneumoniae, L. pneumophila,* and *M. pneumoniae.* Other commonly used drugs for community acquired pneumonia are amoxicillin, cefuroxime, trimethoprim–sulfamethoxazole, and doxycycline. *(Ref. 2, p. 1188)*

1008. (C) Other clues to renal tubule defects include electrolyte disorders, renal osteodystrophy, large kidneys, and proteinuria. Categories of tubulointerstitial kidney disease include toxins (exogenous and metabolic), neoplasia, immune diseases, vascular disorders, infections, and hereditary renal diseases. Defects in urinary acidification and concentrating ability are frequently the most troublesome manifestations of tubulointerstitial kidney disease. *(Ref. 2, p. 1314)*

1009. (B) Ranitidine is six times more potent than cimetidine in inhibiting gastric acid secretion, but there are occasional reports of reversible hepatitis. With appropriate dosing, the two drugs are clinically equivalent. Considering how widely these drugs are used, relatively few serious adverse effects have been described. *(Ref. 2, p. 1369)*

1010. (A) MGUS is vastly more common than multiple myeloma, occurring in 1% of the population over age 50. Patients with MGUS have smaller M components (usually < 20 g/L), no urinary Bence Jones protein, less than 5% marrow plasmacytosis, and no anemia, renal failure, lytic bone lesions, or hypercalcemia. *(Ref. 2, p. 1622)*

1011. (E) Sjögren syndrome is an immunologic disorder characterized by progressive destruction of the exocrine glands leading to mucosal dryness. Pathology reveals lymphocytic infiltration. About one-third develop systemic (nonglandular) symptoms. The most common systemic manifestation is arthritis or arthralgia. If vasculitis occurs, purpura, urticaria, skin ulcers, and mononeuropathy are its most common manifestations. *(Ref. 2, p. 1662)*

1012. (D) The type O donor may contain sufficient anti-A or anti-B to destroy some of the patient's red blood cells, but this is seldom clinically significant. Generally, however, crystalloid or colloid solutions are sufficient for volume replacement until properly matched blood is available. *(Ref. 2, p. 1790)*

1013. (D) Other early changes in mitral stenosis include prominence of the main pulmonary arteries and backward displacement of the esophagus. The chest x-ray changes are caused by enlargement of the left atrium. Severe disease can cause pulmonary congestion (Kerley B lines) and enlargement of the right ventricle, right atrium, and superior vena cava. *(Ref. 2, p. 1054)*

1014. (A) The distribution of muscle weakness is characteristic with early involvement of the cranial nerves, especially the lids and extraocular muscles. Women are more frequently affected than men (3:2 ratio) and the age for peak incidence in women is in the third or fourth decade. *(Ref. 2, p. 2393)*

1015. (E) The risk is life-long and occurs at a rate of 0.5 to 1.0% per year of follow-up. Risk of breast cancer is increased in women with a family history, early menarche, late menopause, nulliparity, and late age at first pregnancy. Obesity, alcohol, and dietary fat are other possible risk factors. *(Ref. 2, p. 1842)*

1016. (D) Patients with minimal or absent gastrointestinal symptoms and atypical respiratory symptoms may be diagnosed as adults. This accounts for 3% of cases. Moreover, more than 25% of CF patients reach adulthood with modern therapy. *(Ref. 2, p. 1194)*

1017. (B) Signs of benignity of a solitary pulmonary nodule are lack of growth over a prolonged period and certain patterns of calcification. Less than 5% of neoplasms in adults are benign. "Popcorn" calcification does suggest a benign hamartoma. A search for previous chest x-rays can provide a definitive diagnosis. *(Ref. 2, pp. 1228–1229)*

1018. **(B)** A period of 24 to 48 hours is usually allowed to attempt medical therapy. Cardiac catheterization and angiography may be followed by bypass surgery or angioplasty. For those who do settle down, some form of subsequent risk stratification (e.g., exercise ECG) is indicated. *(Ref. 2, p. 1084)*

1019. **(A)** Glucocorticoids are not bronchodilators and their major use is in reducing airway inflammation. It is difficult to provide precise recommendations for their use, and a wide range of systemic and inhaled doses are used. *(Ref. 2, p. 1171)*

1020. **(A)** By electron microscopy, focal basement membrane collapse and denudation of epithelial surfaces are noted. The course is generally progressive in adults. It is felt that remission of proteinuria with steroid therapy will improve the prognosis. Cytotoxic drugs and cyclosporine have also been used in treatment. The degree of proteinuria correlates with the likelihood of developing renal failure. The disease recurs rapidly in transplanted kidneys, suggesting a humoral factor in pathogenesis. *(Ref. 2, p. 1303)*

1021. **(E)** Heartburn is a characteristic symptom of reflux esophagitis and may be associated with regurgitation. Odynophagia and atypical chest pain also occur in esophageal disease. *(Ref. 2, p. 1355)*

1022. **(D)** Surgical sympathectomy usually provides only temporary improvement and does not prevent progression of the vascular lesion. Nifedipine is now the drug of choice for treating symptoms not responding to local warming measures (gloves, mitts) and avoidance of smoking and cold. Reserpine, α-methyldopa and prazosin may also be useful. *(Ref. 2, p. 1660)*

1023. **(C)** Freezing does not destroy the virus. Recombinant factor VIII is theoretically the safest product. The use of desmopressin (DDAVP) or ε-aminocaproic acid (EACA) is, of course, not associated with HIV transmission. *(Ref. 2, pp. 1804–1805)*

1024. **(B)** The principal symptom is the pain of acute pericarditis that usually develops one to four weeks following the cardiac surgery, but could appear after months. It can also occur after myocardial infarction (Dressler syndrome) or after trauma to the heart (stab wound, blunt trauma).

The syndrome can remit and recur for up to two years. The acute symptoms usually subside in 1 or 2 weeks. *(Ref. 2, p. 1098)*

1025. **(A)** Blind loop syndrome leads to megaloblastic anemia and macrocytosis. In mild thalassemia, microcytosis is more prominent than hypochromia. *(Ref. 4, p. 456)*

1026. **(A)** The patient has Cushing syndrome secondary to an ACTH-secreting pituitary tumor. Only 10% of such patients have a large pituitary tumor. Over 50% have a microadenoma which is under 5 mm in diameter. *(Ref. 2, p. 1961)*

1027. **(E)** Even with normal levels of lipoproteins the ratio of LDL/HDL is increased in diabetics, thus favoring atherogenesis. Atherosclerosis occurs more extensively, and at an earlier age, in diabetics than in the general population. *(Ref. 2, p. 1994)*

1028. **(D)** The vertebral bodies in osteoporosis may become increasingly biconcave because of weakening of the subchondral plates. This results in "codfish" vertebra. When vertebral collapse occurs, the anterior height of the vertebra is usually decreased. Plain x-rays are insensitive diagnostic tools because up to 30% of bone mass can be lost without any apparent x-ray changes. Dual-energy x-ray absorptiometry and CT scan are more sensitive tests for bone loss, but their exact clinical role has not been clearly established. *(Ref. 2, pp. 2173–2174)*

1029. **(B)** Aspirin is given in low doses such as 300 mg a day, although the initial studies were done with higher doses. Carotid endarterectomy is the best treatment for stenoses of 70% or more. *(Ref. 2, pp. 2240–2241)*

1030. **(C)** Later symptoms of hypothyroidism include loss of intellectual and motor activity, declining appetite, dry hair and skin, and deepening voice. In the elderly, hypothyroidism can be misdiagnosed as due to aging or to other diseases such as Parkinson's disease, Alzheimer's disease, or depression. *(Ref. 2, pp. 1940–1941)*

1031. **(D)** Radiation therapy in stage lA Hodgkin's disease has a very high cure rate. Patients must be followed for hypothyroidism. The long-term disease-free survival is 80%. Mantle irradiation can result acutely in transient dry mouth, pharyngitis, fatigue, and weight loss. The most common long-term effect is hypothyroidism (in 30% of cases), but radiation pneumonitis and fibrosis or pericardial disease can occur. *(Ref. 2, p. 1787)*

1032. (A) Polyarteritis nodosa may be associated with hepatitis B antigenemia in 30% of cases, suggesting immunologic phenomena in the pathogenesis of the disease. Aneurysmal dilatations along involved arteries are characteristic and their presence in small- and medium-sized arteries in renal, hepatic, and visceral vasculature is diagnostic. Biopsy of involved areas can also be diagnostic. *(Ref. 2, p. 1671)*

1033. (E) Cytomegalovirus can also cause neurologic complications from CNS infection. Treatment is with ganciclovir or foscarnet. Relapse rates are high with both drugs, and therefore maintenance therapy is mandatory. *(Ref. 2, p. 1602)*

1034. (B) Most patients have fever, pain, and chills, as well as elevated alkaline phosphatase. Mechanical obstruction is most commonly due to stones, tumors, or strictures. For reasons that are unclear, the serum bilirubin tends to plateau and rarely exceeds levels of 600 micromoles/L (25 mg/dL). *(Ref. 2, p. 1458)*

1035. (B) Malignant melanomas do not usually have hair growing out of them. Dysplastic nevus syndrome may be a predisposing condition. There are four types of cutaneous melanoma: superficial spreading, lentigo maligna, acral lentiginous, and nodular. Stage at time of presentation is the most important prognostic factor. *(Ref. 2, pp. 1868–1869)*

1036. (E) Prerenal azotemia usually has urine osmolality over 500, urine creatinine over 40, and fractional excretion of sodium less than 1. The urinary sediment in prerenal azotemia reveals hyaline casts. In intrinsic renal azotemia muddy brown granular casts are seen. *(Ref. 2, p. 1270)*

1037. (D) The behavioral respiratory control system of the brain drives the hyperventilation, which leads to decreased P_{CO_2} and increased pH. If alkalemia is present with the hypocarbia symptoms can be quite significant. They include: dizziness, visual impairment, syncope and seizures secondary to cerebral vasoconstriction; parasthesias, carpopedal spasm, and tetany (secondary to decreased free serum calcium); muscle weakness (secondary to hypophosphatemia); cardiac arrhythmias (secondary to alkalemia). *(Ref. 2, p. 1239)*

1038. (D) Early ischemic changes are tall, peaked T waves, then they develop into inverted T waves. Elevated ST segments and Q waves also occur early. *(Ref. 2, p. 961)*

1039. (A) Renal elimination of phenobarbital is enhanced by alkalinization of the urine to a pH of 8 with sodium bicarbonate and fluids. Hemodialysis and hemoperfusion are reserved for extreme cases. Short-acting barbiturates are metabolized in the liver, so fluid adminstration and alkalinization are not helpful. *(Ref. 2, p. 2449)*

1040. (E) Excessive risk of leukemia at 1 Gy exposure is 5.2 with a minimum latent period of 3 years. The peak rates occur at 7 to 8 years. Thyroid cancer has an even longer latency. There is no increase in non-neoplastic deaths, but there is an accelerated decline in cell-mediated immunity with aging, and an increased occurrence of hyperparathyroidism. *(Ref. 2, p. 2485)*

1041. (E) Tardive dyskinesia causes involuntary repetitive movements of the lips, tongue, extremities, and trunk, and is especially frequent in patients over age 60. Parkinsonism is a particularly troublesome symptom as well. Akathisia or motor restlessness is also common. *(Ref. 2, p. 2418)*

1042. (D) The loop diuretics inhibit tubular reabsorption of sodium, potassium, and chloride in the loop of Henle and can continue to cause diuresis even during volume contraction. The likely site of action of furosemide is in the thick ascending limb of the loop of Henle. *(Ref. 2, p. 1262)*

1043. (D) Isoniazid acts as a pyridoxine antagonist and causes polyneuropathy in slow acetylators. Both sensory and motor involvement occurs. Treatment with pyridoxine can improve symptoms. *(Ref. 2, p. 2371)*

1044. (B) The first stage of Lyme disease is an acute infection with the spirochete *Borrelia burgdorferi,* usually transmitted by tick bite. It is most common in the summer in rural wooded areas. About 60% of patients who have not received antibiotic therapy will develop arthritis months later. The typical pattern is intermittent attacks of oligoarthritis lasting weeks to months. The knees are the most common joints involved. *(Ref. 2, p. 745)*

1045. (A) Zidovudine (AZT) is beneficial to patients with HIV infection, but the best time at which to commence therapy is still controversial. Common side effects include fatigue, macrocytic anemia, neutropenia, and myopathy. *(Ref. 2, pp. 1612–1614)*

1046. (E) In adulthood, total sleep time changes little with advancing age, although there is less deep (slow-wave) sleep. As well, the elderly awaken more frequently (and for more prolonged periods) during sleep. This means more time is required to get a similar amount of sleep (decreased sleep efficiency with aging). *(Ref. 10, p. 564)*

1047. **(C)** Death rates at all ages have declined, and recently the most dramatic declines have been for those over age 80. This means the elderly are actually living longer. This makes little difference in the age structures of the population, but the increased number of those over 85, who have multiple chronic diseases, impacts powerfully on health and social services. Despite this, the major gain in life expectancy at birth from 1840 to 1980 (about 25 years) is primarily a result of declining infant mortality. *(Ref. 10, p. 17)*

1048. **(C)** The mortality from acute myocardial infarction is greater in women, particularly African-American women. It is unclear whether this correlation is independent of age and disease severity. Ischemic heart disease, not breast cancer, is the leading cause of death in U.S. women. The relative benefit of thrombolytic therapy seems similar in men and women. Estrogen therapy's major effect in decreasing mortality is via its reduction (40 to 50%) in deaths due to ischemic heart disease. Immune-related disorders (rheumatoid arthritis, lupus, multiple sclerosis, thyroid disease, etc.) are usually more common in women. *(Ref. 2, pp. 14–15)*

1049. **(D)** α-Methyldopa has been used extensively throughout pregnancy, with no evidence of harm to the fetus. ACE inhibitors are associated with increased fetal loss. Pre-eclampsia and eclampsia are diseases of the end of pregnancy. There is no evidence that pregnancy affects the course of essential hypertension. Gestational hypertension has a high rate of recurrence in subsequent pregnancies. *(Ref. 2. pp. 18–19)*

1050. **(B)** Postpartum infections remain the most important cause of maternal mortality in U.S. women. Endometrial infections complicated by pelvic abscess, peritonitis, or pelvic thrombophlebitis are the most serious. CMV is the most common congenital viral infection, affecting 1 to 2% of all U.S. newborns. Only a small minority of these infants are abnormal. *N. gonorrhoeae* infection can be transmitted in utero, during delivery, or in the postpartum period. Asymptomatic bacteriuria occurs in up to 7% of all pregnancies. Treatment can prevent about 75% of all acute pyelonephritis in pregnancy, thus screening is warranted. *(Ref. 2, pp. 21–22)*

1051. **(E)** This story of daily attacks of periorbital pain with annual recurrence in a man between age 30 to 50 is typical of cluster headaches. The recurrent bouts last days to weeks. The headaches can be provoked by alcohol and relieved by oxygen administration. Prophylactic treatment, however, is preferred. *(Ref. 2, pp. 68–70)*

1052. **(E)** Wernicke's aphasia involves disease (most commonly infarction) in the distribution of the lower division of the middle cerebral artery. It is frequently associated with parietal lobe sensory deficits, and hemianopsia; motor disturbance is not part of the syndrome. The condition tends to improve with time. *(Ref. 2, pp. 159–160)*

1053. **(B)** β-Adrenergic receptors become less sensitive with advancing age. Higher rates of isoproterenol infusion are required in the elderly to achieve an increased resting heart rate. Clinically, higher doses of propranolol have been shown to be required in the elderly to achieve similar degrees of beta blockade as in the young. *(Ref. 10, p. 67)*

1054. **(A)** Similar blood levels of metaclorpromide in the elderly as compared to the young will provide greater relief of cancer chemotherapy-induced vomiting. *(Ref. 10, pp. 67–68)*

1055. **(A)** Older patients get greater pain relief as compared to younger patients with identical doses of morphine. *(Ref. 10, p. 67)*

1056. **(E)** The elderly have more body fat and less body water. A water-soluble drug such as lithium will have a considerably smaller volume of distribution. Thus dosages should be decreased in the elderly to prevent toxicity. *(Ref. 10, p. 68)*

1057. **(A)** The increased sensitivity for drugs such as aminophylline and digoxin can result in significant toxicity with "normal therapeutic" levels. *(Ref. 10, pp. 67–68)*

1058. **(A)** Altered mental states in the elderly, a predisposing factor for poor nutrition, are often managed with antipsychotics that can exacerbate disinterest in food, resulting in protein/calorie malnutrition. *(Ref. 10, pp. 542–543)*

1059. **(C)** Diuretics promote urinary losses of magnesium, zinc, and of course potassium. *(Ref. 10, p. 542)*

1060. **(D)** Isoniazid can result in pyridoxine (vitamin B_6) deficiency, particularly in malnourished individuals. *(Ref. 10, p. 542)*

1061. **(G)** Corticosteroids impair calcium absorption. *(Ref. 10, p. 542)*

1062. **(E)** Both phenytoin and phenobarbital can cause altered vitamin D metabolism, and can even result in osteomalacia. *(Ref. 10, p. 542)*

1063. **(C)** Both delirium and dementia increase with advancing age. Delirium is particularly common in demented patients. From 30 to 50% of hospitalized elderly patients are delirious (acutely confused). *(Ref. 2, pp. 137–141)*

1064. **(C)** Long-term memory is impaired in delirium and dementia. This can be assessed by asking for items of common general knowledge, e.g., the dates of World War II. *(Ref. 2, pp. 137–139)*

1065. **(A)** Early impairment of attention is characteristic of delirium. It can be assessed by the patient's ability to pay attention to questions and his/her distractibility. Formal testing includes forward and reverse digit span and serial 7s. These test other factors (immediate memory and mathematical ability) as well. *(Ref. 2, pp. 137–139)*

1066. **(A)** Dementia does not impair level of consciousness. The demented patient may not volunteer information but is normally alert and responsive to stimuli. *(Ref. 2, pp. 137–138)*

1067. **(D)** Dementia often results in apathy or disinhibition and is frequently characterized by fear and agitation. *(Ref. 2, p. 137)*

References

1. Wyngaarden JB, Smith LH, Bennett JC: *Cecil Textbook of Medicine.* 18th ed. Philadelphia: WB Saunders Co., 1992.

2. Wilson JD, et al.: *Harrison's Principles of Internal Medicine,* 12th ed. New York: McGraw-Hill Book Co., 1991.

3. Hirsch CS, Morris RC, Moritz AR: *Handbook of Legal Medicine,* 5th ed. St. Louis: CV Mosby Co., 1979.

4. Williams WJ, Beutler E, Ersler AJ, Lichtman MA: *Hematology,* 4th ed. New York: McGraw-Hill Book Co., 1990.

5. Rook A, Wilkinson DS, Ebling FJG, Champion RH, Burton JL: *Textbook of Dermatology,* 4th ed. Boston: Blackwell Scientific Publications, 1986.

6. Rowland LP: *Merritt's Textbook of Neurology,* 8th ed. Philadelphia: Lea and Febiger, 1989.

7. Wilson JD, Foster DW: *Williams Textbook of Endocrinology,* 8th ed. Philadelphia: WB Saunders Co., 1992.

8. Gilman AG, Rall TW, Nies AS, Taylor P: *Goodman and Gilman's The Pharmacological Basis of Therapeutics,* 8th ed. Elmsford, New York: Pergamon Press, 1991.

9. Schlant RC, Alexander RW, O'Rourke RA, Roberts R, Sonnenblick EH: *The Heart,* 8th ed. New York: McGraw-Hill Book Co., 1994.

10. Cassel CK, Riesenberg DE, et al: *Geriatric Medicine,* 2nd ed. New York: Springer-Verlag, 1990.

Appleton & Lange's Review of Anatomy for the USMLE Step 1
Montgomery
1995, ISBN 0-8385-0246-6, A0246-7

MEPC Specialty Board Review: Anesthesiology, 9/e
DeKornfeld
1995, ISBN 0-8385-0256-3, A0256-6

The MGH Board Review of Anesthesiology, 4/e
Dershwitz
ISBN 0-8385-8611-4, A8611-4

Appleton & Lange's Review of Cardiovascular-Interventional Technology Examination
Vitanza
1995, ISBN 0-8385-0248-2, A0248-3

Appleton & Lange's Review for the Chiropractic National Boards, Part I
Shanks
1992, ISBN 0-8385-0224-5, A0224-4

Appleton & Lange's Review for the Dental Assistant, 3/e
Andujo
1992, ISBN 0-8385-0135-4, A0135-2

Appleton & Lange's Review of Dental Hygiene, 4/e
Barnes & Waring
1994, ISBN 0-8385-0230-X, A0230-1

Appleton & Lange's Review of Epidemiology & Biostatistics
Hanrahan & Madupu
1994, ISBN 0-8385-0244-2, A0244-X

Specialty Board Review Family Practice, 5/e
Yen
1994, ISBN 0-8385-8618-X, A8618-9

Specialty Board Review Internal Medicine, 3/e
Pieroni
1990, ISBN 0-8385-8647-5, A8647-8

Appleton & Lange's Review of Internal Medicine
Goldlist
1996, ISBN 0-8385-0251-2, A0251-7

Medical Assistant, 4/e
Palko & Palko
1994, ISBN 0-8385-0197-4, A0197-2

Medical Technology Examination Review, 2/e
Hossaini
1984, ISBN 0-8385-6283-3, A6283-4

Appleton & Lange's Review of Microbiology and Immunology for the USMLE Step 1, 2/e
Yotis
1993, ISBN 0-8385-0059-5, A0059-4

MEPC: Specialty Board Review: Neurology, 4/e
Giesser
1996, ISBN 0-8385-8650-3, A8650-2

Appleton & Lange's Review of Obstetrics and Gynecology, 5/e
Julian, Dumesic, & Vontver
1995, ISBN 0-8385-0231-8, A0231-9

MEPC Specialty Board Review: Otolaryngology, Head & Neck Surgery
Willett & Lee
1995, ISBN 0-8385-7580-3, A7580-2

Appleton & Lange's Review of General Pathology, 3/e
Lewis & Barton
1993, ISBN 0-8385-0161-3, A0161-8

MEPC: Pediatrics, 9/e
Hansbarger
1995, ISBN 0-8385-6223-X, A6223-0

Appleton & Lange's Review of Pediatrics, 5/e
Lorin
1993, ISBN 0-8385-0057-9, A0057-8

Appleton & Lange's Review of Pharmacy, 5/e
Hall & Reiss
1993, ISBN 0-8385-0162-1, A0162-6

Appleton & Lange's Review for the Physician Assistant, 2/e
Cafferty
1995, ISBN 0-8385-0065-X, A0065-1

MEPC: Psychiatry, 10/e
Chan & Prosen
1995, ISBN 0-8385-5780-5, A5780-0

Appleton & Lange's Review of Psychiatry, 5/e
Easson
1994, ISBN 0-8385-0247-4, A0247-5

Appleton & Lange's Review for the Public Health and Preventive Medicine Review, 2/e
Penalver
1984, ISBN 0-8385-5936-2, E5936-9

Appleton & Lange's Review for the Radiography Examination, 2/e
Saia
1993, ISBN 0-8385-0058-7, A0058-6

Radiography: Program Review & Exam Preparation (PREP)
Saia
1995, ISBN 0-8385-8244-3, A8244-4

Appleton & Lange's Review of Respiratory Care, 2/e
Dunlevy
1994, ISBN 0-8385-8414-4, A8414-3

Appleton & Lange's Review for the Surgical Technology Examination, 3/e
Allmers & Verderame
1993, ISBN 0-8385-0066-8, A0066-9

MEPC: Specialty Board Review: Hand Surgery
Kulick
1991, ISBN 0-8385-3558-5, A3558-2

MEPC: Surgery, 11/e
Metzler
1995, ISBN 0-8385-6195-0, A6195-0

Appleton & Lange's Review of Surgery, 2/e
Wapnick
1989, ISBN 0-8385-0220-2, A0220-2

Specialty Board Review General Surgery, 4/e
Rob & Wind
1991, ISBN 0-8385-8638-4, A8638-7

Appleton & Lange's Review for the American Board of Surgery-in-Training Exam (ABSITE)
Stile
1996, ISBN 0-8385-0268-7, A0268-1

Specialty Board Review for Surgery *Written and Oral Examinations*
Hassett
1996, ISBN 0-8385-0061-7, A0061-0

Ultrasonography Examination Review and Study Guide, 2/e
Odwin
1993, ISBN 0-8385-9073-X, A9073-6

1996 First Aid for the USMLE Step 1 *A Student-to-Student Guide*
Bhushan, Le, & Amin
1995, ISBN 0-8385-2597-0, A2597-1

Appleton & Lange's Review for the USMLE Step 1, 2/e
Barton
1996, ISBN 0-8385-0265-0, A0265-7

1996 First Aid for the USMLE Step 2
Go, Curet-Salim, & Fullerton
1996, ISBN 0-8385-2591-1, A2591-4

Appleton & Lange's Review for the USMLE Step 2, 2/e
Catlin
1996, ISBN 0-8385-0266-5, A0266-5

The Instant Exam Review for the USMLE Step 2, 2/e
Goldberg
1996, ISBN 0-8385-4328-6, A4328-9

The Instant Exam Review for the USMLE Step 3
Goldberg
1994, ISBN 0-8385-4334-0, A4334-7

Appleton & Lange's Review for the USMLE Step 3
Schultz
1994, ISBN 0-8385-0227-X, A0227-7

First Aid for the Wards: *A Student-to-Student Guide to the Clinical Years*
Le, Bhushan, & Amin
1996, ISBN 0-8385-2595-4, A2595-5

First Aid for the Match: *A Student-to-Student Guide to the Clinical Years*
Le, Bhushan, & Amin
1996, ISBN 0-8385-2596-2, A2596-3